Ship's Doctor

Terrence Riley

To Marianne Long,
Shipmate & kick-ass
hiker.
Hope you may
enjoy parts of this
sea story. (The intro isn't bad)

Terry
Jan 24, 2014

Ship's Doctor

Second edition

Lee's Summit, Missouri
2006

First Edition and printing, U.S. Naval Institute Press, Annapolis 1995
isbn 978-0-984102808
1st ed isbn 1-55750-721-x

Preface to Second Edition

Gentle reader, the book you are reading was never a best seller. In fact, the first printing in 1995 was followed by a second printing of only a few hundred books a few years later, and is now out of print altogether. In order to have a few copies to distribute to friends, your humble flight surgeon could only afford to print the scurrilous poor tome you are holding. This edition lacks the dazzling photos of the fist edition, covered in impressive hard surface and cloaked in a colorful dust jacket. I assure you, though, the words herein remain the same pungent, musky, irascible, and erudite prose you anticipate. Yea, since the first publisher's insistence on political correctness made me change some of the characters' names – and induced me to tell a fib at the beginning that the whole story was made up – this version is a little bit better. The names are real, and in this volume, which I had to publish myself, I can proudly tell you that everything in this book is true. Please enjoy it. And if you don't really read it, please tell me you did anyway.

Prologue

The nose wheel sliced up horizontally after it snapped and flew straight toward the island. The two aircraft handlers it hit first made loud crunching sounds as they flew up against the island. Metal fragments like burning shrapnel hit four other people after it ricocheted off two tractors.

The plane bounced twice on the orphan oleo strut and snapped the arresting cable under max tension. The cable whipped the skin right off Lieutenant Carson's legs while they were splintering, tore off his left wrist and crashed his skull like a walnut on the hot nonskid.

"Call the Wing Surgeons to the Flight Deck and get Dr Eardley and anesthesia set up now!" I yelled over my shoulder on my way up to the Flight Deck BDS.

Thirty Seconds later, I threw one innocent bystander out of the way to get into the BDS. Carson's legs looked like fresh-skinned drumsticks, with the skin slipped down like loose stockings around his ankles. Blood pumped out of the stump of his wrist. He wasn't breathing. Bill cranked in two large-bore IVs, and I slipped in the endotracheal tube. Dan, the surgeon, arrived just then, clamped down the bleeding stump and handled the loose skin. While Dan took over, I called the bridge, "We need the Deck Edge elevator Now!"

"He's arrested!" Ron called, "No pulse."

V-fib.

"Stand Back!" 300 joules. Sinus.

"We got a pulse. Bill, more fluid."

"Activate the blood bank!" Dan called. "Let's get to the O.R."

Behind the island, two other guys' legs were snapped like twigs by the cable when it whipped back. The Flight Surgeons were triaging the six guys injured from the broken wheel and the metal fragments. One of them had a gash across the left side of his face that tore open his sinus and the left eye, another was unconscious. Deftly covering the open wounds, the team started the IVs, immobilized the spines, and got the casualties into shelter.

In less than two minutes, the casualties were clear and the Handlers pulled the broken F-14 out of the way. We still had 13 airplanes to recover.

INTRODUCTION

This is going to be the personal story of a ship's doctor, a flight surgeon on an aircraft carrier. It's mostly going to be true. I might ramble on here and there, but I'll tell the truth mostly. It may help for you to know a little background first, a little about what military and ships and airplanes and doctors have in common. You can read my story without this part, if you want, but I'd like to set the stage for you.

It would surprise a lot of people that military and naval sciences were so far ahead of medicine for the first millennia, that they almost did not cross paths until the Age of the Reformation. Nobody knew what caused diarrhea, pneumonia, or plague. If the scourges of disease crumbled a city (or disabled an Army), it had to be attributed simply to fate or maybe to conjurers casting spells. Those few aspects of medicine that had any scientific basis at all, and there weren't many, were not demonstrably any more effective for the individual patient or for populations than were spiritual effects. Of course, a lot of people would argue that's still true today, I guess.

After metal, gunpowder, and sailing ships reached certain pinnacles around the 1500s, their progress slowed a bit. Maybe it was one of those technological plateaus or paradigm shifts we hear so much about these days. Arts and the study of nature were catching up with warfare and the study of machines. In this era, Michelangelo, DaVinci, and other artists and scholars began to dissect human bodies. So professors of medicine were more or less forced to look at cadavers too, to try to keep up with the artsy crowd. When they looked they began to learn that not only were there a number of discrete parts inside the body, they surprisingly seemed to fit together in pretty much the same way in *everybody*. This being the case, one could study how those parts functioned in healthy folk and how they looked different in sick or dead ones. Thus was medicine reluctantly dragged into the realm of scientific thought.

Although the scientific method has been sometimes capriciously applied in medicine, once introduced it quickly became downright fashionable. As medicine and surgery began to produce results, armies had to take surgeons along. They couldn't at first really heal many soldiers, but a few could be bandaged up and go back to the front. Just to save as many lives of the other wounded as possible was critical even if they couldn't return to the fight, because the populace was beginning to take note of how many died. Even if an amputee could not return to the front line, if he survived to go home, his fellow villagers would be less angry than if he died.

Medicine and seafaring finally collided in scientific parity around 1617, the year that John Woodall wrote the first text for ship's doctors. Woodall, the Surgeon General for the East India Company, was an accomplished physician in his day. He evidently spent a lot of time at sea, as his treatise speaks of the rigors of sea travel and the effects of loneliness, danger, and hardship on those who sail. In ***The Surgion's Mate***, Woodall extols the importance of behaving like an officer and gentleman, as expected of the physician on a ship. When he left the East India Company, it is unclear whether he left because, as was known, he felt too poorly paid for his level of renown or because of ripping off the Company and junior ship's "surgions" whom he forced to buy the expensive supply trunks and inventories from his personal side market.

Arguably warfare grew more complex in the century after Woodall; it certainly grew more international ... at least colonial. Britain, France, and Spain all sent forces to

America and Africa, warring with one another and the aborigines. Ships surgeons did not all come from academic backgrounds like Woodall. In fact, many were sailmakers or sailors too old and decrepid or too drunk for their original trades who simply apprenticed with an incumbent sawbones at sea. Hygiene and nutrition became as important to the surgeons as did the treatment of wounds and diseases. The simple acts of quarantine and isolation were the only real tools for disease, though. The scientific armamentarium at sea languished for a century.

Aviation began a century later, too, with the first balloons, and physicians, always eager to dabble in somebody's good idea sneaked into the vanguard. Dr. John Jeffries, an American physician, was the first to cross the English channel in a balloon, and he was the first to bring the value of biological perspective to the cockpit. He saved his gondola from crashing by dumping overboard all unnecessary weight: his clothes and about 6 pounds of urine he figured he could spare. In that same year, a French physician, Pilatre de Rozier employed the unique kind of scientific ingenuity for which the medical profession is famous. He reasoned that if hot air could create lift and hydrogen (they called it "flammable air") could create lift, then *hot hydrogen* should be twice as good! His ingenuity went cruelly unrewarded, alas. When he lit the match to the burner to heat up the hydrogen, Pilatre suddenly discovered why it was called "flammable air." Thus a doctor became the first recorded aviation fatality.

Although Naval Medicine progressed very little in the two centuries since John Woodall, in the nineteenth century, the medical revolution came. Biggest changes affected infectious disease, surgery, and psychiatry, the areas most important to doctors who treated soldiers and sailors. The U.S. Navy's first hospital ship, the ***Red Rover***, was commissioned in the Civil War. While America was preoccupied by the Civil War, aviation kept moving on elsewhere, with lighter than air craft and gliders. A French physician named Paul Bert in the 1870s pioneered studies of gas pressures at altitude.

Within thirty years, it became clear that for flight to be really useful to humans, balloons were inadequate. Aircraft would have to be powered and controllable. The airplane. When airplanes were evolving at an accelerating pace their first practical applications seemed to be for the military. The Navy was involved from the beginning, although rather tentatively at first. In November, 1910, Eugene Ely took off from a flight deck built on the scout cruiser ***Birmingham***. Just four months later, he made the first arrested landing, on the cruiser ***Pennsylvania***, turned around and took off immediately. For the next ten years, though, airplanes remained pretty flimsy and short-ranged, so the Navy had little interest in them. World War I, however, woke us up. Airships were bombing London and airplanes were proving major weapons in the war.

Thousands of young Americans wanted to fight the War as pilots. The Army Surgeon General's office designed a set of physical standards and in 1918, the War Department sent doctors from the Air Service Medical Research Laboratory to France to help the squadrons. Doctors became integral members of the flying and fighting organizations to protect the health of the aviators.

The U.S. Navy started an air force, but had no initial facilities for equipment or training, so the first Navy pilots had to go to Canada to train. One of the first was a young Princeton graduate named James V. Forrestal. The son of an Irish immigrant, Forrestal had overcome the barriers against his Catholic middle class background to become a rising star on Wall Street. One of the brightest flight students, Forrestal was not an adept stick and rudder man but good enough to graduate. He became Naval Aviator #154. His greatest skills apparently were as a staffer, so he never flew much and never left the states. Forrestal stayed on duty a couple of years after the war, but soon returned to Wall Street and a very wealthy career. The Navy would see him again later.

After the War, the nation wanted to return to normalcy, (which I guess was a good thing for Warren Harding) and the Admirals wanted to get back to basics, namely battleships. General Billy Mitchell was court martialled for his insubordinate insistence that airplanes could wreck fleets, and the Navy was able to limit its commitment to airborne submarine patrols and airships. Only after being goaded by the more innovative British, the Navy launched its first aircraft carrier, the ***Langley, CV1***, in 1922. All Navy ships are designated by type, class, and sequence. Carriers are "C," fixed wing aircraft are "V," and ***Langley*** was the first of its type, hence "CV1." The Navy sent five doctors that year to the Army School for Flight Surgeons on Long Island, the first Naval Flight Surgeons. Carriers would need doctors.

Aviation and ships grew more complex and more capable. The Navy built the ***Saratoga*** and the ***Ranger***. Higher G-forces, higher altitudes, more psychological stress, all these made the medical needs of the aviator more demanding. The Navy opened a school for flight surgeons at the Naval Medical School on the Observatory grounds in Washington in 1927, just before Lindbergh flew across the Atlantic. In 1932, a Navy doctor, Lieutenant Commander John Poppen, working at Harvard, designed the first anti-gravity "G-suit" to cope with G-induced complications of dive bombing in Naval aircraft.

Since the Army was bigger and they had been doing Aviation Medicine longer, there were pressures to let the Army continue to train Naval Flight Surgeons. The Navy had a different need from its Flight Surgeons, though. For one thing, the flying missions were a little different. But it was the sea that really made the difference. The ships. A Naval Flight Surgeon had all the same medical and physical concerns that the Army doctor did, but he had to practice on a ship. He wasn't just going to be a doctor for the aviators, he had to take care of a lot of other people too in that enclosed but isolated place, and there was no station hospital for him to fall back on as there was for the Army flight surgeon. The isolation and rigors at sea imposed entire dimensions of medical complexity.

The Brotherhood of the Sea was a force in this, too. Being already familiar with that special value of the brotherhood, being a "shipmate," Naval aviators wanted their "docs" to be part of the Brotherhood -- this time, of the Air. If they were real members, maybe they could take better care of us, kind of like Errol Flynn did in that movie when he was a Naval Flight Surgeon. From the beginning of the Navy School of Aviation Medicine at Pensacola, in 1939, all Student Naval Flight Surgeons had to pass all the swimming and survival courses right along with the aviators. This is what set them apart from Army Air Corps flight surgeons: they had to learn to fly. For those who graduated, there were wings of gold, just as cherished among doctors as the Wings of Gold to pilots. If you passed all the courses but did not learn to fly, you would be designated an "Aviation Medical Examiner" not a Flight Surgeon. Good job... but no wings.

The role of aircraft carriers really began to take form in the 1930s. Airships had a period in the limelight too, but did not make the final cut. This was the Flash Gordon and Buck Rogers era, so America loved it when great bullet shaped airships like the Macon could actually perform as flying aircraft carriers. The ***Macon*** could actually land biplane fighters by snaring them with a dangling trapeze and then launch them out as necessary to fight off marauders. By 1935, though, both the ***Macon*** and its sister ship the ***Akron*** had crashed, including Admiral Moffett the father of Naval aviation among the fatalities. Although airships and blimps would continue as patrol craft to hunt submarines, they would never again carry other aircraft. CVs were another matter altogether. In the late 1930s, the United States began to develop aircraft carriers and early concepts of Naval Air Warfare. This seemed particularly suitable for the Pacific, where distances, isolation, and logistical trails seemed designed for a flexible, maneuverable air asset.

When the Japanese carrier ***Akagi*** led the surprise attack on Pearl Harbor, the role of the aircraft carrier would never be questioned again. Within five months, the U.S. carrier ***Hornet*** launched LTC Jimmy Doolittle's Army B-25s over mainland Japan. Then within a month, the Battle of the Coral Sea was the first major naval battle fought primarily in the air. Captain William Davis, the Senior Medical Officer ("SMO") of the ***Yorktown*** was commended for gallantry in the battle as he treated casualties in fires and areas with explosions. On the ***Lexington,*** the SMO was CDR Arthur J. White. Blown against a bulkhead by the explosion from the first of several torpedo hits, CDR White continued treating casualties despite a broken clavicle and two badly sprained ankles. When his "surgery," (what we would now call our Emergency Ward) was blown up he carried patients on his shoulder through hatches and scuttles to get them to safe areas. The ***Lexington*** eventually went down that day, but White kept treating patients for three hours after the first torpedo and later received the Navy Cross. Although usually considered a stand-off, Coral Sea was the prelude for the Battle of Midway, the first major naval engagement where the adversaries were beyond sight of each other, and the turning point of the War in the Pacific.

The Navy had been forced to adapt quickly to this new form of warfare. One of the driving forces was the man who had become the first Undersecretary of the Navy when the post was created in 1940, Naval Aviator #154, James V. Forrestal. The Secretary, a very old Republican named Frank Knox, had left most of the details and fighting budgetary battles to the brilliant young Forrestal and as the War progressed and Knox grew more feeble,
Forrestal took over more and more of the functions of the Department. Known for genius, driven patriotism, and inexhaustible energy, Forrestal was credited by many with virtually reinventing the Navy. A dedicated liberal, the earnest desegregation of the Navy was one of his fondest goals. Human issues were as important to him as efficiency and winning. Strong in his opinions, perhaps even lofty, he was said to dislike what he considered the dirty side of politics, the compromises, the give and take.

There was a haunting dark side to Forrestal also. His marriage had long been difficult. His wife drank a lot. She made vulgar statements and scenes in front of both high society and general public alike. One doctor diagnosed schizophrenia after a brief hospitalization, but she refused further treatment and Forrestal complied with her choice to leave the hospital. Most people thought she was simply an eccentric alcoholic. Whatever the case, the record doesn't show Mr. Forrestal to have eased her torment in any way either. At any rate, Forrestal continued working eighteen hour days throughout the war worrying about the role of politics in government and suppressing his personal life. When Knox died of heart failure in 1944, Forrestal took over as Secretary of the Navy.

The postwar adjustments of the Navy were as demanding as the war had been. Forrestal sparred with Chief of Naval Operations, Admiral Ernest King, a difficult man who chafed under the idea of civilian control. Forrestal had to fight for control over the budget, and the unavoidable reduction in the Navy. On the other hand, while overseeing proper force reductions with the Navy Line, he helped President Truman fight to preserve readiness in the nuclear age in the face of Communist expansion. Along with George Kennan, Clark Clifford, and a few others, he was a member of the clique who urged containment and vigilance about China and the Soviet Union. The concepts of nuclear capability and deterrence were in their infancy. Forrestal was one of the godfathers. In 1947, the individual military services lost their lofty cabinet positions and were reduced to subaltern status in a single Department of Defense. The War and Navy Departments were, along with the new Air Force, now just branches of the Department of Defense. This was a bitter experience to many generals and admirals at the time. President Truman chose Forrestal, now one of his main advisors, to be the first Secretary of Defense.

1948 brought a maelstrom to the Department of Defense that had striking parallels to the ones we face in 1994. The most fundamental views of warfare were shaken by recent changes in the world order and by the atom bomb and the jet engine. Yet at the same time the populace and the politicians demanded drastic cuts in force structure and budget. A Democratic President who had promised economic recovery was being pummelled by Congress and was losing popularity faster than a chaperon at a drive in movie. Forrestal realized that although we had to decommission most of the 33 aircraft carriers, ironically we still needed a bigger one. In the hazardous new world, a deck big enough for a plane that could carry atom bombs for long strategic strikes was necessary. A supercarrier, perhaps as big as 60,000 tons, would be needed by the 1950s when Russia and China could feel their oats. For comparison, the then-newest carriers like ***Franklin Delano Roosevelt***, and ***Coral Sea*** were about 45,000 tons. The Air Force argued then, as they still do now, that their long range bombers could strike any target the nation would need; ships were obsolete. General Curtis LeMay was a persuasive advocate. The Congress had no stomach for the big price tag on a supercarrier. Other challenges Forrestal faced were arguments over bases in the Pacific or in Europe and racial integration of the services.

Forrestal continued to be a star in the Truman cabinet, until, in 1949, something seemed different. He appeared to be fatigued. His concentration began to falter, he overlooked detail. His staff and the others in the Cabinet worried that his wife's illness or the unabated frenzy of high office for nine years were wearing Forrestal out. Finally, President Truman asked for his resignation. Worn out and threadbare emotionally, no solace available in his marriage, Forrestal was eventually admitted to the National Naval Medical Center in Bethesda. One day, he cajoled or ordered the corpsman on duty to go on some errand, and he jumped out his window on the 16th floor.

The supercarrier was finally built. The keel was laid in July, 1951, for CV 59. It was christened ***USS Forrestal***, in 1954. With its slanted deck, huge size, and dazzling speed, I remember seeing reports about sea trials of the Supercarrier completely filling newsreels at the movies in 1955. The crews' motto was "**F**irst **I**n **D**efense," so the big ship was nicknamed the FID.

When I was a neurology resident at Bethesda in 1974, all of us new doctors were tauntingly taken to see a stain on the pavement in front of the hospital, the infamous "this is where Forrestal hit." That was all most of us knew about him, the stain. As most legends about Forrestal, that too was wrong. He didn't hit the sidewalk at all. He struck the roof of the Xray department in the three deck south wing that sticks out from the tower.

The fact is, he remains both a titan and yet a tragic figure. Though wounded and suffering, he left behind the strongest and most adaptable Navy in history. His namesake supercarrier continued the tradition. During flight operations on "Yankee Station" off Vietnam on July 29, 1967, a Zuni rocket was fired accidentally and ignited an A-4 Skyhawk attack jet. Within minutes the flight deck and most of the after half of the ship was in flames. That day 134 ***Forrestal*** shipmates died and 164 more were injured. The heroism of those who died and their shipmates is a naval legend. The Navy had long filmed all flight operations, so most of the conflagration and the fighting of the fire are on film. Most people in the Navy, certainly all who go to sea, study those films in a universal training classic called "Trial by Fire." The film is intended to be a training tool in firefighting and damage control. To people in the Sea Service, though, it's more than that. It is an example of what sailors do and of what shipmates do for one another.

Many in the Navy know of CV-59 only from "Trial by Fire." So the ship is sometimes called "the Forrest'-fire," or "USS Zippo." You will never hear a FID sailor call her that. They don't even joke about the fire among themselves twenty seven years later.

In May, 1988, I received orders to the ***Forrestal***. "Report in July, 1988, for duty in a flying status, to serve as Senior Medical Officer. Duty as Department Head." My wife, Ann, knew that I longed to be back a part of the Navy. We enjoyed our big house in Massachusetts. The kids were in a great school. I had enjoyed my practice, but it had never been enough. For eight years I missed the Navy and longed to come back. Ann told me this was an adolescent longing for "scout camp, " but really she understood -- even if she bristled about it.

I read the book ***Supercarrier*** by George Wilson about a deployment of the ***USS John F. Kennedy***. Intimidated as I was by the book, I discovered that my friend Myron Almond had been the SMO on the cruise in that book. I asked him a few questions. Yes, it was about the hardest job he ever had... but it might have been the best too. I asked him about his experiences with the XO in ***Supercarrier***, a guy named John Pieno who seemed like a supreme hardnosed S.O.B. I dreaded ever working for a guy like that. "Yeah, Pieno was tough. He was kind of hard headed, and he could be a screamer, but, you know, in his way he was fair. That makes up for a lot. He was smart too. But he could be a screamer all right." Myron is a known mellow guy. Maybe he could take it, but with all the other challenges at least I wouldn't want to work for a screamer. That wasn't why I had come back into the Navy.

"One thing," he told me, "when I had a really bad day... when it was over, I'd go out to the fan tail and stand there a while, and tell myself,'only fourteen people in the world have this job.' "

Myron and I were having coffee out of doors in Pensacola. Weighing his advice pensively, I started to leave, but Myron stopped me as he poured himself another coffee. "Did you know that Captain Pieno is the skipper of the ***Forrestal*** now?"

CHAPTER ONE

At 30,000 feet, with nothing to see but ocean and perfect blue sky, it can be very lonesome, knowing that you are somewhere over the absolute middle of the Indian Ocean. At that altitude, you can see the edges of the planet, and there is not one speck of soil or human all the way to those edges.

I was sitting in the back of a US-3 with four other passengers en route from the Island of Diego Garcia to the ***USS Forrestal*** somewhere in the north Arabian Sea. My cranial was too tight. The cranial is a kind of hard hat used by people who work on carrier hangar or flight decks. There are three hard plates that cover the forehead, top, and back of the head, and large hard cup-shaped ear pieces to protect the ears. It's all held on by a big sweaty chin strap. These are better than industrial hard hats because they are lighter and they fit the contour of the head. Since you have to wear them all day long, the cloth composition makes them more comfortable, and to prevent blowing off in the wind and jet exhaust on the flight deck, they must fit firmly against the head. They did not have a "large" size so I had to make do with a medium, and it was beginning to be uncomfortable, especially over my ears, in fact it had been worsening for about a half hour.

Because I was most senior on the airplane, I was allowed to sit in the front line of the seats so that I could look out the wind screen and speak with the pilot and copilot.

The S-3 airplane is an antisubmarine jet aircraft that usually takes a crew of four: a pilot and copilot, an enlisted sonar operator and a TACO (Tactical Command Officer) in the back seat, a Naval Flight Officer. Fleet replenishment squadrons usually use the venerable C-2, a large two-propeller aircraft for "carrier onboard delivery" or "COD" missions. However, at times like this when the ship would be operating beyond the range of the C-2, the US-3 with its longer range had to do COD chores. The S-3, the ship-based antisubmarine fixed wing aircraft, was designed to spend very long hours at sea flying grid after grid hunting for submarines. Its "utility" version was the US-3.

We were going to be flying a total of 5 hours that day, and since we were traveling at about 300 miles per hour or faster, I reckoned we had well over 1,000 miles to go, mostly due north.

After about an hour and a half, my ears and cheeks started hurting from the tightness of the cranial, and I began to realize it was going to be a very long 5 hours. Also, I had a lot of coffee that morning, and I became aware that there would be other reasons for 5 hours to get uncomfortable.

It was too loud in the US-3 to carry on a conversation with my fellow passengers. We made mostly hand signals, and I had on my lap a copy of the book ***Super Carrier*** by George Wilson. Even though I'd read it once before I thought I should brush up on it a little bit since one of the saltier characters, Captain John Pieno, was about to become my Commanding Officer.

There was a kind of bulkhead immediately behind the seat of the pilot on the left and the copilot on the right leaving an opening about 18 inches wide through which I could look to the wind screen or into the cockpit. I had to crane my neck around a little to the right, but I was willing to do that because there were no windows in the fuselage otherwise. I was a little bit surprised to see the copilot with the New York Times spread out over his lap and control yoke, completely covering all the instruments in the cockpit. He was eating a boxed lunch absent mindedly while he read, much like any ordinary employee on a lunch break.

I noted with a little bit of dismay, perhaps jealousy, that they had not provided us passengers with a boxed lunch, but they told us, "Well you will be able to eat when you get to the ship." I craned my neck a little bit further so that I could look up to the pilot and ask him a question or two. He also had a newspaper spread out over the yoke and was reading it. All of the control panel was completely covered, including the gyroscopes and compass, and neither of them had their hands on the wheel. Then I looked up again and looked over the control panel to notice that we were still pretty high. I couldn't tell how high because the altimeter was covered, but clearly the horizon was very far away, and the ocean was so far below that all you could tell was that it was a deep blue. We were high enough you couldn't see the waves. Not a cloud to be seen and, of course, no islands. If there were any way to know we were lost, no one would be able to tell it. What the hell, I thought. If you're lost at sea anyway, what good is it to be in control? To the best of our knowledge, Amelia Earhart had her hands on the control yoke, and it didn't do her any good.

After eight years longing to be back in the Navy, I was finally fully engaged. My promise to Ann and the girls that by returning to active duty, I would have more time to spend at home was not appearing very convincing at the moment, especially since I couldn't really tell them exactly where on the planet I might be right now.

There is a global positioning system (GPS) on the control panel which would help us to navigate, of course, but since the aircraft was on auto-pilot and both our pilots were busy reading the news, there was no way of knowing that we were really on course that way either. I guess I figured we were going more or less north, but I could not see the sun at all, so there was no way to judge that.

The cranial was beginning to hurt me even more, and that other problem, somewhat more biological, was beginning to nag at me as well.

I tried to read the book, but found it hard to concentrate, because of the pain in my ears, the effort it was taking me to remain nonchalant about the two guys reading the newspaper, and that other problem from the coffee. Finally, I asked the third crew member, the Loadmaster, if there was a relief tube, and he pointed to the back of the aircraft, then he spoke into the internal communications system (ICS) to the pilot and then turned back to me and gave me a thumbs-up signal. He had to ask another person who was seated somewhat further back to move forward, and he had to move a bag of mail forward. Although this is a very powerful aircraft, it is small enough that weight and balance need to be kept in line for the people to move around.

Just as promised, in the back of the aircraft, where a person had to bend down somewhat, there was a conical, funnel-shaped device stuck on to a large rubber tube clamped up against the bulkhead. I was able to use it properly to relieve that other nagging problem that I had, but when I went back to my seat the two pilots were still browsing on their newspapers and nibbling at their lunch, and my ears started to hurt even more in the cranial one size too small.

It wouldn't do to let anybody think that I had less than complete trust in the modern Naval Aviator, or to show that I had any worry about personal safety, while we were at 30,000 feet on a 5-hour flight over the middle of the ocean. If you will look at a map or a globe, look directly south from the Arabian peninsula, perhaps a little bit east, and you may or may not find the Maldive Islands more or less halfway between India and Africa, and equally far south of the Arabian Peninsula. In fact, they are so small and so far from any land that they don't even appear on some maps. There wasn't a runway anywhere to be seen if we ran out of fuel. Reflecting on how often in flying my small airplane across the Midwest I had become treacherously low on gasoline, I remembered the time I had to radio a runway, announcing that I had just run out of fuel, and had to glide into a landing because the engine stopped. There I was patted on the back by some of my fellow pilots for a "great job" but received some disapproving stares from older flight instructors who pointed out that running out of gasoline was not conducive to great longevity.

The one thing I had done besides work during the eight years out of the Navy was fly. Instruments, multi-engine, aerobatics, I did as much as I could. I hadn't much spare time other than work all those years, but when I could eke out a free hour I spent in aloft. It simply reinforced the nagging ache to be back in the Navy, to be part of the organization I had missed so much.

At about this point I looked up through the wind screen, and noticed to my satisfaction that the copilot was folding up his newspaper. Short lived relief it turns out, as he then pulled out a paperback book, and opened up one more sandwich, the waxed paper falling away from the sandwich so that it covered up his compass and both our views of the control panel again.

Finally, about 2 hours later, the pilot and copilot both folded up their reading materials, started fiddling with instruments on the control panel, and initiated a descent. There started to be conversation on the radio, and I noticed that there was a cloud bank a few miles ahead of us as we gradually descended beneath it. The perfectly bright sky that had been with us for about 4 hours now gave way to an overcast above us. The copilot reached back to tap me on the shoulder and said, "There's mom."

"Mom" is the title pilots use for the ship. Probably a proper name, and a reflection of the way I felt about the ship at the moment, too, although it was hard for me to think about anything as my ears were killing me, and I could scarcely think about anything else except getting the cranial off. Straining my eyes, I was able to see the ship way off, a small fleck, very nearly on the horizon, and even at nearly 300 miles an hour it did not get much closer very fast. A little bit of drizzle started to form on the wind screen, and just as quickly disappeared. The pilot indicated to the copilot that he was going to let him "take the landing," I noticed again how young the copilot looked. All naval pilots looked young to me at about this time. They were all scarcely teenagers. Even so, this copilot looked a little younger than most of them, and I considered he was probably about the age of my oldest daughter.

We approached the ship at about 5,000 to 3,000 feet, and made one racetrack oval over the deck. The pilot said something about the amount of fuel they had on board. The only activity on the flight deck was a couple of guys running some yellow gear, but there were no other flight operations, and all the other airplanes seemed to be folded up and parked. I had always read how small the aircraft carrier looked from the sky, especially for the first landing. I can't say that I thought it was really minuscule. But then, I remembered a runway in Marlboro, Massachusetts that used to intimidate me because it was only 1500 feet long, when I was trying to land on it at 50 knots. This one had landing area less than half that, with no grass around it, and we were approaching at 200 knots. Finally, we made our left turn-around loop to final, less than a mile out, much shorter than a civilian pattern.

I had waited for this for years. My first "trap." I set myself up. We locked our harness belts in place. Even with the pain in my cranial I looked with anticipation to the first landing. I wanted to savor every marvelous sensation in that experience. I knew it was going to be a sensory explosion. The First Trap was something that every pilot always looks forward to, and is shrouded in much mystique in all aviation lore.

Then finally there we were. In a blur that was so fast, a blink, a speeding bullet, or a bullet train in Japan can't quite describe it, we were coming over the fantail, and just as fast, the entire superstructure of the ship whizzed by. I felt the sudden jolt of the tires on the deck, and the next thing I knew we were back over the water again. A "bolter." Wow, was this fun. On my first approach we were going to wind up getting to do a touch and go, and a "bolter." It was great! We circled around again and began to set up for another approach. Although I enjoyed getting a second go-round, a "bolter" after all does mean a missed landing. Something was off. Either we were too low, wrong speed, failed to hit the 3-wire, or some other wire, or we had been given a "wave off" by the LSO.

Regardless, it was twice coming around, and it was a marvelous thrill. The pilot said something about how much fuel they had onboard, and then told the copilot, "We'd better get down this time." We came around again on final. This time, I decided I would watch the flight deck go by and watch the superstructure,the "island," so that I could always remember that particular experience. Once again, our harness belts were locked in tight, and it blurred by so fast that all I could see was the flashing gray, one person standing over by the superstructure, and then we were airborne again!

Wow, this was great, even two of them. However, it did occur to me now, here we had flown 5 1/2 hours, my ears were killing me, we had a young pilot, possibly making his first approach to the ship, and we were getting low on fuel. In spite of all this fun, we had to get down now, because there were no alternate airports. This time the pilot flew the downwind leg, and I could see we were a little bit lower as we came on to final.

They were speaking to one another a little bit more this time, and I was able to look out through the wind screen and see "paddles" the nickname given to the LSO. Years ago, before radios and fancy communication, and before there were prisms that show a light for landing, the LSO actually stood on the fantail holding paddles in his hand and would direct the plane to the proper glide path.

This time, we hit the deck, and jerked to a stop for my first "trap". As this book goes on, I will describe the experiences of a trap and a catapult shot more. The essence and the ultimate experience of each of them are the stunning suddenness. If I describe in one spot all of the things that go on, it would take so many words that it would blunt the smacking intensity and the suddenness -- and it would be misleading. In no single shot can any person, especially us beginners, experience all the parts. To describe the crammed inventory of a speeding nanosecond to you over three pages would be as inaccurate as playing a sports film in slow motion. Think of a bungee jump from a height of about 15 stories, but not being bounced, just being at the end of a perfectly rigid hemp rope. You reach 200 miles an hour at the end, and in less than part of a second you are snapped to a sudden complete stop. A little bit like splattering on the sidewalk. Nothing springy or elastic about it.

Now, I think of myself as a fast thinker, I'm an experienced pilot, but with all of that happening in such a flash, I was not able to look at the flight deck, the superstructure, or to see ***anything*** except a sudden gray blur when the wire abruptly snapped us back. There is not an amusement ride any place in the United States or any training device extant in the U.S. Navy that gives an experience like it.

While I was indulging in this lusty sensation, I realized that throughout all of it the two pilots had remained busy with the aircraft. While I was still enjoying the experience, there was a guy in a yellow shirt out in front of the aircraft extending his left arm and beckoning with his right while the aircraft was being taxied over to starboard. Just at the same time, the two wings were being folded up by the copilot, and we were taxiing to a place to park. A 41-year-old man, I had waited all these years for my opportunity to land on a flight deck. Images of Van Johnson, Tom Cruise, John Wayne, John Glenn, all came bubbling up, but I did not have time to enjoy them, because as soon as we had turned that corner and traveled about four seconds, the door popped open on the aircraft, and we all started unloading. Since I was the most senior, I was ushered off first. You have to wear a cranial or a helmet at all times on the flight deck, so I was not able to get this thing off my throbbing ears. No sooner had I stepped out of the aircraft than a hand slapped down on my shoulder, pulling me by the survival vest toward the right side. It was a guy in a white shirt with the letters "ATO" printed on the back of his survival jacket. We were all dragged into the "island" on the starboard side of the aircraft, and a large watertight door closed behind us. We were then quickly shunted through a door into what I realized was the flight deck BDS (battle dressing station). Happily, I was able to take my cranial off. Oh, what a great relief! I knew my ears were red and about three times their usual size, but did it feel good to get that off.

So that is how I came to arrive on the Forrestal by US-3 on 29 July 1988. Lieutenant Commander Rausch, the ATO, having jerked me off the flight line into the flight deck BDS, was introducing me around to the corpsmen who were in the BDS, and also to the first officer I was to meet on the ***Forrestal***, Lieutenant Bruce Boswell. Boswell was one of the two flight surgeons assigned to Carrier Air Wing 6 (CVW6). He was a muscular, hyperactive, enthusiastic, mesomorph about 5 feet 7 inches tall. He pumped my hands a few times and said, "We were wondering if you were going to make it here, Sir," which I was to hear from a number of people as the day went on.

Boswell bounced around the BDS, telling me about the ship and his time there. I learned that we had arrived in the middle of a General Quarters drill. There had not been too many of those during the preceding 2 months, because of the high operating tempo of the ship. Since GQ is an exercise every ship must practice periodically, and there is a quota for how many times it has to be done during a cruise, we would have to do it a lot of times for the remainder of the deployment to catch up for the past two months. Because of GQ I could not be taken below to the Medical Department or to my stateroom yet. GQ was the reason there were no flight operations at the present, too. So we were stuck sitting around during GQ, practicing first aid drills, with the ventilation closed, along with a lot of the passageways.

It was probably a fitting time to arrive at the ship, though. Although as a drill GQ is the most boring thing you can do on a ship, it at least gave me time to catch my breath and prepare for taking on the role of shipmate.

CHAPTER TWO. THE FIRST TWO WEEKS

It isn't the first thing you notice about the ship, in fact, you don't notice it until you're away from there. But from the very first, there's a constant underlying hum always in the background. The hum is from the engines, from the electricity, from the activity, from passing through the water. It's just from the ship and it is always there. It was there that day, although I didn't notice it then. It's like the smell of the turf on a football field. You never really notice it, until years after. But now you remember the smell of the turf most of all. I think of the hum now all the time. I miss it.

When GQ was over, we went down a series of ladders on our way to the second deck. The flight deck is four decks above the hangar deck, which is the equivalent of the Main Deck on surface ships. On the first aircraft carriers, a flight deck had simply been constructed on a trellis over the main deck, and so that tradition is continued in the naming of the decks on current aircraft carriers. There are no true stairs on Navy ships, just steep stair-like "ladders." Some of them have actual hand rails attached, but most have chains about waist high that run from the top of the of the ladder down to the deck.

Passing through the hangar bay, at the end of General Quarters, I was impressed, as everyone always is, by the size of the hangar deck, and the number of huge aircraft it could hold. I had been on aircraft carriers before, but always in port, when there were no aircraft aboard. There is a constant melee of activity in the hangar bay. Squatty, short, but powerful diesel tractors are pulling and pushing aircraft and other heavy equipment all over. The tractors have to be short and squatty because they must pass underneath aircraft bellies and wings laden with drop tanks or electronic pods. Technicians wearing green and brown shirts climb all over aircraft 24 hours a day, cleaning them, taking them apart, working on engines and so forth. It is loud with pneumatic and hydraulic equipment buzzing all the time, electrical machinery working, engines turning, hammers banging, and people walking every direction.

More than the activity or the noise, however, one had to be impressed by the attitude and expression of the young men in the hangar bay. Of course, they all looked young and healthy. Yet the vibrance, the attitude, the cheerfulness, the professionalism, these were the most striking. Here were young men, most of them barely past their teen years, who were working 18 hours every day in a stressful industrial plant, in a dirty, grimy place, but they were all paying close attention to their jobs, laughing and joking, virtually all of them smiling. They also seemed to enjoy their work. A young sailor would find something small on the deck and reach down and pick it up. Whenever one worker thought he saw an area with oil dripping from under a wing or a tank, he quickly put a pan under it. When you passed someone on the hangar deck or in the passageways below, they smiled, asked "How are you, Sir?" or had some cheerful comment.

We eventually found our way into the Medical Department, virtually in the middle of the ship on the second deck. I was brought to an amidships passageway that had a brass placard on the door saying "Senior Medical Officer, Captain John Bigbee." We went into that office, which was soon to be mine for the next two years, and I met John Bigbee for the first time. He and I had spoken on the telephone back in the spring when I knew I would be coming to the FID, but this was our first opportunity to meet in person.

John is a tall, lanky fellow with a scratchy voice and an innocent face. Regardless of the situation, he always looks to me to have an expression of innocent bemusement. Although he looks all of his 50+ years, there is an adolescent quality about him as well. He reminds me of a young cowboy named "Sugarfoot" I had enjoyed on

TV as a teenager. In fact, John had been in practice in Oklahoma once. His innocent appearance was deceptive. John was a very accomplished physician. He had come to the FID suddenly, after his predecessor was relieved abruptly under a cloud. In two years, he had restored the medical department to a fine level.

"Well, I see you made it, we're glad to have you. I was afraid you weren't coming."

I learned that the Captain and Executive Officer had been teasing Bigbee about whether I would arrive during the deployment. After a little more than 2 years in the job he was eagerly looking forward to his return to shore duty.

He introduced me first to Lieutenant Rick Combs, the Medical Administrative Officer. During our turnover, there was a huge inventory that I would need to sign for. This included all of the laboratory equipment in the Medical Department, all of the drugs (many of which were controlled substances), along with hundreds of litters, the materials in the four storerooms that belonged to the Medical Department and all of the gear and equipment in the six Battle Dressing Stations (BDS's), each of which could function as an independent medical department with operating room in the event of emergency or ship's damage.

After the short initial tour John said, "There's something you need to know about. I just found out about it today. One of the officers on the Staff is an insulin dependent diabetic. I already brought this up with the Captain, but it looks like it's something you will have to handle eventually." We both knew what that meant. There are a number of conditions that are considered disqualifying for sea duty. Diabetes is high on that list. The aircraft carrier has a large medical department, and of course has insulin as part of the regular formulary of the pharmacy, but for emergencies, not routine care of chronic conditions. Treating an emergency or an unpredictable new medical problem is one thing. A known, and therefore avoidable chronic illness is something altogether different. There are so many potential complications or emergencies with chronic diseases such as diabetes that regulations prohibit diabetics sea duty. So people often hide diabetes and other chronic conditions to protect their careers.

There are a number of things that can cause emergencies with diabetes, such as reactions to insulin, sudden worsening of the diabetes, increased vulnerability to infections, higher risk of heart attacks... even coma. These are situations all of us Navy doctors were trained to contend with, but preventing or avoiding a dangerous situation is always preferable.

That the involved officer was a member of the "Staff" was only a further complication. Aircraft carriers usually travel and function as part of a Battle Group in company with two or more frigates or destroyers, and often a cruiser. Frequently, there are one or more submarines somewhere in the area as well. The aircraft carrier being the largest and most capable vessel in the group is the flag ship for the embarked Task Force Commander and his staff.

The staff is a stable organization, a command itself. People are assigned to it just as though they would be assigned to a squadron or to a ship. Rear Admiral (lower half) Leighton W. "Snuffy" Smith was the Battle Group or Task Force Commander of CCG 6. A gregarious, good-humored, energetic, and immensely likeable man, "Snuffy" Smith was an A7 pilot, highly decorated during Vietnam, well known to be a rising star in the Navy, and liked by most people in the ship's company. By contrast, everybody else on a Staff was usually tolerated. The most hated of all, however, were the Flag Secretary, and the professionally officious Flag Lieutenant. For some reason, the Navy seemed to prefer an arrogant and abrasive, albeit bright, lieutenant to be the Flag Lieutenant, or "Loop," so called because of the gold braid worn looped over his left shoulder[1]. He was short on words like "please," and seldom made requests when commands could fit. Every sentence seemed to begin with "The Admiral wants..." or "The Admiral told me to tell you..." Not so much as though relaying the boss's wish but to remind the listener that you'd better do what I tell you.

So all in all, the relationship between the Ship's Company and the Staff was never cordial, and usually antagonistic. The Staff had their own Mess so that they did not have to join or participate in meals in the Ward Room. The ship's company and wardroom loved the admiral, but kept a guarded but cool professional relationship with the Staff. We were just very careful with them.

So this was the background of the reported individual with diabetes, a member of the Staff, which was a situation promising not to be easily handled, but requiring definite early attention.

Besides walking all over the ship with Rick Combs inventorying equipment and learning about the spaces on the ship, I spent a lot of time that week walking around with John Bigbee. John carried a hand-held Motorola radio with him everywhere he went. These walkie-talkies weighed about 7 pounds, were 8 inches long, and 3 by 4 inches thick. There was a springy 5-inch antenna at the top. They were the familiar radios you see police officers carrying everywhere in the United States. Such a radio is called a "brick" because of its size, shape, and weight. Bigbee had a holster for his that he wore on his trousers like Matt Dillon wore his 45 back in Dodge City. John would never leave his office without it, and in fact usually would leave his radio on when he was in the office. He wanted to be reached at any time, at any hour. He showed me the brick and told me I would need to use it always.

At Formal Dining on my first night, John Bigbee introduced me to the Ward Room, where I was greeted with a round of applause, but less than John received for his imminent departure. The genuine warmth and welcoming from the Ward Room was spontaneous, reassuring, and immediate. Symbolically, John passed on the brick to me and said, "Tonight I give him the brick, and over the next few days I intend to give him the entire Medical Department."

About 2 days later, John saw me one time without the brick on my hip, and asked me where it was. I told him that if anybody needed me, I thought I could hear them over the 1MC, the overhead announcing system, but John told me, "You never know when that could go out, especially in an emergency. You ought to have the brick with you at all times." So I put it back on and carried it until John left a few days later. After John was gone, I never put the brick on again except for special exercises, and through my entire 2 years I don't think anybody ever tried to call me on it. Afterward, I did a study on the subject, and it appears that nobody ever tried to call John with it either.

The day after John introduced me to the Ward Room, we had a meeting in the Medical Department early in the morning, and he introduced me to all of the staff. I had already met Rick Combs, the MAO, and several of the enlisted people, especially HM1 Curt Rosenthal and HM1 Tom Dunwoody, two First Class Petty Officers who, along with the CPO's were the mainstays of the Medical Department. The people on the aircraft carrier belonged to three main organizations: the Ship's Company, all those

---

[1] *The formal name for the loop is "aiguillette," but nobody knows that word except me (and now you).*

people who belonged directly to the ship; the Staff, only about 200 people in total; and the embarked Air Wing. The Air Wing consisted of the eight flying squadrons, their associated Wing Staff, and all the maintenance people belonging to the Wing and squadrons. With the eight squadrons in the Carrier Air Wing 6 (CVW6), there were two flight surgeons, the senior being Lieutenant Bruce Boswell, who would be leaving us at the end of this cruise in another 3 months, and Lieutenant William Flynn, a Yale and Georgetown graduate who would be with us most of another year. On a cruise, the flight surgeons and squadron corpsmen were assigned to the Medical Department. The flight surgeons, however were expected to spend up to 50 percent of their time with their squadrons: giving instruction, looking after the health of the flight crew, and doing some flying themselves to maintain their contact with their charges. Just as there is a traditional friction between the Ship's Company and the Flag Staff, there is often a milder friction between the Ship's Company and the CVW, and this carries on even down to the Medical Department. Flight surgeons are often a little bit unpopular with other members of the Medical Department. For one thing, they're gone part of the time while they're off working with their squadrons or flying, and for another, they are only with the Department underway. When the ship returns to port, they return to the home bases of their various squadrons in other towns. Also, flight surgeons wear wings, and they identify more with their squadrons than they do with the ship or the Medical Department. Some flight surgeons have been described as aviation groupies more than doctors.

In our Department this friction was particularly palpable. On the Forrestal the Medical Department had three officers with very definite opinions about flight surgeons in general, and our two Wing flight surgeons in particular. First was the Warrant Officer Physician Assistant ("WOPA"), Art Forbes. Art was a former Senior Chief Petty Officer, an Independent Duty Corpsman on submarines, who had gone to physician assistant school. Art was reminiscent of Sergeant Bilko in the 1950s sit-com. He knew how to accomplish anything on the ship, seemed to know either everybody on the ship or everybody who could make anything happen, and was in very definite control of his life style. The Warrant Officers had their own community on the Forrestal had their own bank of staterooms on the third deck, and their own ethic. Art enjoyed a particular prestigious position among the other Warrant Officers, and had strong opinions about the way medicine used to be practiced on the submarines, and how modern young doctors had sometimes gone astray of the direction they should go. Flight surgeons were often a frivolous lot to Art, certainly he had not had to contend with them back when he worked on submarines all those years.

Our General Medical Officer ("GMO") was Douglas Kempf, a classics scholar from Georgetown University who had once very nearly decided to become a priest. Doug was tall, spare, meticulous, and exceedingly hard headed. Prussian in his outlook on life, demanding of himself and others, he was fiercely loyal to John Bigbee and to the ship. Doug has no tolerance for frivolity, which he thought was abundant in the person of Dr. Bruce Boswell, and suspiciously likely in anybody who would become a flight surgeon. That is, except for John Bigbee; John was a flight surgeon, but Doug revered him.

Finally our surgeon. Young general surgeons usually hated to go to sea on aircraft carriers. They usually were aggressive young men, as surgeons always are, and they were invariably sent at a time in their careers when they were preparing to take their specialty board examinations. They were plucked away from their surgical practices in Navy Hospitals to go to sea in what they considered a situation worse than Purgatory. Our surgeon on the ***USS Forrestal*** was a bright young, former collegiate wrestler named Rock Tosser. Rock didn't like being taken away from the hospital, where his skills could be used to save lives daily, but he reluctantly recognized that he owed the Navy a lot of money for his medical school scholarship, and if this was the wasteful way the Navy wanted to be paid back, he would comply, although not enthusiastically. What bothered Rock was that the department didn't have the best doctor on the ship be the one in charge, namely the surgeon. Rock thought that Doug Kempf was educable, but doubted that any of the rest of us were. That any serious physician would waste time becoming a flight surgeon when they could be fighting the constant battle against death and disease in the operating room was unthinkable. Likewise, that anybody as old as John Bigbee or I would intentionally still be in the Navy when they could be out doing better for medicine, and doing something more serious in life, proved to him that we were at least lazy, and probably also incompetent.

When John introduced me to the members of the Medical Department the most welcoming and effusive was either Art Forbes, who could charm the warts off a cucumber, or Bruce Boswell, who was as friendly and genuine as "Tigger" in the ***Winnie-The-Pooh*** books. He bounced everywhere, he had an exciting idea almost every day, and he genuinely wanted to be everybody's friend. Doug Kempf was in every respect perfectly courteous, but just as perfectly obvious that he didn't like me, was not going to like me, and was not intending to change for anybody who was not John Bigbee. Rock Tosser shook my hand, said, "Hi," and had a non-committal, almost friendly chuckle. Until proven otherwise, I was a possibly nice guy, even if a little dumb.

John made a little speech about what a pleasure it had been working with all of them throughout the cruise. He pointed out that we were soon going to be in Naples and that he would be catching a flight back to The States from there. He told the Department to welcome me as they had welcomed him, and he talked about how proud he had been to work with the Department and how far they had all come together. Then he said, "It has been a good tour for all of us. We have had no loss of life. That, at least, is something we can all be proud of." No loss of life. That got my attention. Everybody knew that there was at least one death on every cruise. John had been on the ship for 2 years without a single death. I knew that the law of averages would not permit that to go on. What a time to arrive! Anybody who was a good doctor on the Forrestal would not let people die. John Bigbee had set a high standard.

Several days later, we arrived in Naples, the first port call for the ship after 108 days underway. Naples has a large U.S. Navy installation, including a Naval hospital. I would have to make plans as a SMO to visit the Naval hospital, coordinate any patient or specialty transfers, and pay a courtesy call on the Commanding Officer of the hospital.

Because we needed to free John Bigbee so that he could return to The States, because I was new and had to learn a lot about the Medical Department on the ship, and because everyone else onboard had 108 days without stepping on land, during our 8 days in port I determined to have only a couple of days off the ship, trying to free up time for the other doctors.

Aircraft carriers are too big to tie up at the pier in most harbors. So it was in Naples. Inside the harbor proper there was a big breakwater setting off a smaller inner harbor called a "molo." Although we were able to get a lot closer than the ship did in most ports, we were still about a quarter mile away from the fleet landing, perhaps a hundred yards from the breakwater. Beside us on either side were such decrepit and rusted out old tankers, with no signs of life and absolutely no habitation, that you had to wonder how many years had they been there. In fact much about Naples was like that, amidst the flurry of activity and the frenzied pace that Neapolitans set, all around were signs of fallen grandeur, a pride in the artistry and history of Italy, and yet very little evidence of trying to restore any of that. Bob Harris, the AirOps Officer, told me he had once seen a dead horse floating in Naples harbor.

A BUSY SHIFT

I missed all the excitement of pulling into port the first time, being stuck down in the Medical Department. From the moment that "sea and anchor detail" was called away, I began treating people for the accidents of haste and anticipation. Lacerations on the scalp from people who tried to jump through the oval knee-knocker doors on the 0-3 deck, an increased number of corneal abrasions from people who were hurrying their various grinding jobs, a couple of sprained ankles from people who fell while hurrying down ladders while trying to get to the hangar deck to line up for liberty call.

Since the ship could not tie up at the pier, sailors had to take either utility boats, or rented ferryboats to get over to Fleet Landing. The ship only needed about a thousand people onboard to man it, so nearly 4,000 people wanted off the ship within a few hours. Even with ferryboats that could take 200 to 250 at a time, it took 2 or 3 hours to get everyone off the ship. A large ladder was put off at the fantail, to a floating, flat, raft-like platform called a "camel." The ferryboats would pull alongside the camel, and the sailor would step from the camel up to the ferryboat, sometimes with a small ramp, or sometimes negotiating an 18-inch jump. If the water was choppy, there were opportunities for falling, spraining an ankle, or getting stuck between objects, both where the ladder from the fantail came to the camel, or where the camel abutted the ferryboat. The last of these was the most hazardous, because both the camel and the ferryboat would have reciprocal movements. By going opposite directions, they doubled the height of the waves. The camel went down 18 inches and the ferryboat went up 18 inches, all in a split second, like a man-sized mouse-trap. That was the cause of an occasional laceration so I had some suturing to do on shins and wrists as the evening wore on and people came and went.

Beginning at about 2200, the Medical Department became a real growth industry. I was the only physician on duty that night, with a handful of corpsmen, notably HM1 Jackie Branom, and the big walrus corpsman Arden Womple. One hundred eight days without parties and without alcohol was just too big a temptation for a lot of the young sailors, of course. First, came a 19-year-old with a broken nose who was only slightly drunk, bragging "I'll fix that son-of-a-bitch, Doc," but as soon as he said that he vomited all over my shirt, and fell sleep in my arms.

Within minutes, three sailors came down with their younger buddy who looked to be about 15 years old, a fireman on his first cruise, who was only kept awake by his constant retching. After he vomited two or three times, I could not imagine a person as small as he was had enough food left in him to do it again, but it just kept coming, an orange and purple volcano. While I was explaining to his buddies that there was not much we could do for his emesis, the 1MC called "Medical emergency, medical emergency. On the fantail. Medical emergency on the fantail."

I sent away my two emergency response corpsmen who went with a litter and their unit-1, the corpsman emergency medical bag. The seas were getting choppy, and a sailor had fallen off the ferryboat between the edge of the camel and the boat. Just before the edges of the two slapped together and crushed his head, the Chief Petty Officer in charge of the receiving line plucked him out in the last moment, but he still had a big gash on his shin, and had fractured his ankle from the impact. He swallowed a lot of water and was coughing and sputtering, so they brought him to Medical. No sooner had they arrived, about 10 minutes after the call, then another call, "Medical emergency! Medical emergency, on the fantail. Medical emergency."

This time, a lieutenant from one of the squadrons had made it up on the camel, and although drunk and somewhat staggering, had begun to walk toward the ladder up to the fantail. A sudden lurch on the camel threw him down on the ladder, which he straddled, tore his pants, and cut himself in the groin. He could not walk, began to vomit, and was bleeding a lot from the crotch area, frightening the people who brought him up. When he got to the Medical Department, we noticed a large gash in the bottom of his scrotum, and asked if he could void. He was so drunk that for 20 minutes he could not understand us, but it was clear that his bladder was growing larger. Finally, he was able to give us a urine sample, the color of grape juice, clearly indicating bleeding somewhere along his urinary tract, probably in the urethra, the tube leading from the bladder through the penis. We were unable to pass a catheter through his penis, implying that the laceration obstructed the passage of fluid, so we took a kind of X-ray called a urethrogram. This is a specialized technique that would usually not be done in a country doctor's office, but we had devised a technique of placing the catheter to the opening of the penis and injecting a small amount of a contrast material called renograffin and taking a photograph. The X-ray clearly showed disruption in what should be a smooth columnar flow of fluid along the shaft of the penis. There was a ragged, zig-zag pathway of the fluid, although it did pass through between the bladder and the outer wall of the urethra. This would almost certainly need care by a specialist, a urologist. Fortunately, we were in Naples and in the morning when the seas were calm we would be able to bring the young lieutenant to the hospital.

Although gradually waking up, he was still pretty drunk, now reaching the boisterous, laughing, uninhibited stage. When we explained his injury to him, he said, "Just my luck, no score in town, and then I broke my dick on the way back to the ship."

HM1 Rosenthal, who was making the record of the case, asked me, "What should write down for his diagnosis, Captain, 'Broke dick'?" This became a cause celebre through the Medical Department over the next hour while people seemed to repeat for the fun of it the diagnosis of "broke dick." None of us had ever seen that particular injury on returning from liberty before. Two hours later, the identical injury happened to a young sailor, so we had two "broke dicks" in the same night.

Around midnight, Jim Bowersman was brought in by three of his buddies. Bowersman was a 40-year-old Petty Officer who had made rank three or four times and been busted back to Seaman each time after some fight or other misadventure. Tonight he was tearful and morose, clinging to his buddies, scarcely able to stand.

"You're gonna have to help him, Doc. He keeps sayin' he's gonna do himself in. He was trying to cut himself on the edges of a bottle." In fact, there were some scratch marks on his chest, his shirt was torn, and there were some ragged, very unartistic scratch marks on the underside of his forearm. His friends said that he had tried to cut himself or stab himself with a broken beer bottle. "It's no sense. This is the only thing I can do. Leave me alone." He occasionally would make some feeble effort to push people away, then he would swear or just slump down like he was trying to fall asleep. My job was to try to console him, and to assess whether he was really suicidal, or just impulsively drunk. We had to go off to my office so that he and I could have some privacy and try to work through this problems. His buddies started to wander off like they were either going to go back to their racks or maybe back to the beach.

"Oh, no you don't, you guys sit down right out here." We needed to keep a buddy nearby in the event he would have to be escorted off to the hospital, or in the event we were able to send him back to his rack. A buddy would need to stay with him throughout the night. Bowersman and I went into my office, where he slumped down in my chair, looking at his feet in a surly manner, at this point having nothing to say. I sat quietly nearby trying to give him time to talk, maintaining eye contact, but not trying to prod him. At these times, in medical school, we were taught to just nod knowingly or to say something soothing like, "Tell me more," or "Go on."

Bowersman and I sat in that position, him nodding off or muttering something about how life had been unfair to him, me wishing that the night would hurry up, for what seemed like a couple of hours, although I guess it was only about 15 or 20 minutes. We were interrupted by a loud noise out in the passageway, sounding like a wrestling or boxing match. When I looked outside, there was a tall, skinny sailor fighting with the four people trying to bring him into the emergency room. Three of them were Shore Patrol in their white uniforms, all stained with blood. Another one was probably his buddy, also matted with sweat or beer, and some blood stains on his shirt. The protagonist, being pretty agitated and obviously also loaded, had a large zig-zag cut on the right side of his face from his eyebrow down to his chin, and a smaller one stretching across the left side of his forehead down to the middle of his check. About this time, Doug Kempf came back from liberty. Doug, of course, was absolutely sober, and as usual was pretty cross. Although Doug was planning to become a psychiatrist, he prided himself on suturing, especially on the face, and he offered to take care of the sailor whose name we found to be Jimmy Fulford. The skin on his face was filleted and hanging over to the right side, flapping every time he moved. When momentarily he would hold still, it was obvious that he had a third cut running under his chin, penetrating most of the way through the mouth.

Doug found a couple of corpsmen, plus the two shore patrol to help hold Fulford down. Because he was so drunk he could not be given a sedative, but he intermittently would fall asleep.

I did the best I could, patiently sitting and talking with Bowersman, who was gradually sobering up and becoming a little bit embarrassed about what he had done. Obviously all of his wounds were very superficial, and once we had assured that they were clean with peroxide and adequate scrubbing, at about 3:30 or 4:00 in the morning, he assured me he was safe. I had made his buddies stay nearby, and although they had fallen asleep on the bench in the passageway, they were with him now to go back to his rack and look over him to make sure no further shenanigans happened all night.

Almost 2 hours had gone by now, and I stuck my head into the suturing room where Doug was still working on Fulford. Deep sutures had been required to put together the soft tissues of the cheek, to close the floor of the mouth and the chin, and Doug was now putting the finishing touches with tiny little silk sutures on the last closure on the left side of the face. Fulford was asleep most of the time, but periodically would twist his head or twitch in such a way that Doug would throw his arms up, being careful not to put too much tension on any of the sutures. When you looked at the suturing job, despite all the bruises on his face, it was truly a work of art, something that Doug was justifiably pride of. The fellow had obviously taken quite a beating. Besides the cuts, he had obviously been pummeled by a far superior force, his face was pretty purple besides the cut. Finally, when Doug was finished, he admitted Fulford to the ward so that he could be properly restrained, because Doug was afraid that he would have further troubles if he went out.

"Captain, I'd like to put this guy on Liberty Risk, because I don't want him to go out and pull the damn sutures the first thing out tomorrow." Liberty Risk was a program prohibiting individuals with behavior disorders or something else wrong from leaving the ship. We found out subsequently that Fulford had been in a fight with some civilians in town, had done some local damage to a civilian bar, insulted several Neapolitans, and before he had his clock cleaned had charges pressed against him by the local police, the carabinieri. At least we knew would not get into any further trouble in Naples, after the XO agreed with us to keep him confined to the ship on class A Liberty Risk.

The next morning, Sunday, the only day I would be able to go into town, I received a call from the Officer of the Day at the Navy Hospital Naples. The Commanding Officer, Captain Bullis Butts, would like to come and visit the ship. Could I arrange for a tour and a visit between the Commanding Officer of the hospital and the Commanding Officer of the ship? He would be able to arrive at about 11:00 in the morning.

This was my first time ever to visit Italy. My only day off during this port call, and I had hoped to take a trip to see Mount Vesuvius and Pompei. Now this character was going to come at about 11:00 o'clock. I took some smug pleasure knowing that the both the CO and XO were going to be off the ship. I said good-bye to John Bigbee that day, and waited around until 1100. Then 1200. Then 1300. Then, finally, at 1500, I heard him announced with the bell and the 1MC, "Bong. Bong. Naval Hospital Naples, arriving." Commanding Officers from other commands were always "bonged" aboard, just like our own Captain or Admiral. On the small boys, all captains or above got "bonged" on, but on the carrier there were too many captains. Ships company captains, other than the CO, only got bonged off at their last departure.

I went up to meet him at the quarter deck, and there he came, trying to imitate George Washington crossing the Potomac, a typical hospital Navy doctor. A somewhat portly guy with an ill-fitting uniform and only three ribbons, the skipper of the Navy Hospital was standing awkwardly in the bow of the small boat. He was wearing his own version of the famous MacArthur cap. His naval cover was flopping down on the edges, something that naval officers never do. Maybe in the movies people take pride in a "salty"uniform, but naval officers when visiting other ships try to have everything as spiffy as they can. The gold braid on the visor of his cap was tarnished and worn, looking more dusty tan than gold. This was "salty" all right.

When he came aboard, he confessed that he had never been on an aircraft carrier before. He had been Commanding Officer of the Navy Hospital Naples for almost 2 years, during which time a number of carriers had come into port, but he had never come to visit them. He had never gone to sea personally either.

I tried to show him all around the ship, from the fo'c'sle to the Medical Department, to the flight deck, and offered him lunch in the Ward Room. With his studied nonchalance, he nodded knowingly about everything I had to tell him about the ship, as though he had seen it all many times before. This, despite our discussing that he had never been on a carrier before. If I had called the fantail a goldfish or the fo'c'sle a fladderap he wouldn't have known the difference. Finally, the boredom overtook both of us, and it was time for him to leave. I noticed dusk was coming, to guarantee that I would not have to worry about a day of liberty on my first and only time in Naples. I was happy to show him off the ship, thinking under my breath something along the lines of "Good riddance, you old. . . " not realizing that my most unpleasant encounters with the famous Captain Bullis Butts were yet to come.

That evening the seas were a little calmer, and we had nobody falling down ladders or off the camel, although we had a few torn or bitten ears to sew up. The next day was busier though.

On that day, the Morale, Welfare and Rec Department on the ship put on a big picnic at Carney Park. It's a park utilized by Armed Forces of all the NATO countries in the Naples area, resident in a volcanic crater just outside town. Although a number of sailors had too much beer to drink, athletics were the main order of the day. These were not only people who had not been on dates or had any drinking for 108 days, but they had also not played any sports, except for calisthenics and running on the flight or hangar decks. No softball, no running or sliding in the dirt, and no soccer. It looked to me like they had tried to catch up all 108 days (on out-of-shape limbs) in one day. Four different people had ankle or lower leg fractures, three had fractures of the wrists or forearms, and a number had black eyes or broken teeth, just from the sports.

Fractures of the lower extremity required casts, of course, and the cast itself hampered mobility, so that anyone with a fracture or cast on his lower extremity could not be permitted to go to sea. All of those people, even if treated on the ship, had to be sent off to the Navy Hospital at Naples, later to be transferred back to The States and had to be replaced in the ship's company. We referred to this day from then onward as the "Carney Park Massacre." Seven people had to be shipped off from the FID that day, one of whom was in continual traction at the Navy Hospital Naples. Finally, not having any liberty that day, and having been awake most of the prior night taking care of drunks or people with facial lacerations, I crawled into my stateroom near midnight.

I was awakened the next morning with banging on my door. "Sorry, Captain, we have an emergency up in the flag spaces." It was Curt Rosenthal. "There's a guy passed out up in his cabin, Captain. It may be that guy with diabetes Captain Bigbee told you about."

I dressed as quickly as I could and followed Petty Officer Rosenthal up the four decks to the 03 level where three senior officers were huddled around a figure slumped over the edge of his bed. On the desk in the room were two bottles of insulin, one of them empty, the other half empty and cloudy, and three insulin syringes on the table.

The patient was a fortyish-year-old, very frail looking individual. His pulse was 115 beats per minute, and he felt feverish. He was very sweaty, and he had the kind of fruity aroma suggestive of ketosis. The insulin was of two types, NPH U-100, labeled on the half-filled bottle, and another with the label mostly off.

"We haven't seen him for about 3 days, Doc. We thought he was out on liberty. Somebody was just looking for him today, and found out he was in here."

"Commander, how long have you been sick?" I asked.

His answer was groggy, but he was clearly conscious and could understand the question.

"Been sick for about a week. I thought I was doin' okay until about 3 days ago. I'll be all right. Just let me rest, and leave me alone for a little while."

"Commander, I'm not going to try to hassle you, but your fever is hot as Hell. Something is wrong. When you get an infection, you know, your insulin requirements change. I can tell by your pulse rate, and by the smell of your breath, that your diabetes is out of control, do you know what ketosis is?"

"Yes, I know, I've had it before, but this isn't it."

"Look, Commander, you're sick, at least we all can agree on that. At least let us take you down to medical, let us check your blood sugar, and get you back into balance. You've got a high fever, we have to make sure you don't have pneumonia or something a lot worse. Blood infections can happen to guys with diabetes, too, you know."

"It's probably a bladder infection. I get those sometimes."

Great! The guy knows that he's prone to bladder infections, he has had ketosis before, and yet he hides away with his insulin here on the ship. That's just great. This is the worst kind of nightmare we could imagine. For God's sake, the guy could have died if somebody hadn't just stumbled into the room.

He refused to be carried down to medical, and walked mostly under his own power, although with support by his buddies, other senior officers on the Flag Staff. It turned out his blood sugar was 560, he had ketones, breakdown products of fat, in his urine and blood. On what we call a "sliding scale" of insulin, we were able to get his blood sugar back in balance within 15 hours, but as usual, his level of alertness and concentration lagged behind the body chemistries by about another day. He had pyelonephritis, evidenced by tenderness over his kidneys and his back and abnormal urinalysis tests, as well as slightly elevated BUN and creatinine.

I told him he would need to transferred to the Navy Hospital, and he really would have to be transferred off the ship.

"No, I don't think the Admiral would agree to that."

"Don't worry, Commander, I'll go talk to the Admiral about it."

I went ahead and arranged to transfer him to the hospital which was of course the right thing to do even though we were able take care of his ketosis on the ship, and to start him on proper antibiotics. The causes of pyelonephritis need to be found, though. Although diabetes predisposes, if there were some structural abnormality in the kidney, or some other illness, we sure needed to find it, for example, a foreign body or stone in the kidney. Admiral Smith is very concerned about his people. He recognized, of course, that medical necessity was the overriding concern, and he agreed immediately with transferring Commander Leen to the hospital. He said we could deal with the situation later after Leen recovered.

I was at least relieved by the outcome of this. Diabetes is a controllable, although still dangerous, disease. The worst nightmare, though, was the possibility that somebody would try to manage it himself and not tell you about his condition. Worst of all, that somebody would confine himself to his own stateroom, quietly wasting away, either not taking his insulin at all or taking too much of it, and dying simply because he would not communicate with the doctors. This was one paradox a Navy doctor feared more than any other. A patient who was more concerned about the bureaucratic ramifications of treatment for his illness than he was about the complications of the disease itself. A guy who would think like that might not only be responsible for his own demise, but could bring the doctor down with him. It's not the way a doctor is supposed to think, but this was an entirely preventable disease, or possibly preventable death -- besides worrying about the patient, a doctor couldn't help being a little angry, too.

We got underway uneventfully the next day, Jimmy Fulford's cuts healing up well, under the careful view of Doug Kempf's daily evaluation, and all the sailors on the ship still joking about the two "broke dicks."

THE FLIGHT DECK AND OTHER DECKS

On the first day out of Naples, the ship was headed west towards Spain, and I was about to get my first flight off the ship, this time on an H-3 helicopter, the aircraft flown by HS-15, the "Red Lions." Before the flight, I trundled up with all my flight gear and survival vest, up through the passageway in the forward port side of the ship just above the fo'c'sle, to the Ready Room for HS-15. The passageway leading into their Ready Room was along the port side catapult run by steam. The passageway was as hot as a sauna. By the time I arrived at the Ready Room, which was well air conditioned, I was soaked all the way through my flight suit.

Before every flight in a naval aircraft, there is a detailed brief for all flight crew members. Although as the flight surgeon you usually have very little to contribute, you are, after all, part of the flight crew, so you have to sit through the brief. In the brief, the mission and the weather conditions are reviewed. Communications procedures, the use of all the various radio frequencies, how the call signs will be used, with whom the crew will speak, how they will talk to the ship, and how they will talk to other aircraft are reviewed. Emergency procedures including how to egress under water are reviewed in the same picky detail for experienced flyers as the first flight. Then the mission of the flight is discussed in some detail and how the exercises or training will be done. The H-3 is antisubmarine helicopter as its main mission, although it has about five other auxiliary missions including rescue. They have a large sonar dipper that is suspended or "dipped" from the belly of the aircraft into various depths under the ocean to emit sonar detection for submarines. In addition, sonobouys can be propelled from the aircraft, to float at preset depths in the ocean, trailing an antenna that floats to the surface. The sonobouys send out and receive sonar images looking for submarines, and then transmit back the reception they get to a receiving station on the helicopter. In this manner, one helicopter can have a number of sounding stations, and can pinpoint a submarine. If two or three helicopters are functioning at once, they can look for submarines at some distance from the ship. The helicopters are also used as "plane guard" whenever flight operations are going on. Whenever fixed wing aircraft, the jets, are taking off or landing from the aircraft carrier, there is a helicopter in the air at all times, so that in the event of an aircraft mishap, they can go and rescue any survivors.

Finally, after the long brief, my flight suit was partially dried, and we began walking up to the flight deck. Once we got to the aircraft, I took my seat in the back of the helicopter, because both the pilot and co-pilot were necessary for controlling the aircraft on a takeoff. There is a wait before you can get clearance to take off just like at an airport. Because the helos need to be in the air throughout all other flight ops, they are the first to take off and the last to land during any scheduled flight operations. I plugged into the ICS, the intercom, and listened as the pilot was speaking to the tower. They talked about this clearance and that clearance, the weight of the aircraft, the wind across the deck, and the amount of fuel in the aircraft. Then I heard something about "man overboard," then something about we would have to abort the flight, and at first I thought there was going to be a man overboard drill conducted below. As the talk went on further, I realized it wasn't a drill. Oh-no, man overboard! If they were to find him, of course, there would be first aid to be done, or a corpse to be taken care of.

I broke into the ICS, "Commander, this is the Doc here in the back. Is that a real man overboard?"

"Roger, Doc. Seems like a guy was either blown off the fantail or the starboard side."

"I'm gonna have to get off, Commander. Can I?"

No answer for a while. It looked like the pilot and co-pilot were speaking to each other, then they came up on the radio to the tower, "Boss, 602. The Doc says he has to go down to Medical in case they pick up the man overboard."

I hurried off the helo and ran down to Medical as fast as I could. About the time I got to the catwalk on my way, another helicopter was just landing on the deck. It appears that they picked up the man overboard about the time he hit the water. I got down to Medical about the same time the victim did.

It turns out that Stan Mitchell, a 19-year-old Plane Captain from Plainsfield, Pennsylvania, had inadvertently stepped behind an A-7 and was blown off the fantail on the starboard side of the ship. It is a 9-story drop to the water. At that height, the mere impact with the water can cause injuries. There is a drill all of the people on the flight deck go through, practicing curling themselves up into a ball so that they impact on their feet and buttocks when they hit the water. AN Mitchell did everything perfectly. He calmly pulled the beads on his survival jacket, and inflated his vest. He put out his dye marker immediately, and was picked up within 2 minutes, and back on the deck of the ship within 7 minutes. His only complaint was soreness in his left wrist, which was pretty tender. When you hit the water from 9 floors up, it may break a wrist or an ankle just the same as hitting the ground.

Down in Medical, I examined him and found that all his parts were moving, his eyes were clear, his lungs were clear. He had full movement even of his wrists, the left one being sore. We took an X-ray and it was clear.

I called the Captain, who was relieved to learn there was no injury. He put out the notice on the 1-MC that the man overboard had been retrieved and was not injured. You could hear clapping and shouting throughout the ship. This was pretty satisfying to everybody, knowing that if somebody really was blown off the Forrestal, we would recognize it and find him within 7 minutes.

There was as mixed blessing in all this, in addition to the fact that I had not been able to take my flight. On the one hand, Rock Tosser had not butted into the care of the patient, but on the other hand, it was not like Rock to stay out of the case. I began to ask around where he was.

"I think he may be in the OR, Captain." I went up to the Emergency Room, and to the door leading to the operating room. It was locked. "Where is Branom?"

"I think he's in there with Dr. Tosser," said HM1 Dunwoody, clearly hoping he wouldn't have to get into the fray. "They have a guy with appendicitis."

You can't do an operation on the aircraft carrier without the permission of the Captain. It's one thing if you're taking casualties and everyone knows that people are injured and dying. Under those circumstances, you have to do what you need to, to save life and limb. While an appendectomy may be an emergency, it never has to happen within 5 or 10 minutes. Even if I were about to take off on the helicopter, Rock could have reached me by radio to discuss it. I could have come back to the deck. I have to approve all operations, and I have to get them cleared with the Captain. However routine an operation like an appendectomy might be, induction of anesthesia and violating the human skin could always lead to an unexpected tragedy or complication. It was a hard and fast rule that the SMO had the prerogative to be involved with any decision to do an operation, and had to clear it with the Captain. This was something Rock had trouble with, figuring that only a surgeon had the ability or right to make decisions about operations.

I would have just killed him. However, I figured it might interrupt the operation. It could look unmedical to leave open an unattended surgical opening in the patient while I pounded the holy hell out of the surgeon. Besides, this was also a chance for me to exert that leadership and persuasion I had been working on, so I thought I would try to rise above my anger. That would not be easy.

I went back to my own stateroom, got out of my flight suit, and showered so that I would be cool and calm when I had to talk to Rock about doing an operation without conferring with me. Knowing I had in fact been in an aircraft at the time made me feel a little bit cautious or defensive, I suppose.

About 15 minutes later Rock came out of the operating room. The individual did fine. I asked to see the appendix, which was not at all inflamed.

"You can't tell by just looking," Rock said. "It needed to come out."

"From now on, can you let me see the patient first?"

"If you're where I need you to be, that's fine, but I have to do what I think is right."

"Rock, I'll never ask you to do whatever isn't right, but you and I both know, you didn't need to start that operation before I got back. You know you could have got me on the radio for a real emergency, and also that I have to clear these things with the Captain."

"There is only one surgeon on this ship," Rock said. "I can only do what's right."

I think at that time I was about to punch his face in, but we were interrupted by the 1-MC.

"Medical emergency, medical emergency. Seven-tack-seventy five-tack-six. Medical emergency, seventh deck." Petty Officer Ramirez was our Emergency Response

Corpsman that day, and he came running into the Medical Department about the same time as the 1-MC announcement, "Man down in the seventh deck. Brian Haack is giving him CPR right now!"

Tosser and I ran immediately to the scene, on the port side, through a watertight door in the passageway. We looked straight down to about the sixth deck, where we climbed immediately, diverting slightly to the left and then down one more ladder. Meantime, some of the other corpsmen were bringing the life paks and other emergency response bags.

Brian Haack was giving CPR to a tall skinny fellow in the corner, and two sailors were standing by in another corner.

I got up to where Haack was and looked down at the face marked like a baseball. It was Jimmy Fulford.

"What happened?!" Haack kept doing CPR.

No answer.

"What happened!"

One of his buddies said, "He just started shaking all over, like a convulsion, and then he fell down. He kept shaking on the ground, and then he just quit breathing."

At about this time, Ramirez arrived on the scene, too, breathless, just like the rest of us. He was carrying the emergency response bags, all of the contents for CPR and advanced cardiac life support. "He wasn't breathing when I got here. I was never able to feel a pulse."

On the deck near Fulford's feet were two empty cans of solvent spray.

About this time Bill Flynn arrived on the scene and picked them up, trying to read the contents of the cans. He looked suspiciously at the other sailors standing in the corner.

CPR was continuing. "No pulse. No respirations." Haack was relieved by another corpsman.

By now I had the paddles set up for the defibrillator. This kind of life pak enables you to read a cardiac trace on a monitor from the paddles before you give a jolt.

"Here, let me take a reading," I said. Flat line.

"Everybody stand back." Two hundred Joules. Body jerked. CPR continued. No pulse.

"Everybody stand back." Three hundred Joules. His body jerked up again. Still no response in the ECG. No pulse.

"Everybody stand back." One more jolt. Again the body jerked quickly, but no pulse.

Rock was at his head. "Okay. Intubate." Rock slipped the endotracheal tube in deftly. He put an ambu bag over the end of the endotracheal tube and began ventilating while I listened to Fullford's chest with a stethoscope. Full breath sounds bilaterally. "Good breath sounds, continue ventilating him." CPR continued on his chest. Bill Flynn was putting in an intravenous line in the antecubital fossa.

The code was proceeding just as smoothly as it would in any major hospital in The States. Still there was no pulse. We gave epinephrine intravenously, then we gave lidocaine, repeated Lidocaine and epinephrine. We gave more shocks. Still no pulse.

It turns out Fulford and his buddies had been sniffing freon from those solvent cans. Apparently, they had been using freon down in this space throughout the cruise periodically. They would have a very good high from it, very much like sniffing glue. No chiefs or officers had known about it, but furtive glances among some of the sailors suggested it may have been more than a three man secret.

While the code continued, Bill got out one of our toxicology books and read the complications of freon inhalation. Ventricular fibrillation and cardiac arrest, or asystole, were known complications, and were resistant to CPR, apparently. We continued with the code for about 45 minutes, following everything just as it was in the book. Finally, Rock suggested, "We've done everything we're supposed to do. The only other possibility is if he had a cardiac tamponade. I know it seems unlikely, but we're not getting anyplace otherwise." I agreed. Rock used a cardiac needle to try to see if there were blood in the pericardial sac. There was not. Finally, after we had been going almost 1 hour, I had to call the code off.

"That's it. He's dead." So that was it. A 20-year-old, slightly rebellious, but vigorous young man was dead. John Bigbee had said "No loss of life" in over 2 years while he was the SMO. I had been the SMO for less than 2 weeks and already one of our boys died.

The corpsmen stayed behind to clean up the mess. Someone called for a body bag, I climbed up the top of the ladder to the second deck, and there was Captain Pieno. I realized when I got there that my cheeks were wet, and I told the Captain, "We did everything we could, Captain." I think he patted my shoulder and said only, "I know you did, Doc, I know you did." As bad as I felt about it and all of our corpsmen did, clearly the Captain felt it at least that much. He walked back with me, on his way to the bridge, so that he could send the message to Jimmy Fulford's parents.

After we finished up all the paperwork, I had made my records, and I prepared the medical details for Captain Pieno to send off the ship, I walked back to be alone on the fantail. It had been a busy couple of weeks. I looked off at the wake in the night, and remembered what Myron Almond had told me. There were only 14 people in the world who had my job.

CHAPTER III. BENIDORM

It's important to deal with death. In a closed community like an aircraft carrier, words, emotions, and attitudes all spread faster than in any small town... which after all is what a ship is, anyway. Death is just as hard for the medical folks as it for anybody else, and in a way worse. A lot of guilt goes along with losing a patient. This is a painful and difficult thing for health care workers of any age to learn, but as Bigbee had pointed out, this was something the Forrestal hadn't seen for at least 2 years. It was the first encounter with death for most of our 30 corpsmen, whose average age was less than twenty.

Once we had taken care of the scene, and delivered the body to the cooler, I made all members of the Medical Department who were not asleep to come to a meeting in Ward 2. Only about a dozen people had been directly involved with the resuscitation effort, but really everybody was involved one way or another whenever somebody died. In a department as small and tight as one with only about 40 people, a death is felt just as keenly among the Medical Department as it would be among a family. About 30 of us were there that night. Even corpsmen who had been asleep when the code began came. Some of them had been awakened when they heard there was a medical emergency. Others weren't awakened until somebody shook them to say a guy just died.

Among the 12 or so who had been involved in the Code, their buddies were particularly attentive now. They might have their arms around the guy's shoulder, bring him a cup of coffee, offer him their seat or a place to sit on the rack. Except for these signs of deference though, facial expressions could not tell which members had been involved in the Code. There were a few wet cheeks in the crowd, but everybody in the room was pretty sober.

"I wanted all you guys to come here right now so that we could spend a little time together working this out and for me to tell you a few things." I had been involved in dozens of Codes over the last 15 years. Some of them were at Bethesda, some at other hospitals. This was my first one on a ship. I had never seen it done more professionally, better, faster, or with more deliberate excellence than that night on the FID. The teamwork and love shown by those guys was as powerful a demonstration as I had ever seen in any hospital. Rick Combs was there, and although he was as shattered as the rest of us about the loss of a young man's life, he was tearful, frankly, because he was so proud of what his boys had just done.

At this time we were steaming west in the Mediterranean, conducting air operations daily, and exercising with members of the Southern NATO Fleet. Flights ops began shortly after dawn, of course. The morning routine started as usual. Just like every other morning, people were busily walking up and down the fore and aft passageways on the second deck, airplanes were moving in the hangar deck, hundreds of people were eating in the mess decks, and occasional joggers were running back and forth between airplanes in the hangar. Early that morning, the Captain came on the 1-MC, something he did almost every day, but usually in the afternoon. "This is the Captain speaking. We are 300 miles west of Sicily, steaming west, and we have just finished our morning cycle. We will be heading on down to our next port call in Benidorm in a few days. The weather there is good. It's a beautiful Spanish coastal city.

"I want to talk to you guys about the tragedy that happened last night. A young sailor died on the Forrestal after inhaling fumes from an aerosol can. Most of all, I want to point out to you that his shipmates contributed to this. Two other guys were down there sniffing that stuff, too. Guys, this is not the way we stick together. A lot of you know that sailor, his name was Jimmy Fulford, and he worked in E Division. Tomorrow morning we are going to have a special service for him on fo'c'sle. You are all invited."

The Captain came on the 1-MC every day to give the guys news about what was happening, how well we had done with prior exercises, to announce messages about children being born at home, special events happening in the news. Captain Pieno was known to have a temper, and to be a hard driver. The sailors loved him, though. He had a down-to-earth quality. He was said to have had a pretty wild adolescence, which was another thing the sailors generally liked about him. They liked being told what the ship was doing and why, but most of all, they liked it that they mattered to the Captain; that he knew how much it mattered to them to be informed. Every sailor on the ship knew about Fulford's death last night, well before the Captain's announcement. They didn't need the announcement to tell them what had happened; they just needed to hear the Captain's voice, they way we all need sometimes to have a parent's presence.

The rest of the day all of the activities went on as scheduled. The crowds bustled up and down the passageways, we started Sick Call as always at 0730 in the morning. People went to the mess decks as usual, and all the ship's business and all the flight operations continued. It was different, though. Instead of the general buzzing level, people were a little quieter. There was less joking, people walked a little slower, not everybody spoke to everybody else.

There was plenty to do, so really nobody on the ship had time to sit around and stew about it, although it was on all of our minds as the day went on. Sick Call started every morning at 0730. On a few ships, Sick Call was held twice a day for the convenience of the crew, and even occasionally three times a day for people who worked at night. On the Forrestal we only had one Sick Call, with the understanding that any time a person was sick they could come to the emergency room to be seen.

Sick Call was basically the walk-in clinic. Ward II was used for Sick Call in the morning, muster meetings, special functions like immunizations, and sometimes for the guys to hang around after hours. I tried to curtail the hanging around, however. We wanted medical spaces used only for medical stuff, whether by us or others (like the XO). It was set up, like Ward I, with bays of the racks parallel, two or three in a stack, and they could be folded and clamped back against the bulkhead so that a bay then could be made into a small 6 by 8 cubicle.

These beds were like many other things that could be folded up and clamped in an upright position on a ship. They had to be clamped very carefully because under rough seas or unexpected movement, if the bed came crashing down, it weighed a couple of hundred pounds and could put an ugly gash in an arm, shoulder, or head. Even so, these were the lightest of any of the things you could find bolted down on a ship. We will talk about the hatches and scuttles later, but they were heavy, and if you ever looked at them and thought about how your finger would feel crushed by one of those, it could keep you fretting for 20 or 30 minutes. I was always worried about how somebody might be injured somebody by a door or hatch.[2]

Inside these little cubicles of the bays on Ward II, we could pull the curtains closed, the curtains that were used for privacy if you ever had patients, but they could

---

[2]*Hatches are the ones that open and close on decks, that is, the horizontal ones. The things that open in bulkheads, that is the vertical ones, are just called "doors." Even if they weigh several hundred pounds, are oval shaped, and have wheels for dogging them down to be water-tight, if they are vertical, they're not properly called "hatches," they're doors.*

make each cubicle into a small office/examining room, and this is where we did our clinic work during sick call.

Back out on the starboard passageway, on the inboard side of the passage was the X-ray suite. Our X-ray suite, like in any small hospital, had a table that could tilt up and down, an X-ray machine that could take pictures while a person was standing up, elbows out, chin up on a film, up against the upright film holder for chest films, or a whole series of films taken while lying down. Behind the patient room was the X-ray tech's working lab, a perfectly black little black room, with a small red bulb as needed, and automatic film processor. In the olden days, ships did not have automatic X-ray processors, and the corpsmen, if they ever took an X-ray, would simply move it from one basin to another by hand, perhaps holding it with paperclips. We can process a film and have it out and dry nowadays in about 1 minute, probably faster than a Polaroid, but with a conventional X-ray picture.

There was more we had to worry about in our X-ray suite. HM3 Eddie Hastings was the moody little technician who ran our X-ray department. He seemed so efficient. He could take the finest X-rays, with the angles just the way you would need them, with such great efficiency and concern for your patients, that you would be impressed from day-to-day with his clinical function. As with every other person on the ship, though, the X-ray tech had to do more than just the apparent "primary" job. Eddie Hastings also had to make sure that all the X-rays were filed perfectly. He had to make sure that the requesting doctor would put a summary report on paper, so that it would be filed with the film so that there would be a record of what the diagnostic impression had been of the X-rays. The Navy had a policy for the past few years that all X-rays had to be read by a specialist radiologist also. All of us are well trained in reading X-rays, especially those sent to isolated duty like on a ship, where our ability to read to films may be critical immediately. Nonetheless, there are specialists in radiology for very good reasons, so that all of our X-rays had to be read over by a radiologist as soon as the ship would return to port, or go to a port where there was a qualified Navy radiologist. It would be Hasting's duty to see that all these films were kept in sequence, properly carried to the radiologist, and the reports brought back to the ship.

There was another job Eddie had, taking care of the radiation badges. All X-ray techs and radiologists wear a little badge, with a film that is a little bit like X-ray film, detecting whenever and how much they are exposed to radiation over time. It is an example of the myriad safety and health surveillance programs that the ship had. This one we customarily think of as primarily a medical issue.

There were other people on the ship who had to wear radiation badges, too. These were mostly in the Weapons Department. The Navy's policy was, and remains, to neither confirm nor deny the presence of nuclear weapons on any given ship. About two years after I left the FID, the United States decided to cease carrying nuclear weapons on any of its carriers. In those days, though, the Navy could "neither confirm nor deny" that there were any nuclear weapons onboard the ship, so we who lived there could neither "know or not know" either. All we did know was that some people in the Weapons Department, who worked in an area in the ship heavily guarded by the Marine detachment, wore these radiation badges, and Eddie Hastings was responsible for them. You can understand that the Navy would want people in all Weapons Departments to wear the badges, whether needed or not. Otherwise, bad guys would be able to tell that ships where sailors did wear badges must have certain material, and ships where guys didn't wear badges didn't have that category of material. Hastings was supposed to take readings on those badges periodically, save the badges, keep excellent records of them, and pass them on at the end of the cruise to the proper regulatory agency. Well, we were to find out later that Eddie sometimes did not pay attention to certain details, and this was one of them.

The next morning, we had the memorial service for Jimmy Fulford. The Chief Engineer and Jimmy's Division Officer spoke about him. It seems he was something of a hellion. A number of people liked him, however, especially for his enthusiasm and sense of adventure. After the CHENG and DivO had spoken, the Chaplain, CDR John Gundlach, spoke. The fo'c'sle was packed. A few people were able to sit on chairs that we had set up in the middle, but most of us packed in around the sides and around the capstans.

Gundlach was in his mid thirties, a well-scrubbed guy with good posture and wide open sincerity. There was a captivating **cleanness** about John, a midwestern intensity in his round welcoming face that told me he had always known he would be a chaplain, somebody who could be both as minister and a scoutleader full time and all the time. He spoke some reassuring words and read a section from The Scripture, but then his tone changed and he stopped being wistful and soft. The chaplain lashed out about shipmates looking out for each other. He began to speak about how other shipmates had let the young man down by joining in the behavior, sniffing the fumes, how they had led him into trouble in port, so that he had too much to drink, how they had failed to help him cope with the stresses at sea. Gundlach's voice began to rise, he got angry, and he spoke about the "damnable" attitude that permitted one shipmate to let another shipmate get into trouble.

After John's talk, we sang the Navy Hymn "Eternal Father." It's an emotional hymn, anyway, but with several hundred people singing this special hymn about a lost shipmate, voices cracked and a lot of us were choking on tears. We filed out slowly. The ship did have a chapel, a very nice one, with a little alter in the front, nice paneling and wallpaper. The chapel, though, would be crowded with even 30 or so people. It was really not large enough for ordinary Sunday religious services or for a service like the one we just had. It was somehow more fitting, more proper, to have the funeral in the fo'c'sle anyway.

People went back to work that day, pretty much choked up, but better off for the ceremony. We needed to speak to each other about the episode, air our emotions. Saying good-bye is not completely satisfied by just a couple of hours of people standing around talking, but it helps. It provides an open forum for dealing with the emotions. Certainly, one of our emotions was our collective outrage about how Jimmy had died, along with our regret of having lost a shipmate. Kind of unstated was the underlying, contagious sense when somebody dies at sea about the vulnerability of the rest of us. Dealing with the situation in a funeral, ferreting out the causes, these help with the coping.

Preparations now had to go on for the second port call of the cruise. Naples is a dusty, grimy, busy place. In Naples there had been a lot of work to do. Some painting had to be done on the side of the ship, stores had to be replenished, we had to meet with a bunch of folks. Benidorm was going to be different. Benidorm had been a sleepy little fishing village on the southern point of Spain up until about 30 years ago when the emerging financial recovery, and the rolling back of Franco repression permitted the evolution of a real bustling and forward looking tourist economy. We were on our way up to an exercise called "Northern Wedding" around the Arctic Circle later. That would be a little unusual for a 6-month cruise. Usually a ship would be stationed in the Mediterranean or the Indian Ocean, occasionally both. To spend a few months in the North Arabian Sea, and on the same cruise have a substantial commitment up in the Arctic Circle, was a little wider than the usual cruise. It had also been unusual to spend

108 consecutive days underway without a port call. Sixteen-hour days, 7-days a week, usually port calls every 40 or 50 days. Every day beyond that adds geometrically to the potential strain, and to accidents. This was an unusual ship and an unusual crew, who seemed to prosper and thrive with a kind of an operational pace that would wear others down. Even so, Captain Pieno wanted to give them a few days' reward, especially with the looming prospect of several tough weeks of more heavy operating up in the Arctic Circle.

Before coming into any port, all of the department heads and certain other key players having to do with the docking operation have a conference up in "CVIC" to make sure that the procedures are all properly planned.

Because of the kind of intel activities that go on in the CVIC, the fancy computers, the classified information, and so forth, there is a cipher lock on the door leading into the area, a security manager seated right inside the door, and then another locked grate-door just beyond that. The security manager identifies the individual coming in. He verifies against a list all the proper security clearances, and then pushes a button to enable you to pass the grate door to get inside. Everybody was assembled inside, and then Captain Pieno entered. At this meeting in CVIC, all of the nitty-gritty details about the tides, how we would make the approach to the harbor, procedures about dropping the hook (anchor) would be discussed.

The person presiding at the conference was the 'Gator, the short term for Navigator. That was Bill Bodenweber, a very tall, broad-shouldered guy A7 attack pilot. He preferred to be called by his call sign "Bohunk." Some aviators preferred to use their call signs all the time, others did not. For example, Captain Pieno's call sign was "Cajun," of which he was duly proud, but people always called him "Captain," at least in his presence[3].

Bohunk showed us the maps leading into the harbor at Benidorm, then the "weather guesser" told about weather and tides and the Assistant Navigator("A-Gator") discussed protocol observations, which American Counsel we would visit, what colors we would fly, and so forth. The conference was long but bearable, and we all got very excited about the coming port call. The next morning Benidorm was in view early. I went down to the fo'c'sle for the approach. The approach to a harbor is an interesting and precise exercise, even reversing the pitch on the screws on the bottom of the ship. It takes a long time to slow down and stop a 75,000 ton floating vessel. Over a number of hours the vessel has to be slowed down, but it has to stay above a certain speed in order to simply maintain steerage, that is, the ability to guide it and direct it by rudders, faster than about 5 knots to simply be steerable. Then the quartermasters and 'gators have to decide how far they are from the point that they are going to drop the hook, and time everything precisely. I decided I would have plenty of opportunities to watch the precise approach from the bridge in the future. Coming into Benidorm, I wanted to see all of the excitement I had heard about the fo'c'sle when they would drop the hook.

The fo'c'sle is kind of a hangout for the Deck Department. The forecastle was a little box or castle in the front of old sailing ships from the Middle Ages. It was called the forecastle because it was the castle in the front part of the ship, from which galleons

---

[3] *You don't get to pick your own call sign. That is done for you by your shipmates in the "rites of passage" early in your aviation career. Ethnic identifiers like Cajun and Bohunk were unusual. Usually the call sign came from a personal flaw or a humiliating experience. One fighter pilot was named "Eagle," the kind of name you might expect a fighter jock to like, but I discovered he got that name because he wore a toupee, and he was called an eagle because of a physical trait other than eyesight.*

could fight others, cannons could be kept, and people could keep lookouts. On surface ships, the fo'c'sle is a weather deck, that is, it is exposed to the sky and the weather. When aircraft carriers were first made, a flight deck was simply put on a trellis up above the main deck, and the fo'c'sle was still out in the open air with the forward part of the flight deck simply on top of it. Beginning with carriers in the 1930's and in World War II, the fo'c'sle tended to be enclosed, as it was on the Forrestal. The fo'c'sle more or less belonged to the Boatswains Mates, the rates in the Deck Department. They used it for their meeting place. They took pride in the cleanliness and the clean paint. A fo'c'sle is a place of chains, paint lockers, grease. Like a big garage, a fo'c'sle tries organically to become grimy, littered and dirty, if allowed to. All of that Boatswain Mate stuff is in there, chains, ropes, capstans. Up in the very pointy end of the fo'c'sle was the ship's gym, the Nautilus equipment, rowing machines, stationary bicycles, and stair climbers. The fo'c'sle was also used as the main auditorium on the ship. You couldn't use the hangar bay, because it was so full of airplanes all the time. We used the fo'c'sle for church services, assembly meetings, formal occasions, Captain's Mast, any event that needed a large space. Because the fo'c'sle could not permit other machinery or other "work stuff," it was always available as an open place.

Dominating the fo'c'sle were the anchor chains, of course. The chain lockers, the containers in which the chain was curled up when the anchor was stowed, were huge cylindrical wells about 120 feet behind the pointy end of the ship. The chains stretched from those wells forward, coming at an angle toward the front where you could look down a hole and see the anchor clinging to the side of the ship. The anchors weighed many tons, were about 1 1/2 stories tall. About 20 or 30 links on the chain were exposed lying along the deck each about 4 feet long and 12 inches thick. Each link weighed about 300 pounds.

Gradually as the ship slowed and slowed the fo'c'sle became busier. Everybody was required to stand at certain positions way toward the back of the fo'c'sle. At a certain point the ship obviously was no longer moving, and the First Lieutenant was standing there with his brick. He heard something on the brick, turned to the First Class Boatswain Mate standing by with a sledge hammer who then smacked some metal thing back out of the way of the capstan, and all of a sudden, you couldn't see the chain links anymore. The chain seemed to jump up and down and vibrate. All of the dust in the whole world obscured our view, and I felt like I was standing in a dust storm. Even wearing the Mickey Mouse ears hearing protectors, as well as internal ear plugs, it was the most deafening, stupefying thunder I had ever heard when those chains bounced along kicking up all the dust in the world, and letting out anchor. The chain itself gets heavier than the anchor once you let some of it out. The old legend goes that the anchor only holds the chain, and the chain holds the ship. The anchor hits the soft bottom and folds out so that two sharp prongs more or less dig into the bottom, but it is not those sharp prongs that hold the ship. They simply hold the first couple of links until the pile of anchor chain grows. It is not the anchor that holds the ship, but the amassed tons of anchor chain on the bottom. My ears rang for probably over an hour during which I could not hear ordinary conversation. Shortly after I could hear again, I heard on the 1MC, "Shift colors." When the ship is at anchor or in port, the National Ensign is shifted from its position up on the island and near the stack back to the fantail. You only keep the flag back there when the ship is stopped.

I guess it stays sunny and beautiful in Benidorm all the time. Certainly it was the whole time we were there. The first day there I was busy and could not leave the ship all day. Finally, late on the first day we were in Benidorm I was able to make a trip to the local hospital. I came armed with an armful of Forrestal ball caps. There was no fund for paying for those to give out, so the SMO had to pay for them, but it was well worth the price of four or five ball caps to make friends with medical colleagues in another country, and advertise for the ship. Someday, some Americans might see those docs wearing a ***Forrestal*** ball cap. Benidorm was the first Spanish hospital I ever saw, and it was to set the tone for an impression that kept getting reinforced. The Spanish hospitals were not merely professional and cleaner than most American hositals. The people and the staff seemed familiar. In my first encounter with Spanish people I was impressed how much their styles, mannerisms, and demeanor seemed more American to me than European. That wasn't a value judgement At the hospital, I met the head doctor, invited him to come for a tour of the ***Forrestal***, and arranged for emergency care of any FID sailors if needed in town while we were there.

I was not able to go to the "admin" that night. An "admin" is a rendezvous, a lodging point, a "base" in a liberty port. The concept of the admin started as a squadron idea years ago. Whenever a ship would go to a liberty port, a few guys from a squadron would go out and rent a hotel room so that officers would not have to come back to the ship at night. This, of course, was done in the event that the seas were rough and boating could not be permitted, or if there was a late party. There was no question that a naval officer would be unable to return to ship for any reasons of incapacity. Aviators have always been, and continue to be, a little more flamboyant, a little more imaginative than the surface Navy, known as "black shoes" or "shoes," because surface guys wear black shoes with their khakis rather than brown like aviators.

Over the years, however, even the "shoes" on the aircraft carrier began to see the merit in having an admin. It takes at least 20 minutes to take the boat from the ship to the shore. Sometimes an officer who does not have duty, just spending a night off the ship can be a welcome diversion. So each department tended to have an admin, as well as each squadron. Also, the department heads, mostly being in their 40's, liked to get together for a Department Head Admin. It allowed them to let their hair down away from their men, talk about their current problems, and have some social time on liberty away from the ship. The Department Heads did not have an admin in Naples because we had been so busy, and everybody had a lot of things to attend to there, but Bohunk had arranged for us to get an admin in Benidorm. Usually, Captains did not stand watches on the ship, but being new onboard, I still wanted to become more familiar with my department, and since all the doctors who worked for me had gone those 108 days without liberty, I thought they needed liberty more than I did. So I stayed onboard the first night. I was looking forward to getting to know the other Department Heads better, though, so I planned to go to the admin the next day.

An aircraft carrier may look big from the inside, and it looks even larger when you see one from the pier. But the two best views of an aircraft carrier are on final at a few hundred feet above the threshold or looking up at the great gray expanse from the gunwales of a small boat. It is such a proud leviathan. Rising up so rigidly to the many stories above the water, the great gray angularity exudes a confidence and a power that is both intimidating and assuring.

That evening as I came back to the ship, I saw that view for the first time. You can look at it in photos a dozen times or read about it just as many, but that view is different, the hull wider, the deck higher, from the surface of the ocean in a small boat. No wonder we sailors are so arrogant.

Apparently the first night in town the Captain and the 'Gator were obliged to meet with the dignitaries in town as often was the case in foreign port calls. The next night, though, I was flattered when Bohunk the 'Gator, told me that he and the Captain invited me to join them for the evening. We would first go to a Hail and Farewell party to say goodbye to the SuppO, Joe Kinsey and a couple of other guys, but then I was invited to join them when they went out to the local casino and then a couple of drinks afterward.

First I had an opportunity to go to the Admin, finally, a nice hotel room shared by the couple of dozen of us. The Admin overlooked the main boulevard that ran along the beach. It was ribboned by a manicured park with palm trees, flowers and benches. Even though I hadn't been deployed as long as the others, it had been several weeks since I had been able to run on dry land, so I had a chance to run for about an hour.

After the dinner at a very patient restaurant in Benidorm, I was pleased to join the 'Gator and the skipper in their car. This was heady stuff, now, don't forget. I was still awed by this crowd, and here I was going out on the town with the two main guys in the ship's company. The Navigator was driving the rented Mercedes. (In Europe, Mercedes appear to be as common as Ford Escorts in the States). I would have figured the safest person to whom I could entrust myself in an auto ought to be somebody like Bohunk, a forty year old man whose life profession was the control of complex jet powered vehicles and whose current job was the navigation of a 75,000 ton aircraft carrier. Wouldn't a reasonable person expect somebody like that to handle a small automobile as well as anybody? What a surprise! Bohunk had not been in an automobile for over four months, it was dark, and he probably had not slept more than four hours in the past four days. It was the most terrible ride I'd had in thirty years -- since riding with drunk teenagers! Whoa -- we zigged -- we tailgated. "Hey, 'Gator! You OK?" I asked.

"Don't worry, Doc, I'll get the hang of it."

"Gator, if you get us arrested in a foreign country because of your driving, I'll kill you," the Captain said. "We don't need any international incidents here."

There must have been nearly a hundred guys from the FID in the casino. Everybody was having fun and were happy to bump into one another. Bohunk and I stood around and laughed at several guys pumping the slots one after another. Bohunk was tired. He and the Skipper needed the port call. They spent hour after endless hour together on the bridge, and this being only their second port call in over four months, they needed rest. We saw the Captain chatting with some sailors over by the Baccarat table, and we ambled ourselves over to the Black Jack area. The Gator lost about $15-$20 in short order. "That's it for me, Doc, I've had enough," the 'Gator said. He went to sit on a bench near the door to nod off as he watched everybody else.

I was having better luck, and in fact was up $40-$50, when Tod Graef the Senior Dental Officer and my semi bunk mate on the ship, came by. He was accompanied, as I would learn he usually was, by an attractive young woman. "Hey, Red, say hello to Persepone. She's English."

I said something pleasant, but probably also sarcastic about how Persepone should not spend time with sailors, and it made both of them laugh. For the next two years, I would frequently be introduced to attractive young women who were just meeting Tod. I always told them something bad about him, but that just made them like him more! They would always laugh and squeeze his arm harder. "You should try the roulette table, Red, I made some money over there." [giggles from Persepone].

Bohunk the 'Gator was asleep on his bench over by the door at this point. I couldn't see the Captain, but figured he was over in some other area with some of the crew. So, I edged cautiously over to a roulette table, my first time ever. Hedging first only small bets on two or three combinations, I won gradually up to several hundred pesetas, about $200. Figuring that was good enough for a first time at a casino, I decided to stop, and besides Bohunk was sound asleep and needed to go.

"Hey, Gator, wake up, it's time to go."

He woke up easily enough, and said, in the requisite style of Spencer Tracy in "Captains Courageous," "OK, Doc, we go bock sheep." We couldn't find the Captain and decided he must already be back at the car.

Sure enough, when we got out to the car, the Cajun was sound asleep, his head lying on the window ledge in the right front passenger seat. Both the Skipper and Bohunk were sleep-deprived. They spent more than the number of hours a day contains on the bridge, both of them. Coming into a port is especially demanding when the ship's never been there, and our operating schedule had been murderous for the two of them. No wonder the 'Gator had fallen asleep right in the casino and the Captain had come out to the car to sleep. We couldn't wake him.

"Hey 'Gator, I've got an offer you can't refuse."

His eyelids at half-mast, the 'Gator asked what it was.

"Frankly you didn't distinguish yourself driving over here, 'Gator, and you can scarcely stay awake even now. Why don't you let me drive us back to the ship?"

"OK, Doc. Bock Sheep." He gave me the keys.

Backing out of the parking spot I immediately smacked into the Mercedes right behind us. Smashed its tail light right out with a loud cracking sound that means the same thing in every language. Made an ugly contour in the two fenders, too, one vaguely recollects. I have to admit that it crossed my mind whether in this one itsy bitsy, never again, exceptional case, maybe I should just drive away. Two things decided me to do the right thing. My conscience of course, was one. But what really convinced me was the spanish cop standing right there.

Fortunately, none of us had been drinking at all. Imagine the embarrassment if we had been! The FID of course was about the biggest news in Benidorm that week, and here was a car with its Commanding Officer sound asleep in the front seat. Could have a questionable appearance. So I got out and handed the policeman my identification. He didn't speak English, nor I Spanish. He saw the Captain asleep. From the back seat, Bohunk was saying, "Yo, Doc, we go bock sheep now, buddy." He would sputter something now and then and fall back asleep. Lot of help. Impressed the policeman.

This was difficult for the policeman too. He didn't want an international incident over a tail light, but he wasn't supposed to encourage this sort of thing either, especially with a car full of sleepy foreigners, one of them the reputed commanding officer who was snoring audibly. The officer looked around furtively and then waved for me to get back in the car and drive away.

The Captain was now snorting and sputtering little bit. I turned the car toward the Admin and somehow, the Captain woke just enough to merely mumble, "No, Doc, we've got to go down to that other place. I promised some of the guys I'd come and have a drink with them tonight."

"Captain, are you sure? You look pretty bushed to me."

"I'll be all right. We won't stay long."

It was late already. Midnight or later, but the skipper insisted we go down to the club where most of the sailors were. The 'Gator and I went to sit over by the bar, where he kept sleeping and I tried to stay awake too.

But the Captain wasn't sleepy anymore. It was like somebody had sneaked in a remarkable impersonator. The same guy who was sound asleep a minute ago was now the life of the party. FID sailors flocked around him, introducing their new friends and young Spanish, English and German tourists who wanted to meet the Captain of the big American ship. A klatch of young college age women, like a sorority group, all asked him to dance with them. He thought he was just being an avuncular celebrity, but you could tell the sorority sisters thought differently. After about an hour, the 'Gator's snoring was telling me we might never wake him up, and I was getting sleepy too. The

Captain, though, was more festive than ever. Finally, we somehow persuaded him to go bock sheep, and I drove us very gingerly back to the Admin

CHAPTER IV. FOUR WEEKS OF VARIETY

The first several days after we left Benidorm the weather was beautiful, occasionally with small amounts of haze in the morning, and the routine on the ship was not too busy. We had flight operations going every day. The first day out I went up to "pri-fly," which is the equivalent to the tower on an airport. Pri-fly was a narrow, but long compartment looking down on the flight deck from the island. It stuck out aft on the island, and about a half deck higher than the captain's bridge. A little bubble at the after margin was where the Air Officer and Assistant Air Officer sat in twin leather thrones. They were called the "Air Boss" (more often "the Boss") and the "MiniBoss" (more often "Mini"). There were other kinds of "bosses," especially the Weapons Officer, who was called the "Gun Boss," the Communications Officer, sometimes called the "Signals Boss," but whenever somebody referred to "The Boss" they meant the Air Officer[4]. The Boss during my first year on the Forrestal was Ray Laturno, an S3 NFO. The Mini, who was to become one of my best friends, was Larry Osborn, an A7 pilot. He sat in the right-hand chair, just like a copilot would. Both the Boss and the Mini had just completed CO tours on squadrons assigned to the Forrestal Air Wing just before getting their current jobs, the Boss to the VS28 "Gamblers", and the Mini to the VA105 "Gun Slingers," one of the two Light Attack Squadrons in the Air Wing.

Behind the Boss and the Mini were airmen who marked on big Lucite graphs with grease pencil the names and numbers of airplanes, listing the weight of the aircraft, the name of the pilot, and the amount of fuel onboard. In one column was the name of the tankers flying around to refuel airplanes who needed it after taking off or just before landing. Over the Mini's and the Boss' heads, in the panel above the windows were compasses and gauges that would show the direction of wind. The Boss and the Mini held microphones that they had to speak into, but also two banks of communicator telephone squawkers. They spoke frequently to the Captain and carried a continuous dialogue with pilots in the pattern and with the LSOs down on the port side of the ship just past the 3-wire. Periodically the Boss or the Mini would reach up and grab some other microphone so that they could speak on the 5-MC, the loudspeaker system for the flight deck, and selected other parts of the ship, for example, the Medical Department.

On the 5-MC they would give directions that were necessary for performance on the flight deck, or call to announce certain emergencies. The Mini had a propensity to grab the microphone and shout down to some yellow shirt who was not wearing his cranial, or remind somebody else to put on his goggles. Whenever the ship would turn, the Boss or the Mini would speak into the 5-MC, not to tell the people on the flight deck that the ship was turning, but to remind that the flight deck would tilt one way or another. One of the things that distinguishes a "ship" from a "boat" is that a ship tilts away from the direction of the turn. So when the ship would turn to the port side, the flight deck, especially on the after end, would heel over toward the starboard side. For flight operations, the ship had to turn into the wind. So as the ship would begin turning into the wind, if it had to turn to port, the Boss or the Mini would warn people on the flight deck, "Heel to starboard, heel to starboard." This would warn anybody on the after end of the flight deck to watch out for what could be a rough unexpected motion and a list, and maybe prevent somebody from falling overboard.

---

[4]*This "Boss" talk was carried to extremes of cuteness. For example, the Dental Officer was sometimes called the "Gum Boss," or the Chaplain the "God Boss."*

The Mini was kind of a renaissance man. There were a few of those among aviators, although they were more often to be found in the VAW or VAQ communities than among the single seat attack guys. The Mini was a scholar, and a musician, but of note in this job, where he held a microphone, he was something of a vocalist, and an orator. With a melodious baritone voice and a glib gift for the microphone, it was obvious that he enjoyed communicating with those who worked on the deck or in the cockpits. On the other hand, maybe that's not entirely it, maybe he just enjoyed speaking into the microphone. Enjoy it he did, though, and I enjoyed hearing him enjoy it too. Before each flight cycle, the Mini had a paragraph of precise instructions. "On the Flight deck! It is time for the cycle to begin. All unauthorized personnel must clear the Flight Deck at this time. Now all personnel don your equipment..." The patter went on to remind all the people to check their survival vests, cranials, "Now put on your goggles, and make sure your sleeves are down." The words and their sequence were identical each time. I knew that there must have been a required script in order to guarantee that every topic was covered. If it had been repeated in an obligatory monotone as some clergy do with a litany, or some Minis do on other ships, they guys would also be bored with it and never pay attention. Our Mini saw each iteration as a pleasure, though. His inflection was almost musical, so obviously did he enjoy it. He made the rote recitation of those instructions sound new and different each time he said them, because of a little different nuance or syllabic emphasis. Sincerity too; how he could make it sound as though he believed in buttoning up those life vests, and tightening those boot laces!

Either in the morning before the launches began, or in the afternoon, before all the aircraft returned to the flight deck, we had the FOD Walkdown. Then would come the launch part. The last group of airplanes were still up flying around, and they had not yet returned overhead. In order to clear the deck for them, the current launch had to be sent out. The first aircraft to be launched would be the H-3 helos, who would fly around in the "starboard delta" pattern for the entire flight in the event a search and rescue mission were necessary.

The next aircraft to launch would be one of the tankers. Some of the A6's were configured with a large extra flight tank in the belly, in addition to extra drop tanks on the wings. These would be up there to replenish anybody who needed more fuel, either at the beginning or the end of the cycle.

Pri-fly was a busy place. On the ***Forrestal*** it had a special atmosphere because of the magical teamwork, starting from the symbiosis of the Boss and the Mini. For one thing, they made it all look so easy, so much fun, so *under control.* Also, the two of them worked together as smoothly and cheerfully as a pair of disc jockeys on a morning radio show ... where I suspected the Mini longed to be at times anyway. Cheerful, light banter, witty repartee, they were obviously having fun. Yet their eyes never left the Flight Deck or airplanes in the pattern. The Boss and the Mini were always welcoming, and despite the high-pressure tempo of their job, they were always eager to show a visitor what was going on, and the complexities of lining up the aircraft. About the time half the airplanes had launched, other airplanes began to circle overhead and continued circling until the last plane was launched. Within moments after the last plane launched, the conversation between the Boss and the Mini on their various speakers seemed unchanged, but their gaze now shifted away from the catapults to the after end of the ship, one or the other of them would pick up binoculars, and they would look at airplanes coming in to land. Over the head phones at this point one could hear the LSO saying, "Power. . . power. . . come left. . .glide slope. . ." as they guided in the landing pilot. Periodically, the Boss or the Mini would snatch out at a microphone, and curtly pronounce, "Wave off," usually thereafter you would hear the LSO's voice over the microphone saying, "Wave off," and the airplane on final, just about to touch the threshold, would accelerate and begin to climb. For some reason he had not been set up correctly, and the Boss or the Mini did not want him to land if he had a poor configuration. Sometimes, eschewing the microphone, one of them would say something like, "Dumb son-of-a-bitch, I told him he had to stop that." Or they would make a comment that somebody had to go down and speak to the skipper of that guy's squadron. More often one of them would affectionately pass a cheerful joke or pun to a flight crew. Succinctly though. Not much chatter on the radio. Sometimes just a terse, "nice job 'one-oh-three'." After the last plane in the pack was landed, there was supposed to be a 30 to 60 minute lag before the next cycle started, but it really always seemed only 10 or 15 minutes. It was 30 to 60 minutes between the last trip and the next launch but a lot of airplanes had to be readied, spotted, and moved in the interim.

"Vultures Row" was sensually more exciting, though. Down on the O-5 level, one or two decks below pri-fly, and only a deck below the Captain's bridge, there was a catwalk on the port side (inside) of the island, right over the flight deck where you could stand and watch the airplanes take off or land. It was louder than the inside of Hell, though, and had winds always at least 25 knots, even before the planes threw out their exhaust. You had to wear good ear protection, and it was best if you wore heavy outside Mickey Mouse ears in addition to inner ear plugs. From there you could watch the jets, always blurred and angular at this speed, and real big, as they would reach gradually up to the threshold of the ship, and seem gently to stretch their wheels down to touch the flight deck, with the tail hook dragging. But then, as soon as those wheels touched the flight deck, they didn't seem to be floating anymore, but going faster than light. With the crashing thunder louder than anything you have ever heard, the airplane seemed to snap forward and jerk to a halt as the hook would grab the wire. It all happened so fast. Nobody had time to catch a breath, because just as soon as the airplane stopped, a yellow shirt was out there beckoning him on, bending a left arm to taxi the airplane off to the starboard side, as the cable called "a wire" was slowly retracted back into place to catch the next airplane. In less than 60 seconds, and sometimes as short as 30 seconds, another airplane would be stretching out its wheels to touch down on the flight deck and crash right into that same position, then another and another, each a little quicker than the last.

There are several reasons for the diagonal flight deck. The first is that if an airplane has to bolter, like on my own first approach, with the runway a little bit at an angle, if things aren't working, the plane can fly or skid off to the port side of the ship, and not carom into all the airplanes that might be in front of it. A traffic pile up is bad enough on a freeway. It would be downright ugly on an aircraft carrier. The second reason for the slanted deck is that with air coming across the flight deck, the island sticking up on the starboard side of the ship causes a disruption of air flow over the flight deck. The resulting little "burble" distorts the wind coming across an airplane's nose at the most critical time and speed in flight. With a canted deck the ship can steam a little to the right of the oncoming wind, so a quartering port headwind comes down the angle of the deck. The landing headwind is unaffected by the island, and provides a direct headwind for the aircraft arriving at an angle to the ship's course, but directly into the wind.

By the time World War II broke out, our airplanes were all-metal monoplanes, and they were much heavier. All the bombs and bullets (which were supposed to be used up before you came home) made them even heavier at takeoff than at landing. Simple deck launching, just using the deck as a runway, did not provide enough air speed to get reliably airborne. This became even more critical when jets were developed in the

1950s. Every jet on the Forrestal was heavier than anything but the biggest bombers in World War II. They needed air speeds near 200 knots to take off, so the catapults had to be enormously powerful. The acceleration is legendary among flyers. Movies can only hint of the feeling. It's something all real Americans want to do before they die.

FLIGHT IN THE INTRUDER

My first flight was in an A6 Intruder, the two-seat, all-weather bomber belonging to the VA-176, "Thunderbolts." VA-176 was commissioned about 35 years ago flying the A-1 Sky Raider. The Sky Raider, an enormous propeller driven aircraft, was the last piston powered aircraft to fly off Navy carriers. It was developed in the 1950s as an all-weather, "medium attack" airplane and it continued as a rescue airplane in Vietnam even after the A6 stole away its bombing mission. When, in the early 1960s, the VA-176 transitioned from the single seat A1 to the A6, they kept their logo, squadron, and heritage, but changed in the most fundamental way for a tactical squadron. They now had a second occupant, an NFO, the bombardier-navigator, or "BN" not only in the Ready Room, but right there in the airplane. A cockpit for two is a team, not just an airplane with an observer. The BN didn't just "help" the pilot, he did other stuff, working complicated computers and gadgets that put ordnance on target. the BNs delivered that which made the A6 different from just an airplane.

At the appointed time, more than 2 hours before scheduled departure time, I came to the VA-176 Ready Room. I was going to go on a tanker mission. The pilot would be Lieutenant Commander Bob Slowik, "Slow Bob." He was one of the few Academy graduates who would retire as a Lieutenant Commander, sometime in about a year. A remarkably easy going guy, he obviously had thousands of hours in control of the aircraft. He played the guitar and sang folk songs.

Before going on any flight, just as we had with the helo, we had to sit through the flight brief, the weather recording over the closed circuit TV and the Operations Brief, also over the TV. Since our mission this day was to be the tanker, it was OK to have a novice BN in the right seat. There had to be a lot of training in the airplane before I could go on any bombing runs. The A6 in its bomber configuration is a very busy two-person aircraft. The right seater in this airplane -- and NFOs in any airplane -- are not copilots. They wince if you call them that. To prove they're not helper pilots, there is not even a set of flight controls on the right side. The BN would tell you the flight controls over on the left side are just there for the chauffeur anyway; they would get in the way of the important stuff if you tried to put them on the right side too.

On our mission today, we would be circling around not too far from the ship to help airplanes refuel right after taking off, and to be available toward the end of the mission. The big jets guzzle fuel ravenously. Some of the airplanes have afterburners, on our ship those were the F-14 Tomcats, the biggest airplanes we had. Afterburner on takeoff and climbing with a full airplane (all the bombs and bullets still aboard) burns up more fuel than just flying around. So some airplanes, especially the fighters, may need to top off their tanks right after and need to top off a little bit while waiting their turn to land. Finally, if some pilot has some trouble getting down to the deck, because he bolters, because the deck is cluttered, or any other reason, that extra flight time forces him to ask "Texaco" for a drink.

"So this is your first cat shot?" Slow Bob was very understanding. I think he had been stuck with flight surgeons on their first flights before. He knew that I had been checked out in oxygen masks and so forth. All fight surgeons have to be certified in ejection procedures and survival techniques such as escaping from the shrouds of a parachute underwater, treading water with boots on, and crawling into the life raft. As part of the routine brief, though, he had to run through all of those things with me. We talked about the procedures we would use if we lost communication. You wouldn't be able to hear one another in the cockpit if the ICS failed.

Every crew always reviews ejection procedures before a flight. With a novice in the crew it gets special attention. You can eject by pulling a ring over your head, or one down between your legs. There are two different rings because if the aircraft is tumbling, or under a high G-force, or if one of your arms is blown off, you may not be able to reach one ring or the other.

When crews work together, trust one another's judgment, and have been through danger together, they usually trust each other enough that they use "crew eject." Most airplanes have two different ways to handle ejection. One is "crew eject." If either guy pulls his ejection handle, both shoot right out immediately. If left on "manual" you only get out by pulling it yourself. If you are badly injured you might not be able to pull yourself out fast. If something is happening too fast for you to see it coming, your buddy might. "Crew eject" lets him save both your lives. On the other hand, it's an unpleasant image to think of a fruity or skittish new guy in the right seat who pulls the loop too quickly, or accidentally pulls the ejection loop when he simply meant to reach down and untie his laces. If he just blows himself out when he shouldn't, it ruins a good canopy and that day's mission, but at least if the pilot didn't get ejected, there's somebody inside who can bring the multimillion dollar airplane home. Ejection can be dangerous, so no pilot wants to eject when he doesn't need to. An inadvertent ejection by a naive right-seater can cause the expensive loss of an otherwise perfectly good airplane. So with a new guy on board, they seldom use the "crew eject" setting. These considerations are not completely reciprocal, though. Everybody in the right seat should prefer crew eject. If the pilot chooses to depart, and leaves you behind, there is no good reason to stay in an airplane you can't fly. We would use manual eject on our flight that day. I was ambivalent; glad not to worry about accidentally shooting us both out of the airplane, yet not able to count on Slow Bob getting me out, either.

He laid out the procedure, "I will say eject three times: 'Eject, eject, eject.' When you hear me say it, you pull your ring on the second 'eject.' because if you wait for the third time, I'll be gone." Now, I've heard that particular speech a number of times either in movies or in instructional briefs. Perhaps you have heard it that way too. Believe me, the first time you hear a real live guy in a flight suit looking you right in the eye as he says it before you get into an airplane, it comes across in a much more meaningful way.

We hurried down to the parachute loft to put on our G-suits, torso harnesses, survival jackets, and the straps that automatically snap ankles back under the seat during ejection. In the rocket forces of ejection, the feet can flail out. If they do, they can be sliced off by the wind screen, or get stuck on the control panel on the way out. The straps slap the heels back into the seat.

The ejection sequence blows the canopy off the airplane, so that you won't hit it. You may remember in the movie "Top Gun" that the guy in the back seat had his neck broken because he hit the canopy on his way out. That was because he hit the canopy frame, I presume. The fact is that many people eject right through the glass in the canopy. Some airplanes are even designed that way. Just like a dancer popping out of a big birthday cake.

Later that year, I would meet a 50-year-old pediatrics professor from some research committee who came to the ship on a fact-finding tour. In a chat late one night, he told me that 20 years ago he had been a flight surgeon, and in his first flight off the flight deck in an A6, there was engine failure right off the pointy end, and he and the pilot both ejected. On his first A6 flight he wound up using every part of the brief. It's not just in movies. Flight surgeons have done it often. Of the experienced aviators on the ship, probably a third or more of them had been in a real ejection sometime in their career. I took all this stuff pretty seriously.

All the flight gear puts an awful lot of parts on you. The G-suit is like leggings or chaps that fit tightly against the calf and thigh, but also well up into the abdomen. There is a big tube sticking out the side like a dangling appendage hanging obscenely off the left side of the body, then it plugs into the anti-G apparatus in the cockpit like a pneumatic umbilicus. The torso harness is a network of very heavy canvas that goes under your buttocks and thighs, and locks you both to the seat and the parachute. The torso harness, which becomes the "seat harness," has to fit tightly because if you ever eject, the ejection seat pulls you entirely out of the airplane, and the torso harness is what holds you into the seat and also into the parachute.

It is hot in the parachute loft, so by the time we left there, wearing all that gear, I was sweating pretty well. It was August just south of Spain to begin with. We walked up to the flight deck which was a little smokier, a little hotter, and much more exciting than it had ever been to me.

The A6 looks like a big airplane from the flight deck, but it looks much bigger when you start climbing up on the ladder to get in. It has a big bulbous nose sitting out in front, and so to the uninitiated this big, round fronted jet looks somewhat ungainly, less pointy, and to some people perhaps a little bit less sexy than the other jets. When you see the silhouette in the sky, though, it's transformed. The wings taper back from the broad shoulders of the intakes and those bulbous eyeballs of the canopy are so ominous and menacing. It is a vicious looking airplane. It may be big and ungainly on the deck, but it's sleek in flight.

After we climbed up into the cockpit and got strapped in, I nonchalantly tried to stick my G-suit plug into the oxygen outlet, twice, three times. Wrong plug. Not cool. I was glad it was Slow Bob with me. He patiently reached over to help me plug each tube into its proper receptacle. They all have different shapes, probably with the faint hope of protecting flight surgeons from the kind of mistake I was trying to make. The great shaded bulbous visors on the helmets had to come down. Then we got strapped in. Slow Bob showed me the things he wanted me to do, when to push the lever to spread the wings out, the things I was not supposed to touch and the circuit breakers I was to help him to give the run down during the preflight inspection. Faster than I could savor everything that was going on, there we were taxiing into position. The helos lifted off, so the tanker was next. It was our turn. We taxied up to the bow cats. There are four catapults on the ***Forrestal,*** two on the bow and two others near midships, the "waist." The waist cats are shorter and since they have to reach the same speed in a shorter distance, they're rougher, so they aren't used as much. During a busy launch sequence, having four launching positions in sequence instead of two increased launch rates exponentially. There were four jet blast deflectors, one behind each catapult to protect workers in the flight deck from the searing heat and tornado winds of the jet exhaust as it spooled up to launch an airplane. Somehow, you didn't see them all, but there were around a hundred guys working up there during flight ops. It was only a couple of weeks ago that AN Mitchell had been blown overboard.

Suddenly we were very busy. Bob was doing the preflight checklist, reading off items aloud with me participating at the places where he told me to, checking circuit breakers, looking around on the flight deck for the things he told me to look for. One of the flight deck crew came up to the left-hand side of the airplane and held up a slate giving the weight and how many pounds of fuel in the airplane, and Slow Bob gave him a thumbs-up sign. He used these weight calculations to be certain that the catapult was set correctly for our aircraft. All of these things happened in about five seconds.

Two guys rolled under the airplane checking the landing gear, and then just as quickly rolled off to the sides. The "shooter," an aviator himself, was standing in the middle of the flight deck waving his hand above his head while pointing at Slow Bob. Slow Bob looked at him. The shooter saluted. Bob said, "Are you ready?" I told him I was, and Bob returned the salute. The guy held up one finger, two fingers, three fingers, shook his fingers, then he kneeled down suddenly, touched his fingers to the flight deck, and then pointed them straight ahead like a bird dog. Bob had showed me how to bend my neck slightly forward so that it would not snap back too suddenly into the seat, there was a little thud when the trellis grabbed the front of the airplane. Then ... Oh!...mmmphhh...gone!

Ever since I first saw William Holden fly off the deck in "The Bridges at Toko-Ri" I had looked forward to this, but as I already said, movies can't feel it. It sucks your teeth right back to your throat, and your eyeballs back to your elbows. The flight deck, all the guys, the antennas, everything -- blurred by faster than you can see them. Then suddenly you're out in space, the catapult lets go, and it's like stepping gently off a cliff. Roaring under about four G's through a keyhole into a quiet weightless float. You're flying.

Too much sensation, too much experience, in less than one second to realize all of it the first time, maybe even the first dozen times. This all happens in the time it takes a tennis ball to fall from the hand to the floor. It is so fast and so rich, that you must notice one aspect or another each time in order to gradually see all of them. Just as quickly as we were thrown out into space, I looked over and noticed that Bob had been working that whole time. So much had just happened to me in the last part of a second that I wanted to revel in it, but I saw he had been busy the whole time. He spoke something into his oxygen mask that I could not hear, presumably to the Boss. I looked down to watch the ocean as we flew by, remarking on how low we stayed as we went perhaps a half mile, two miles, some distance, and then started to climb. First we had to build up speed. Then our climb came rather rapidly. We were at our assigned altitude of 10,000 feet within just a couple of minutes.

We started a slow turn to the left, and Bob pointed out toward that side where there were a couple of F14's. "There's our traffic," he said over the ICS, the intercom. I had not heard them speak to us on the radio, nor him to them, so I asked how they knew where to find us. After all, these are war planes, and one way the bad guys can find you in a conflict is to listen on their radios. So procedures were developed down through the years letting everybody know what to expect. On your way back at the end of a flight sequence, you know where and when to meet the tanker. That was part of the reason for all the instructions and briefs we had in the Ready Room before taking off. Likewise, on the rendezvous up in the air, the two pilots did not need to speak with each other. It was always the thirsty one that would have to fly formation on the tanker.

Formation flying is a skill that all pilots learn in basic training. It's a lot harder than it looks on film. Both airplanes are flying at around 200 miles an hour. The tanker slowly dangles out a hose with a conical basket on the end, trailing it out 50 or 100 feet behind the airplane. The other airplane sidles up from behind and gently sticks the refueling probe into the basket. Looks easy, but have you ever tried to ride up and take a hand off from one bicycle to another at just 25 or 30 MPH? When opened up in flight, the basket is probably about 24 inches in diameter, but while you're up there it looks only about 6 inches across, and the airplane has to hit a certain spot right in the middle. All this is done without any radio communication and only hand signals between the pilots. A light goes on in the control panel, and a digital indicator near the light begins to click off numbers at a dazzling rate. After about 2 or 3 minutes, the fueling aircraft pulls back just a bit, the basket lurches forward, and the two airplanes are simply flying in formation again, no longer attached by the long tether. The pilot of the F14 that came alongside on the right to take the fuel touches his fingers and thumb together in a kissing gesture on his mouth and flips the hand, fingers open, toward us, the "kiss-off" sign. Just then, he banks steeply away and flies off away and slightly downward in a graceful pirouette that no eagle could equal. His wing man then slides up underneath our aircraft to take his place, like the next calf to the cow, and within moments places the probe right in the basket and repeats the entire exercise. Minutes later, he, too, gives us the "kiss-off" sign and then flies away.

Our first two "customers" were the only fighters from the prior sequence. Being the heaviest airplanes, and likely to have also been the most acrobatic, of the flight, those two needed fuel just to sustain them in the pattern waiting for our launch sequence to clear the deck so they could land. Our next customers were airplanes from our own launch who needed to top of before getting on with their sortie. At that point, we continued to circle over the flight deck at our present altitude while we watched the planes from the prior sequence come in to land.

The view was obviously a lot different from this high. The choreography of all the different airplanes following in their assigned sequence on the landing was fascinating up here where we could see all of them and watch the ballet from above. Radio silence was maintained for both security practice and safety. If all the pilots were chattering on the frequencies at the same time, it would be just like civilian airports where landing traffic sometimes has trouble "getting through" to the tower. There were well over a dozen high performance jets, all buzzing around the ship like moths around a porch light. If each one had to have an individual conversation with the Boss, they couldn't execute the tight landing sequence bringing one plane after the other to the deck less than a minute.

Each type of airplane had an assigned altitude coming in, based on fuel consumption and capacity, air speed in the landing pattern, and where each plane would be parked when the sequence was over. The recovery cycle took 15 or 20 minutes. The first airplanes would be coming back in about another 25 to 30 minutes, so we had about a half-hour to fly around. Slow Bob could not show off in the airplane too much since we were heavily laden with loaded drop tanks on the wings. Besides, this airplane, like most of the A6s on the FID, had first flown in Vietnam. She was too old for any athletics. There was a project underway to replace the wings on a lot of the A6s, but it had not been done to many of airplanes, certainly not this old KA6, so we mostly just flew around looking at the scenery and the clouds.

The ship was close enough that we would pass through the Straights of Gibraltar the next day, so we flew over The Rock, which looked surprisingly small. Prudential Insurance had been fooling me for a long time. The Straights looked just as narrow as I had ever imagined. Morocco looked just as tan and barren compared to Spain's green as it did on my Rand McNally maps.

Shortly, we had our first customer from the next recovery, an A7 Corsair II. The refueling probe in the A7, as in the F14, fits into a groove along the side of the aircraft. In the A6, it permanently sticks up in front of the canopy eyeballs, like a big ugly stinger or a hooked nose. The A-7 had a big, gaping mouth of an intake right under the nose. It was a little ungainly and somewhat ugly on the ground because of this flat, gaping mouth, and it looked a little bit like the F8 fighter of the fifties. Possibly because of that similarity, A7s were often called "fighters" which they were not, they didn't even have a gun. Like the Intruder, the A7 became beautiful in flight. It had a beautiful planform with its short, swept wings and relatively slender fuselage, but this was really recognized fully only when you could see it from above or below.

When the A7 finished drinking, he slowly rolled over on his back, and fell away descending, gradually rolling over in a maneuver called a "split S." As he fell away, the wings arched out gracefully from the plane, he looked like a diver gliding into a half-gainer. One after another, airplanes came up to pump from "Texaco" to sustain them through the pattern. We watched our own recovery cycle to the deck just as we had the one before us, and finally there were no airplanes in the pattern except the helos that were off on the starboard side of the ship and us. Bob took us down to pattern level and described all the next steps gradually. We flew one racetrack pattern over the ship, flying in from behind at pattern altitude, directly over the flight deck. Then abruptly into the "break." That's the point where the airplane breaks away sharply from over the flight deck and banks suddenly to the left into the downwind leg. In civilian airplanes we do this with a gentle, rolling, banking turn toward the left. As Ike and Tina used to say, Navy pilots like it rough. Abruptly yank the jet up on its left wing, and curl you around at a couple of G's. The alleged reason for the high-G tight pattern is to stay as close into the deck as possible when landing. If the engine stops, one prefers being as close to the ship as possible. In an ocean of ice water or sharks, every hundred yards can be costly.

But the <u>REAL</u> reason pilots do it is because it <u>feels</u> so good.

Just before turning to final, the gear comes down, the airplane yanks again to the left, curls around toward the deck, wings level right at the threshold.

Out on the ends of the A-6 the wedge-shaped air brakes pop up. All of this happens faster than it does in our civilian airplanes, but if you watch fast you can grasp it. The rest starts going too fast to follow, though.

Suddenly, the airplane is over the flight deck, that blur happens again, the wheels bang, and the tail hook grabs the wire. This is my first time sitting in the front. The blur is just too quick. One or two of the flight deck crew and some yellow gear are visible, off to the right just before the wheels hit, but everything else whirls by in a tangled streak. The slam into the neck and chest surprises me as much as it did the first time, but it's even faster this time.

Faster than it started it was over.

Had it happened at all? Before I could be certain, it was over, the airplane was turning, Bob was gesturing for me to put the ejection seat on safety and pull the wings up. The canopy was already rising. I pulled the right lever and looked out timidly, reassured that the wings were folding back as they were supposed to.

The helo was coming in to be spotted at the position on the waist just in front of where we had been. As the canopy came up, the blast of hot Mediterranean air reminded me it was August. I realized that the air conditioner on the A6 must have been working pretty well. As calmly as turning off a Ford, Slow Bob shut down the engines, and it was time for us to climb out of the aircraft. I disconnected the G-suit tube better than I had plugged it in, and I checked my flight suit to make sure it wasn't wet anywhere that it shouldn't be (it wasn't). Climbing out of the airplane, I noticed my legs were a little wobbly, and I had to be careful as I jumped down the three feet from the bottom rung of the ladder to the flight deck.

THE TOMCAT

A couple of days later, we were out of the Mediterranean and headed north. I went down to the Ready Room of the "World Famous Red Rippers." VF-11 is the oldest surviving, continuously commissioned flying squadron in the U.S. Navy. On the bulkheads of the Ready Room, panelled in simulated oak, were photographs of various generations of airplanes over fifty years. There were open cockpit biplanes, piloted by toothy leather-helmeted men with white silk scarves. The old planes were adorned with the same emblem of a snarling red, heavily fanged boar on the F14s that belonged to the

Red Rippers now. There were F4Fs from World War II, and F9s from the 1950s. The Rippers had a grand old tradition, and they had decorated their Ready Room accordingly. All the Ready Rooms had closed circuit television, VCR for watching movies late at night, and a nice stereo system. They all also had those famous "Ready Room chairs."

I figure the first ready rooms on the Langley or the Ranger back in the 1920s were furnished with surplus barber chairs or chairs from an old Pullman railroad car. Thereafter, all other ready rooms felt they had to use something similar. The pilots were given tall-backed, cushioned chairs with funky metal arms, all of them having an ashtray mounted in them. I guess back in the old days pilots were expected to smoke, probably either Lucky Strikes or Camels. Almost no pilots or NFO's smoked anymore, but all the chairs had those dysfunctional metal arm rails, with the semi-comfortable naugahyde upholstery. Probably up and through World War II, the upholstery had been leather. The same yellow-tan pablum color was used in ready rooms throughout the fleet, and certainly in all the ready rooms on the Forrestal. The chairs were semi-comfortable, but whether they were comfortable or not, they looked the way ready room chairs are supposed to look. When my daughter Abigail first saw a Ready Room, she recognized the setting instantly. "Oh yeah, this is where the guy says, 'Gentlemen you are the Best.' "

They say that every aviation community has a personality, and an hour or two in the Ready Rooms would surely bear that out. Aviators in general are more flamboyant, more spontaneous, and a little bit more raucous than the "black shoes." Within the aviation community, though, there are further distinctions. Fighter squadrons are a little more aggressive, have a little bit harsher edge on their sarcasm and in their taunting of one another. Current Navy fighters have two seats, the pilot in the front, and the NFO Radio Intercept Operator, or "RIO," in the back seat.

Fighters live to chase and kill the enemy, to interdict other airplanes. Air to air combat is still their main mission. Of course, a secondary mission might be ground support or bombing also, but they are hired to look an enemy in the eye and kill him.

The attack aircraft, by contrast, are for "attacking" targets on the ground or ocean so the Navy calls their bombers Attack aircraft. It is their job to be deliberate and accurate in seeking out a target, and hit only that target, but hit it accurately. Bombers aren't so much interested in killing a specific hated adversary one-on-one like the Red Baron. Their job is to fly out someplace, have a good time, and bomb the Hell out of something. So attack pilots and attack A6 crews maybe are a little bit more analytical, a little bit more deliberate. If aggressive, like all pilots, they are at least not quite as stinging among one another as are the fighters.

Helo pilots tend to be people who would do whatever it takes to get the job done, they stick together, and yet might be somewhat more independent. In general the helo pilots tend to be more flexible, more adaptable. Because the heritage of Naval aviation has traditionally focused on the "go fasters" and the jets, helo pilots sometimes are just a little bit defensive. They quickly stop having fun if you forget that the H3 is a very large aircraft. Helo pilots often say, "If you can't hover, you ain't shit."

The A6 Intruder and the F14 Tomcat are both two-seaters with one pilot and one NFO. the role of the NFO in the two crews are different, though, and this difference is important. In the A6, the BN sits side by side with the pilot[5]. In the F14,

---

[5] *In fact this is not exactly true. The BN sits ever so slightly lower, and just a little bit further behind in the cockpit than the pilot. But for the most part they are side by side in the aircraft, right next to each other.*

the pilot is up front, and the NFO in the back. In both aircraft, there is only one set of flight controls. But in one airplane, the NFO sits in the back[6], and in the other, side by side (and just a little behind).

A6 BNs, single seat pilots, and F14 pilots all enjoy speculating on what this means. The F14 NFO seldom enjoys this kind of conversation.

The brief for the flight with the F14 had the same format as the brief for the A-6, but the mission was a lot different. We were going to go out and fly combat air patrol, or CAP, then do some "dog fighting," one-on-one Air Combat Maneuvering (ACM). Then we would come back and have some strafing practice before landing. I would ride with "Bullet" Richardson, the Commanding Officer of the Red Rippers, one of the best pilots in the Air Wing. He was said to be a shoe-in for Captain, and probably on the fast track for Flag.

The F-14 was probably the prettiest airplane on the flight deck. It was certainly the biggest and the longest. Two great big cylindrical jet engines stuck out the back with nozzles that opened and closed depending on whether the afterburner was working. The wings did not fold up like they did on the S3 or the A6 but instead had an adjustable sweep. For slow flight or landing, the wings would fold out, and the airplane would look like a turkey does in flight. The faster the airplane went, the more the wings were swept back by the computer, and the sleeker and faster it could go. The slower it went, the more the wings would come out toward a nearly perpendicular position. This particular movement of the wings was similar to what the Air Force F-111 used, and one or two of the Russian Migs. When parked, the plane would sweep the wings as far back as they would go, taking up less space in the hangar or on the deck.

Sometimes in dog fighting, in order to turn tighter corners, or to maneuver in a particular manner against an adversary, the airplane might slow down, so the computer would bring the wings forward. Fortunately the pilot does not have to think about controlling the wings, while he's busy doing other things. The computer takes care of that for him.

I tilted my head forward about 45 degrees as I had been instructed, and prepared for the shot. This time, my second cat shot, I vowed that I was going to pay attention to the "Shooter" and the flight deck crew while we shuttled down the catapult, and not lose everything in a blur. I saw the "Shooter" point toward the airplane, wiggling his hands overhead in the air. Bullet saluted him to say we were ready. I held tight with my right hand, and then slam, the catapult drove us down the shuttle. Just as before, everything streaked and smeared; all I could see was just one sailor over in the catwalk on the port side. Smushed tighter and tighter back into the seat, suddenly -- like squirting my entire body through a keyhole and then dropping down into space -- VARROOOM -- off the flight deck. Flying.

Imagine sitting on the hood of a car that is driving along at about 150 miles an hour and then suddenly off a cliff. No more acceleration and yet not slowing either. Thunder to silence instantly.

In the movies, airplanes dip down below the flight deck after take-off before they pick up and climb. Modern jets have to gain speed to climb well, but they don't sink off the deck. Just as in the Intruder, we accelerated for a half-mile or so, before we began to climb, much faster in the F-14, though. First we formed up on our wing man, and then up to meet the tanker.

---

[6] *Where, by the way, the pilot has his back to him.*

Flying up on the right side of the tanker, our probe slipped out from the side of the aircraft, and Bullet drove up as smoothly as parallel parking at a shopping mall. He slipped the snout of the refueling probe immediately into the basket on the first try, and within 3 or 4 minutes our fuel tanks were full and we were gone.

The dog fighting was no different from dog fighting in a T-34 or small airplane, although distances were miles instead of hundreds of yards and we were much faster! We scrimmaged with another Tomcat from the squadron. Passing each other nose-on at a closure rate of nearly 800 knots, within seconds we were miles apart and craning our necks back and left to try to keep the sweeping adversary in sight. If you forget your airspeed, you'll find yourself spinning out inverted, or at the top of an arc without enough speed to angle back at the enemy. They call that conserving energy. It can mean life or death in a fight. Wearing the G-suit, every time we pulled two or three G's, I was aware of the suit's bladder pushing in on my belly and my thighs, but the being upside down and then suddenly closing at closure velocities of nearly 1,000 miles per hour was sensually more exciting than the movies had ever been able to convey.

Just before the end of the ride we went out for strafing practice. For a target we used the wake behind the ship. Bullet did a little jig maneuver, yanking to the left and the right, with a sudden dive, which would have been used to elude ground fire if this were a real mission. Then he shot off a bunch of rounds from the machine gun. I have forgotten how many rounds per second the gun fires, but the sound describes it better than a number would anyway. It doesn't make a "rat-a-tat" sound like you expect. The gun fires so fast that it makes more of a buzz, the "PPFFTHZZ" sound that you make when you stick your tongue between your lips and blow to imitate certain biological sounds. That's the way the machine gun sounded. I asked Bullet how many bullets we fired when we did that, and he said, "Oh, a few hundred."

Bullet had given me certain jobs to do on final, including reading off to him the altitudes as we came onto the final. He left the ICS on so that we could communicate in case there was anything he needed me to do, or he had to tell me to eject. This was an uncomplicated daylight landing, without any hazards. Even in this setting, with this experienced pilot, listening was educational. His breathing had been virtually inaudible throughout more than an hour of flight up until now. As we came to the down wind, the 180, and then on final, his breathing got faster. I counted 20 and then 22 breaths per minute. The wings groped out sideways as we slowed, the nose came up, and the wheels smacked down on the flight deck, the tail hook grabbed, and BOOM, the arrest. My head jerked forward, and the belts jerked my shoulders and abdomen back. This time I was able to look at the flight deck a little bit as we landed, and things blurred just a little bit less because I could note the stripes and the landing markers whisk by beneath us. If I had not been locked into my seat with the torso harness, my face surely would have tumbled into the control panel.

************** ****** ******** *******************

After we left Spain, we had almost a week sailing north up to the Arctic Circle where we were going to begin participating in the NATO exercise "Northern Wedding." I had to take advantage of that time to satisfy some of my own "Qualifications" in being a member of the ship's company. All members were required to fulfill certain Qualifications in Damage Control and in "3-M" Materials Maintenance Management. The Damage Control requirement was the same for about everybody, regardless of rank or position. 3-M depended on your job. If you had a job that used a lot of gear or supplies, or if you had people working for you, you had higher requirements.

Damage Control is obviously important on any ship, but especially a ship of war, and DC training is required at some level for everybody in the Naval Service, even those not likely to go to sea. Even those who think that they are not going to go to sea, may have to someday in the future, even reservists.

Firefighting is a specially important part of DC, a world of its own, almost. The FID tradition, of course, knew that well. Everyone at sea needs to have a periodic refresher trainer in shipboard fire fighting every 4 years, regardless of how many times they have done it in the before. Fire Fighting is a 2-day school, several hours in the classroom, and several hours practicing fighting fires, avoiding burn injury, and learning some first aid. The classroom sessions seem always to involve one more viewing of the film "Trial by Fire" about the ***Forrestal*** fire of 1967. Some sailors have seen it so many times, they shout out some of the narrator's lines just like groupies at "Rocky Horror Picture Show." At the Certified Fire Fighting Training Centers, there are mock-ups of ship superstructures and spaces. Oil fires, wood fires, smoke inhalation, and the use of oxygen breathing apparatus ("OBA's") are all part of the training. In fact, the training can be pretty frightening, when you're down in that enclosed metal space scarcely able to see your hand in front of your face. Knowing that the fire was artificially started doesn't make it any less scary. It's a real fire, and it's real smoke. You can't see where you're going, and if you put your hand out, the fire can sizzle your fingers like a hamburger.

A hundred years of evolution have produced some pretty clever gadgets and nozzles. The standardized, well rehearsed lecture series and the obvious importance of the material make the firefighting classes pretty effective. They are physically demanding though and hot.

On the ship, there is a lot more to learn. Where are the individual fire mains on that particular ship, how to do shoring, how to patch pipes that leak, what teams to belong to, what signals to listen for on the 1-MC, and how to make good your escape from various places on the ship. One of the drills is to escape from the living quarters to an outside weather deck or a place to abandon ship in less than 2 minutes. It takes a little practice, but most people are able to escape from their berthing area even while blindfolded within just a couple of minutes. There are also two kinds of breathing apparatus everybody has to master. One is a little plastic hood kept right by the bedside, and in every work space. These are Emergency Egress Breathing Devices, or "EEBD's." They slip over the head and tighten around the neck, still permitting vision out the front. They carry a little oxygen cartridge in the back of the hood because filtering out the smoke isn't all you need in a big fire. It's not just fumes and particulate matter that will kill you, fires also burn up all the oxygen. The EEBD provides a few minutes, long enough to make that blindfolded escape everybody had to practice.

Although there are more EEBD's than there are people in the crew, the other gadget, the OBA is mostly for the use of Damage Control teams or particular rescue individuals. The OBA is a peculiar-looking contraption, like cross between a SCUBA tank, an accordion, and a mask for the Creature from the Black Lagoon. A little green metal canister fits inside the black rubber compartment over your chest or tummy. Reminds one of the power pack that Commando Cody used when he flew around on Saturday morning serials during the Depression. This chemical canister, when activated, releases free O_2. The reason for not using plain old oxygen tanks is that oxygen, of course, feeds fires. Heat and flame that could either make compressed gas expand, and explode, or could leak oxygen to build up the fire.

In Fire Fighting School we all had to learn to use the OBA, but there were more practice drills on the ship.

One day I was attending my D.C. class when a corpsman had to come up to the lecture room way back in the after part of the ship over on the port side, to tell me that Dr. Tosser had said I should be notified that he was starting an operation.

"Darn it! I asked him to consult with me before he started an operation." I ran down from the training room to the Medical Department as fast as I could, down about four decks, and forward a little over half the length of the ship. I was breathless when I got there, after a few minutes. Nonetheless, they had already started the operation. I put a mask over my face and cracked the door to the operating suite slightly, "How's everything going in there?" I thought that was a pretty diplomatic way of saying, "What the Hell is going on!"

"Everything is goin' fine. We just started an appendectomy," Rock said as though it was just the finest day in the world.

"When did he get sick?"

"Yesterday morning. He has had a high fever and has been getting worse ever since."

"When did you first see him, Rock?"

"About an hour and a half ago."

I closed the door to the O.R. then and walked back to my office, hoping none of the people who worked for me would see how red my ears were, trying not to sputter or foam at the mouth. We had gone over this several times since that day after we left Naples. The question of appendicitis never needed an operation within 5 or 6 minutes. I had only left the department about 40 minutes ago to go to the lecture. Since this case had been known an hour-and-a-half ago, I should have been notified, and could have examined the patient. While I had no reason to question Rock's diagnostic skills, I was beginning to get a little worried that he was more aggressive with the scalpel than I liked. I signed off a few of the reports I had to finish that week in my office, and then I went to the ward to make rounds. I was still worried about Tosser's eager scalpel and how I might avoid a dangerous confrontation. This would have to be watched I knew.

We only had five people admitted to the ward that week. One was an individual with suppurative eczema on his feet and toes, in others words infected athlete's foot. We saw a lot of that. Many of the young men had only one pair of boots and they wore them everyday. It was hot in the engineering spaces or on the flight deck, they sweat a lot, and if the boots never had a chance to air out, they stayed moist inside, and if there was a fungus in there, it had a perfect home. We occasionally had to put a sailor with very bad athlete's foot on the ward. We kept him bare-footed, usually kept his foot dry, sometimes with a lamp shining on it, and soaked it periodically with hexachlorophene or iodine. We usually treated it with a steroid creams also.

Two other patients were post-op cases, one recovering from an appendectomy, another from a hernia repair. The fourth patient, FN Tommy Burns, had stomach cramps and diarrhea. Doug Kempf admitted him because he was afraid that Burns might get dehydrated. When he became sick 2 or 3 days before, he stopped eating and drinking because, he said, "My mama told me once when you have the runs, if you don't put anything in your mouth, the runs will stop."

It may have seemed logical to FN Burns that if no fluid went in, none could come out. Wrong. Although the body in its healthy state has ways to conserve fluid, when it starts to get dry, once it gets out of balance, the adjustment mechanisms can't catch up. Even without exertion, most people exhale over a quart of water just in breathing. A lot of our sailors could sweat out over a gallon a day, especially guys on the flight deck or down in the engine rooms, like Burns. Diarrhea would waste even more fluid, and exceed the amount a sailor had been in the habit of replacing with normal eating and drinking habits. So a young man like Burns might be in precarious fluid balance already, but by not drinking for even a day, he could find himself dangerously low in total fluid volume and some of the important electrolytes like potassium, chloride, or calcium. Burns' pulse was a little fast, but the rhythm was good. His skin turgor was diminished and his blood pressure low when he stood up, all signs of relative dehydration, but he didn't seem to be in any danger at the present.

Even a single case of diarrhea could be the first sign of a food borne epidemic, a warning that we had to take some drastic action on the mess decks to prevent a further case. Or a single case could be the first case of even a viral outbreak like the one they had experienced a few months before I arrived. FN Burns had been crying all day. A big muscular snipe, he had probably never been sick in his entire life, so this experience was especially difficult for him. When I came on the ward, Tommy had just been brought back to his rack by the corpsman after having been helped up to the head for about the twenty-fourth time that day. He really was not significantly dehydrated. His pulse was normal, his blood pressure was normal, and he had been receiving intravenous fluids, plus taking a fair amount of fluids by mouth also. The corpsman, HN Bowker was tired of getting up every 5 or 10 minutes to help a whiney Tommy Burns to go to the bathroom yet one more time.

"Doc. . . " Burns called out to me tentatively, "Doc, can I ask you a question?"

"Sure, FN, go ahead." I came over and took his right hand with my right hand and put my left hand on his elbow. I tried when talking with the patients to sit down at their bedside rather than standing over them and to hold their hand or put my hand on their shoulder whenever I could.

"Sir, do farts have lumps?"

"No," I told him, "just air."

"Oh, no. Then I think I just crapped in my pants." Sure enough, a very unpleasant aroma seemed to spread through the ward just then, and Tommy's diarrhea got the better of him.

After we cleaned him up, we increased his diphenoxylate, the medicine for controlling diarrhea. I made sure to spend a little extra time with him that night, and we asked some of his buddies to come by and visit with him too.

Because of the operational tempo of the ship for the first 108 days, we were behind in the number of GQ drills. In order to reach the quota for the cruise, then, we were going to be doing a lot more of them for a while. We got in several during that week.

GQ as a training exercise ... The objective is not simply to see whether everyone wears the proper garments and closes the hatches the right way, but those people who have battle functions to be done during GQ have to exercise them. First aid was a requirement for everybody on the crew. Besides teaching basic first aid and first aid principles, there was a central core of the famous "Five Basic Wounds," that everybody at sea had to be able to treat promptly and correctly. The wounds were: fractured jaw with facial injury, a sucking chest wound, an open abdominal wound with extruding viscera, an amputated hand, and a compound fracture of a lower extremity. During GQ, then, Medical sent first aid trainers from one station to another, giving refresher training on the Five Basic Wounds and throwing down a flopper to test people on their proficiency. First aid lectures were part of the regular D.C. curriculum, the subject of both commercially prepared films, and live instruction over the closed circuit television. We also had pamphlets that we published right there on the ship about a number of the first aid techniques, and we distributed those to all hands. But the most intense first aid training was done by the roving teams during GQ.

Those first aid sessions were the only break most of us had from the suffocating boredom during GQ! The engineers and DC teams had lots to do during GQ, checking water mains, water-tight seals, and so forth. The rest of us just sat around for hours, manning our battle stations, and staring at one another. My station was in the Main Battle Dressing Station -- the main medical department. Tod Graef, The Gum Boss, had the same station, so when we exhausted the training catechism with our corpsmen and dental techs until catatonic saturation caught up with our collective boredom, we spent the time in front-porch conversation. Tod was a fascinating guy. I always thought he looked like Clark Kent, but somebody had once told him he looked like Clark Gable, and he liked that comparison better. Sure enough, Tod was a big guy, a weight lifter and a fanatical bicyclist. His voice was a little graveled, although not truly Gable-esque. He used to call me "Red," which at first I figured was because of my hair, although it never really was red. Since then, I've lately realized he was probably referring to my neck, an oblique implication or what he suspected to be my political beliefs. A Truman New Deal/Fair Deal liberal, I was usually way outnumbered in political discussions with the predominant conservative Republican population on the ship. Tod liked to imply I was only faking, and must really be a Rednecked reactionary Missourian.

We joked about a lot of things, including the shower stall and head that the two of us shared between our state rooms. The cold water knob wheel worked correctly, but there was no handle for the hot water. By the way several layers of paint covered the faucet hub, it was clear there had been no handle on the hot water knob in that shower for years, perhaps even generations. To make the hot water work, one had to reach up almost eight feet and turn the wheels on the hot water main coming into the whole room in order to regulate the hot water. Tod and John never told me about it, or how to make it work, but by tradition, nobody ever told them, either. You just had to figure that out for yourself. Tod had enjoyed a good relationship with John, whom he had clearly respected. He told me that shortly after he arrived on the FID, Rock Tosser had taken him aside to warn him that John was "weak" as a physician. An experienced oral surgeon and Naval officer, Tod had been able to recognize for himself that Bigbee was an excellent physician. So his warning from Tosser told him more about the surgeon, he figured, than about the former SMO. Interestingly, on my second or third day on the ship, Rock had told me something like that about Tod, too. I figured he'd be saying it about me before long.

Something we maybe should have joked about a little less was flushing the commode. Old Clark too often forgot to flush. We joked about it, but truthfully I used to hope he would figure that it was just my tactful and indirect way of asking him to do better. When he left the FID a year later, I had one of the flushometers, that's the shipboard name for the chrome flushing toggle switch, mounted on a nice mahogany plaque for him as a going away gift. I was hoping it would embarrass him, but he still thought it was part of our serial repartee.

******************** ********************

After a few days the weather began to get colder, and the sky was overcast most days. We were up north of Scotland by this time, and we had been busy working on first aid drills and drilling Mass Casualty scenarios a number of times. One morning I was making rounds in the ward, and I noticed a pale young man with NG tube sticking out his nose. Bill Flynn was making notes in his chart, so I asked Bill to tell me about him.

"He has been sick on and off for the last couple of weeks, with a lot of belching sometimes, and occasional stomach cramps. He has lost his appetite, has been pretty listless, and somewhat constipated. I've been treating him as an outpatient for a few days, but he has developed an ileus, so I put the tube down this morning, and I thought I would watch him on the ward for a couple of days." His name was Sam MacDonald, a

Second Class Aviation Electronics Technician. Thirty-four years is a little bit old for a Second Class Petty Officer, but he had entered the Navy late. It looked like the NG tube would take care of things, but it was a little bit unusual for an acute gastroenteritis to cause an ileus in a person his age.

The next day Sam MacDonald was still on the ward, and he still had an NG tube. I asked Bill about him again, and Bill said that he seemed to be doing fine, except that he still had not had a bowel movement, and that his abdominal films still showed a lot of gas in his bowel. We talked about the possibility of a bowel obstruction, and asked Rock Tosser to see Sam, also. Rock thought his treatment was proper, but share our concern that the ileus continued, even after the NG tube was in place.

On the third day, the ileus was not resolved, and Bill and Rock thought we needed to do an exploratory laparotomy. We debated all the various options, at this point we were outside the range of any of our aircraft to send him to a European hospital. I had to admit, he had normal blood counts, no laboratory abnormalities, his belly was not tender, and it was hard to explain why a man in this condition should have an ileus. For the first time since I arrived on the ship, I had an opportunity to discuss a case before the individual wound up in the operating room, and remarkably enough, this time I did agree (although a little reluctantly) that an operation was necessary. Cautioning myself about Rock's eagerness to operate, I went up to see the Captain on the bridge and explained to him that we had to find out why gas was being trapped in the young sailor's bowel. I explained about how viruses or other forms of irritation of the organs could cut down on movement of the intestine, but that with an obstruction like this we had to look for some form of blockage, a place where the bowel could fold back upon itself, or even the possibility of a tumor, although that seemed pretty unlikely in a 34-year-old man who had been healthy right up until this point. The Captain asked if there were any alternative treatments we could recommend, and I told him that at this point, even if we were on the beach, without any relief by now from conventional treatment, that a laparotomy was necessary. Maybe if we had a CT scan or the opportunity to do a barium enema, we would do that first, but ultimately with a continued ileus and no explanation, he would probably have to be decompressed. Out of everything we discussed, the possibility of a tumor was the most alarming to Captain Pieno. "If he has cancer, I want him off the ship."

"Yes, Sir." I took his direction that if a cancer were found in the operation, which I knew would not be the case, that somehow I was expected to get him off the ship. I did not control the aircraft nor the flight schedules, and there was nothing I could do for the present about our being outside the range of any of our aircraft. Furthermore, we would not want a guy with an abdominal incision to take the G forces of a catapult shot for several days. Helicopter evacuation might be acceptable because of the fewer G forces, but we were even further beyond the range of helicopter transport to land. In short, the Captain wasn't interested in a two-way discussion on the subject, so there was no sense in opening a complicated discussion right then. Besides, this was a young guy, and although we were forced to relieve the bowel obstruction, cancer was not a very realistic concern... even if the Captain was sensitive on the subject.

Within minutes after the incision, Rock had discovered a mass in the colon. It was about the size of a plum and had all the characteristics of a malignant neoplasm. Cancer. Rock removed the tumor, leaving Sam with a colostomy. I found myself reluctantly trudging up the seven decks to the bridge to tell the Captain that one of his patients, a 34-year-old man had a probable malignant cancer of his colon.

The Captain was not surprised. He should have been... it wasn't reasonable to have expected a cancer. I suspected the Captain was one of those folks who have a semimystical fear of cancer or even the word cancer. He asked how the patient was doing, how he had tolerated the operation, when he would be able to have visitors, and if there anything else we needed to do at the present. I explained that the operation was very well tolerated, but that they were just at that point closing the wound, so he was not out of anesthesia as yet. The Captain said that he would be down to visit him that evening, and reminded me what he had said earlier, "We've got to get him off the ship as soon as possible."

Sam did well after the operation. There was no evidence of metastasis at the time of the operation, but a lot of tests remained to be done to see if he had any spread of the tumor and to get started on whatever treatments he would need. Our first job was to be sure he healed well from the operation, that he was well stabilized now. The next job was to deliver Sam as quickly as we could to good cancer treatment, although at this point it wasn't the kind of emergency that had to begin within one or two days, and get him to his family in New England.

We were arriving at the Arctic Circle now. Days were getting colder, men had to wear jackets or double layers on the hangar decks and heavier garments up on the flight deck. Sam couldn't take anything by mouth for a few days after the operation, until his peristalsis would return and the colostomy work. His wound was healing cleanly though. Aside from the Captain's wishes, for purely medical reasons as the SMO I wanted to send Sam to the Air Force Hospital in Lakenheath, or preferably back to the States as soon as we safely could. He was safe and well-cared for here. A healing belly wound can be jostled a lot on a helicopter, and can't tolerate the G forces of a catapult shot at all. So we wouldn't want to send him too soon. In addition, his Attending Physician was Rock Tosser; not me. The Attending should have a central role in deciding when to transfer a patient. There should be a special relationship between the Attending Physician and the patient that any hospital, including this one, should always endeavor to protect.

About the second day after the operation, I raised the subject. The talk wasn't easy, because Tosser had been cool toward me ever since our first discussion about the appendectomy after Naples. Always a diligent worker, he kept up his office hours and the training he had to do with the corpsmen, but he left the Department immediately whenever his work was done. It was obvious he wasn't interested in any spare conversations with the SMO, and it was becoming clear he didn't have much regard for my medical judgment, either. "Rock, when do you think we can begin to talk about Sam's leaving the ship?"

"Oh, never, not 'til we get back. He's riding the ship home."

"But we've got a month left, Rock. He's got to get home and start getting treatment."

"He doesn't need anything yet. I'm keeping here until we get back to Mayport. He can get his oncology at NHJax."

"Rock, his family's in Newport, not Jax. I know we can't send him off right now, but in a week or so, we'll be in England, and we can let him walk off and then fly back in a regular Medevac flight to the states."

"I'll think about it."

In my opinion, Rock was medically incorrect, but on both general principle, and for the purpose of keeping harmony in our department, I didn't want to take away his role as the Attending. What Rock didn't know was that a couple of times a day, in addition to the morning and evening briefs that I presented regularly, the Skipper would call me or step in my office to ask about Sam... and to ask when I was sending him off the ship. "Captain," I would say, "he's just not stable enough to take the vibration of a helo or the G forces in a COD cat shot."

"But you said he has cancer. He needs treatment doesn't he?"

"Not necessarily, Captain. But you're right he does need some testing and scans. Those can wait a little while, though. Certainly until he's stable."

"OK, but I want him off when we go to Portsmouth."

I felt some of the camaraderie I built up with the Captain in Benidorm might be slipping.

Up in the North Atlantic, we exercised with the Brits, the Danes, and the Norwegians. The Norwegian pilots got especially high marks from our Air Wing. One day, I got a chance to go flying with the Red Lions. They promised we could fly up around the fjords for some site-seeing and take Admiral Smith over for a conference on the ***USS Theodore Roosevelt.*** We had to wear an extra piece of survival gear, a watertight suit covering toes to neck. Hypothermia, which can kill you in five minutes or less in the Arctic Ocean, is forestalled a little if you stay dry. The suits have to be personally fitted and swaged together, getting into them is an athletic feat, and they are insufferably uncomfortable. After a while, I got used to it, though. It was never quite as bad as that cranial I had to wear from Diego Garcia.

The trip to the TR was great. We left the big barn door in the back of the helo open. Admiral Smith showed me how to fasten the Gunner's Belt around my chest instead of my waist to enable me to walk around in flight and lean out the door to look around. When we landed on the TR, it was my first time on the deck of one of the ***Nimitz***-class nuclear carriers. This new ship, just a couple of years old, was only ten or fifteen percent bigger than the FID, but it looked more than that. I felt like a country boy who just came to the big city for the first time. Stepping into the island, I might not have known I was on a ship. They had a real **ceiling**, not an overhead! The bulkheads didn't have pipes and rivets, and cables -- it looked like the walls in a fancy office building.

Stepping into the Flight Deck BDS, I felt a little more at home. Two corpsmen, aged and dressed just like my guys back on the FID, were surrounded by all the IV bags, bandages, lights, and sinks in a small emergency treatment room just like ours. As I stood there, though, something was very different. I couldn't tell then what it was, but gradually later it came to me. Not the bulkheads, or the overhead, or the size. Not just the more modern appearance. This ship didn't have the hum. It didn't have that smell, a kind of metallic steam and a distant memory of petroleum fuel. I guess it might be like playing football on Astro Turf. It's still football, I guess, but if you don't have the smell of the turf to remember, how can you miss it?

For a couple of hours while Snuffy was in the conference on the ***Roosevelt,*** we flew in and out of a bunch of the fjords. There were roads here and there along the mountainous coastline connecting the red, brown, and white cottages and villages, but I never saw a car or a truck on any of them. The craggy grey and wooden countryside was even more beautiful in three dimensions from 300 feet than in all the paintings and photos I had seen all my life. The rustic simplicity of the fishing villages impressed me most in the apparent cleanliness and orderliness that one could recognize even from this altitude.

When we returned to the FID, I stopped in to see McDonald. There was beginning to be some accumulation in his colostomy bag, showing that peristalsis was returning. Rock had let him have a little custard and some fluids by mouth. I thought once he could start eating, Rock would be more comfortable and we could think about sending him home when we got to England.

The Northern Wedding exercise was going well according to the Ops Department. We would be coming to Portsmouth, the largest British naval base, in just a couple of days. The CCTV was giving background information for the Port Call and telling the crew where to sign up for tours.

The Captain sent word that he wanted me to come up to the Bridge. It had to be that he was tired of waiting for me to send Sam off. Bracing for trouble, I hurriedly went by to exam the patient and check over his chart and current lab reports. Then I huffed up the ten decks to the bridge.

I always tried to catch my breath before going to see the Captain. It wasn't just good manners, either. Of course, you shouldn't begin a conversation with **anybody** out of breath, so manners were part of it. It was self defense, too. Captain Pieno was a take-charge guy. He was going to dominate any discussions we had, of course, after all he was the boss, but I didn't want to give him any more advantage than he needed. At least up here in the North Atlantic it was a little cooler than it had been a few weeks before. At least my khakis weren't stained with sweat by the time I reached the Bridge. After stopping for a little rest before asking the OOD, "permission to enter the Bridge," I was still breathing deeper than I wanted to. The Captain was all business that morning. Uh-oh, I thought, here it comes.

"Doc, have you seen this message?" The Captain handed me a message that arrived the day before. Relieved that I had read it already, and especially relieved that this discussion wasn't going to be about MacDonald, I found my breathing slowed a little. The message was from CINCLANTFleet. Apparently there had been some medical waste and plastics washed up on the shore in North Carolina from the Coral Sea. It had attracted some very unfavorable press coverage, and Admiral Kelso, who was CINCLANTFleet, was outraged. The message emphatically said we would no longer dump any plastics at sea, and especially medical waste. We were henceforth to store all medical waste and all plastics until we were in port where it would all be treated in accordance with standard practices from that locale. The message was dated 29 August, 1988. We had received it yesterday, the 30th, and Rick and I had begun grappling with what steps we would need to take to comply. It would be difficult. Virtually every container of any product on the ship was plastic. In medical, almost all the trash we had would be either plastic or had some biological fluid. Little of it could be incinerated, so we were going to have to find some place to store everything. We were on top of it, though, I reassured the Captain. "Don't worry, Sir, we've got it under control."

"Good, Doc. This is going to be very important. Make sure we don't have any problem with this, OK?"

Of all the things the Commanding Officer of this enormous vessel has to worry about, I thought it a little curious that he should be so interested in medical trash. Not a big problem in the big scope of things, I thought. Sure, it would take some work from all of us in the Medical Department, but it seemed funny the Captain would be so interested in this. Captain Pieno had a way of focusing on some topics that he thought were particularly important. One had to admit, though, that he did have an uncanny sense of what would become dangerous or important. Maybe it was a survival instinct. It made him react to hunches more than he should, though, I thought. This interest in the syringes was an example of that, just like his agitation about Sam MacDonald.

A couple of days later we arrived at Portsmouth. It seems like it was overcast and drizzly the entire time we there. It was my first time to visit England, but for some reason, the gray damp seemed right. The whole crew was in great spirits. Portsmouth was a popular port of call. The Brits and the Brit sailors welcomed Americans as enthusiastically as fond relatives. The local language was similar enough to our own that the guys were able to carry on conversations in which they understood entire passages.

The morning we arrived, Sam MacDonald had taken a full breakfast, and his NG tube had been out for over a day. Rock and I had a long talk about his plans, and he agreed that once the skin staples were removed the next afternoon, Sam would be out of any immediate post-op risks. Candidly, I told Rock that since the Captain was so concerned about this case, it would be important to all of us to send Sam home as soon as it would be safe to do. No cutting corners, but no delay, either.

"I think he wants to finish the cruise with his shipmates," Rock argued.

That's not what Sam had told me, but I didn't dispute the surgeon on that point. "Rock, we have to think about his family and the crew's apprehensions. They're all worried about him, the Captain especially. And I know it's not an immediate emergency, but really we shouldn't wait an extra three weeks to get on with his oncology work-up."

Finally, Rock reluctantly agreed. He expected to take the staples out the next day and we could send Sam over to the Air Force Hospital in Lakenheath the day after for transport back to the States, "But only if he's ready. We can't just forget about the patients because the Captain is superstitious." I let him have the last word. Pieno was **far** from superstitious, and I disliked Tosser's implication. ...Yet, reluctantly, I had to admit Rock was right on this point. We really **wouldn't** send Sam off unless it was clinically safe, but of course the Captain wouldn't want that anyway. Rock's tone irritated me, but I didn't want to make him more argumentative, so I let it go. We had an agreement, and that was good enough for now.

Other than one sailor who somehow stole off with the log book from the Mary Rose, the old ship that had been Henry VIII's flagship, we had no major problems or drinking incidents in Portsmouth. We were treated to VIP tours on the Isle of Wight, just across the bay, and several formal dinners with English Naval officers. On our third and fourth days in port, I went to spend a day in London and an evening off the ship in the Admin. Sam was up walking around, eating well, and Rock promised me he would arrange for his evacuation trip back to the States. HM1 Rosenthal, who was every day proving to be a stalwart, promised me that he would assist Dr. Tosser to **be sure** it all happened.

After a whirlwind single day seeing the sites in London, I took the train back to Portsmouth and joined a bunch of Forrestal officers at a pub near the Admin. One guy named Redgie Gutshall seemed to know a lot of rock n' roll trivia, a challenge I can never miss. He and I battled back and forth, nearly neck and neck until I smashed him on a question about the Hollywood Argyles (the answer is Glenn Campbell played lead guitar). Redgie was from Kansas City, too, so we talked a little about our hometown. A former enlisted Air Traffic Controller, Redgie was a part-time professional actor, and had appeared in the movie "Brenda Starr," which alas still has not been released as this is written.

The next day, the ship was scheduled to get underway at noon. Seas were so high that boating had to be suspended for several hours, so I couldn't get back to the ship until just before the Sea and Anchor detail was called away. As my boat pulled up to the camel behind the fantail, Rick Combs was waiting for me, hopping back and forth from one foot to the other like a little kid who has to potty. We started to greet each other when the 1MC interrupted us, "Senior Medical Officer report to the Captain's In Port Cabin immediately." An unheard-of announcement. That kind of announcement not only meant that the Captain was mad, but that he didn't care that the whole ship knew it.

"That's what I came to warn you about," Rick told me, not that I hadn't already figured it out. Rock had decided the seas were too rough to let Sam leave in a boat. The British did not permit Flight Ops here at this anchorage, so we couldn't fly McDonald off. The Captain was angry that he was still on board.

When I arrived at his office, the Captain didn't even look up from his papers. "Nice of you to grace us with your presence, Doctor, since we're getting underway."

I didn't know what to say, so I said nothing.

"I thought I told you to get him off the ship!"

"Yes, Sir, but since he's still recovering from the operation, Dr. Tosser and I didn't feel it was safe for him to be climbing in and out of boats, and the boat ride in these seas could be hazardous for him."

"Would have been nice for you to tell me that, don't you think?!" (I was remembering a little of what Myron Almond had told me about the Captain. The Screamer part)

"I want you to get him off today, before we are out of helo range! Is that clear?!"

It was clear all right. When I got down to the Department, though, Sam was having a bad day. He had been nauseated all morning. None of us wanted to put him on a helo while he was sick. "He's not leaving today," Tosser said... as though nobody on the ship had a say in the decision but him.

"It's a twenty minute flight to Lakenheath," I insisted. "He can handle that. We're overstepping our limits here. If he doesn't go home now, he's stuck with us for the whole crossing."

As soon as I said that, seeing Tosser's grim smile, I realized he had manipulated just this very outcome. He had wanted MacDonald to stay under his care all the way home. It wasn't Sam's return with his shipmates that Rock wanted, it was his **own** return with his cancer patient.

"I can't permit that," he announced.

"It's not up to you to permit or not permit. You just lost your vote."

Frankly, I wasn't enthusiastic about sending Sam off while he was sick, either. Yet, it was only 20 or 30 minutes by air to Lakenheath and the man did need to get on home to his family and his workup. Curt Rosenthal took me aside to tell me that Sam did go into town the night before and spoke with his wife by telephone. She seemed to accept the situation, Sam said, and since she could speak to him, she was not too anxious.

Wait a minute. If it was acceptable to Dr. Tosser for Sam to go in a boat to the phone, why didn't we just send him on to Lakenheath by driver? "I just didn't think he should drive that far," Rock said.

I contemplated telling the Captain the whole story; in other words, putting Tosser on report. What would be the use, I figured. After all, I'm still the SMO. I'm the one responsible. Getting the Captain angry at somebody other than me won't get Sam on that helo any faster.

When I went to see Rich Strickler, the XO of the Red Lions, about sending Sam off, my hopes were dashed. Only two aircraft were "up" for this afternoon, and they both had just developed problems. We wouldn't be able to send one of our own helos until about ten hours from now. By then, it would be dark, and NATOPS (flight rules) forbid flying anybody not aircrew rated over water after dark. By tomorrow, we would be out of S3 range.

Quickly I ran over to the ATO and AirOps offices, both of which were on the O-3 level like the Red Lions Ready Room. No, there were no deck qualified American helos in the area that were not already involved in other ops. We called the British local air ops. They let me talk to a senior British flight surgeon. While they could send a helo for a true medical emergency, the case of sending a guy who had been here all week, and who didn't have an actual emergency at the moment, would not really qualify. Sorry, they couldn't send a helo either.

I went up to explain the whole situation to the Captain. I didn't tell him that Sam had been on the beach the night before, but I said only that he had spoken with his wife and she was OK. That made the Captain feel just a little bit better, but not much. MacDonald would be with us for the crossing. He was not happy about it, but there was nothing else to do. Still, it was clear he had given me some clear orders I hadn't done the way he wanted. Having developed respect and fondness for the Captain, I regretted losing his confidence.

I went on back down to Medical about the time I heard the 1MC announcement, "Shift the Colors." The deck shuddered and moved a little.

We were on the way home.

CHAPTER V. CROSSING THE ATLANTIC TO GO HOME

By the time we left England, I thought I was getting the hang of it. Day to day routines of the ship and the department were becoming familiar -- to the degree that anything in this tempo and these 18 hour work days could ever be routine. Now that I thought I had the job description in its most concrete terms under control, it was time to start working on the "Big Picture." We needed to improve customer service, fix it so that people did not come and stand in long lines for sick call, for example. I wanted FID sailors to feel like the service in their Medical Department was as personal and attentive as they would get in a private doctor's office. We needed to get our records on a data base, too. My other goal was to improve our preventive medicine and surveillance programs, and tracking patients. We would not be able to do that without a computerized data base, I was sure.

Putting our preventive medicine and surveillance programs on a regular, continuing schedule instead of mammoth once a year marathons would improve quality, and could reduce the size of lines sailors would stand in. Every member of the Navy had to have certain things like HIV tests, TB skin tests, and flu shots every year. The tradition throughout the Navy in the past had been to line up everybody on the ship on a certain few days and draw blood from everybody, stick them with their TB test needle, and give them whatever shots they needed. Like a massive "round-up" to brand cattle. My, but it was ugly, though.

Massing everybody together created crowds and lines that spilled into space well beyond just the Medical Department. Tables and equipment had to be set up in the hangar decks and mess decks to accommodate the masses. Every department on the ship was interrupted or involved. Operations dictated when space could be available in the hangars, and mutual adjustments in both our schedules and meal hours had to be made for the mess decks. Worst of all was the indignity for the sailors. It hadn't changed since those photos from WWII, or for that matter WWI. Grim, expressionless young men were herded like beef on the hoof through impersonal lines of robot-like medical humanoids, also expressionless, holding some medical thing with a point on it, poised to puncture the beef in its arm. Huge long lines. I *hated* lines!

Jamming hundreds of people together for all their shots and blood test set up a grand opportunity for errors too. If we could only get the whole system into a computer data base we could be more accurate schedule more rationally too.

Somehow, besides getting the mass and preventive medicine programs straightened out, if I wanted to make the customer services better, I would have to win over Doug Kempf. Doug held forth on his own over in the Emergency Room. He saw patients more or less "on referral" from sick call and just kept the charts on his private patients in a drawer in the ER. He did have his own exam room over on the same side of the passageway as my office, but it was so filled with stuff -- his trunk, piles of amorphous clutter, neck ties, old mail, and hideous stacks of unrecognizable clutter -- that he really couldn't see patients in there. I always thought somehow I should tell him to clean up his office. If telling a teenager didn't work, though, I figured telling a grown up doctor wouldn't work either. Besides, it didn't seem right somehow to tell a Naval officer to clean his room. I once asked HM1 Branom, the LPO in the ER if we couldn't just return Doug's charts back to the Medical Records file room with all the other records. "Oh, no, we can't do that. Dr. Kempf wants them to stay here." Even though I was the head of the department, Doug's authority over this private practice was a different matter. It didn't occur to Branom, or in fact to anybody but me, that I might have a vote in the matter. Dr. Kempf wanted the records to stay there. That was that.

What if somebody needed treatment in the ER during Dr. Kempf's treatment times?

Hmmm. Nobody ever thought of that... It doesn't happen. That's Dr. Kempf's time in the ER.

Well, could it happen? What if somebody needed treatment?

That was not an easy one to answer. Maybe they'd have to come back later when Dr. Kempf was finished.

Maybe Dr. Kempf would let them use the other table, if they'd draw the curtain.

Doug had not hesitated to speak his mind the first week I was on board. I could tell he was not comfortable with me yet. Not comfortable? He just didn't like me. In time, I planned to talk with him about his 'private practice' in the ER, but now wasn't the time for that. He was clearly the stalwart in the department along with Art. I had a lot to learn from the two of them and I needed to win their confidence and their friendship a lot more than I needed to sell my newcomer ideas. Doug already saw me as an invader, I thought, and not a very smart one at that. Somehow I would have to win his confidence.

The second morning after we left England, Lonnie Pizza came to Sick Call and said the Captain wanted me to come up to his cabin when I was free. The Skipper and I had not spoken since we left Portsmouth. He had clearly been angry that day and I was afraid he still had more to say on the subject. I braced myself, but there was no escape, of course. About an hour later, when Sick Call was finished I arrived. "You asked to see me, Sir?"

"C'mon in, Doc. Have a cup of coffee. How are things going?"

I mumbled a little about the flu shots, but nothing very coherent. The Skipper was obviously busy this week, and I didn't expect him to have time to sit around and chat very long before he delivered the whatever it was I was expecting. He spoke about going home, asked if Ann would be able to come down to meet the ship. Told me he and Carolyn would like to meet her if she did. Shortly I was feeling more comfortable, but now I was a little perplexed about why the captain wanted to talk.

Gradually, I realized what this visit was about. He didn't invite me up here for idle coffee talk. What we were really talking about was our last meeting, the day we left England. John Pieno was not an apologizing guy. Neither of us would think he had anything to apologize about anyway. We finished our coffee and each had to return to work, but I understood. I had just been told, by my shipmate ...sorry I yelled at you, Doc. Maybe you were right. Let's drop it.

From Pieno it was more sincere than if he had said the words and it was OK with me.

That's why he was the Captain.

The Crossing was a convenient time for people from the States to do all the inspections a ship had to be put through every year. They mostly had to be done while the ship was underway and while the entire crew was onboard. Doing them at the end of a cruise hit the crew at their most experienced peak, in a way, but people were also beginning to get tired then, and equipment problems were accumulating after six months of hard use and limited repair opportunities. Civilians would have hard time comprehending all the inspections. The Secretary of the Navy wanted inspection data, so did Congress, the DOD, and the Naval Occupational Safety and Health Agency. Even though the word "Naval" might be in an organization's name, they were not on your side any time they came for an inspection.

One big inspection was the 3M inspection, the Maintenance and Materials Management system. The 3M inspection was one of the most taxing inspections, had to be done every year, and tied up every sailor on the ship at one time or another, some of them for hours.

The 3M system covers every piece of hardware on the ship, and every job that any member does, virtually down to the paper clips. For every piece of hardware or equipment there is a line in a master log prescribing the preventive maintenance cycle, and a card like a recipe that outlines the steps in inspection and maintenance. A multi-member team of real grouchy and finicky guys comes aboard the ship once a year to check the records in every department. They also nab four or five sailors in each division and test them on how well they do a maintenance job. When they do the test, how closely the sailor follows the card and how well he knows the 3M rules counts more than whether the gear itself works or the sailor operates it right. The 3M inspection is not only important because the score goes into some unfathomably obscure data base someplace in the Navy. The real reason seems to be that scores on the 3M inspection are a big part of the competition for the Battle E. The Battle E counts.

In 1987, the ***Saratoga*** won the Battle E as the East Coast carrier, edging the FID by just a few points. In the heartbreaking defeat, the FID had a low score on the 3M inspection, so Captain Pieno, in his final year in command, wanted to win. He wanted very much to win. Captains never would say that they cared about things like Battle E's, though. Captains said things like, "Who cares about that? All we can do is strive to serve the United States in the best way we know how, and let others worry about awards." Captain Pieno believed it when he said things like that, but ... he wanted to win, too. He liked winning. This year, we had scored 100 in nearly every Compex. We were a little ahead of the ***America*** on points, reportedly (***Saratoga*** was in the yards in Norfolk for an overhaul). The 3M inspection was the only obstacle apparently. So as the 3M inspection neared, we crammed for the test. Ed DeMartini, a Shoe who worked in the Maintenance Dept, was put in charge of the 3M training task force. Like every self-respecting Blackshoe, Ed would have preferred to be on a cruiser or destroyer, doing Shoe stuff. The exciting jobs on carriers go to aviators. Some things, though, are in the purview of basic shipdrivers, the Shoes. Aviators, like Ozark, could work hard on 3M business, but everybody knew that Shoes are the best when it comes to this kind of grinding detail. Well, maybe Bubble Heads (submariners) are *really* the best at mind-numbing arbitrary minutia, but Shoes are better at it than aviators. Ed made some really very entertaining film clips, with Ozark and others adding humor to entice the sailors to watch. He also assembled a Tiger Team of people who went department by department to give classes and coaching. When the 3M team came, we would be ready.

One afternoon, early in the Translant, Commander Kit Hennesy, the CO of the HS-15 Red Lions came in for his annual Flight Physical. An Academy graduate, he had been an aviator for about 13-14 years, and he ran a squadron with high morale and a great reputation. He was in fine physical condition, but for the first time, his visual acuity had been a little below 20/20. Looked like he would need glasses for the first time. Glasses do not disqualify pilots anymore, if they already had their wings, and could be corrected with glasses. Kind of like occasional impotence -- needing eyeglasses wasn't something they thought **other** people should be ashamed of, just a simple, natural, physical phenomenon, not a matter for either panic or shame. "Oh, no, I wouldn't mind wearing glasses if I **had** to," Kit said. However, he just didn't really think the test was accurate in his case. "You know, I was flying a lot the last couple of days...I've been tired. Never been below 20/20 before, Doc. Could you check it for me just to be sure?"

Sure enough 20/25 both eyes, just a little myopic. Myopia often gets worse in the dark, right when marginal vision is especially critical, particularly in the big H3 helicopter.

"Well, don't you think this can be just because I'm tired, Doc? Maybe if I could check it again after we get back."

I just smiled. Vision is kind of symbolic to aviators. The heritage of that goes back to their first few hours in the culture, when some of their first comrades years ago couldn't cut it because of vision, when some had to become NFOs instead of entering the pilot pipeline because of needing glasses.

"We can check it again after we get back to the States. You can get it done over at Jax or it might be easier if you come back here to the ship where we've done the rest of your exam.

"You know, though, that I have to give you a down chit until either you get glasses or your test is 20/20, right?"

"What about the Fly-Off? That'll be in daylight and we have two pilots in the cockpit."

"As the CO, you can decide to fly with a down chit, but you know I have to give you one."

Kit knew that of course, and we didn't argue about it. I knew he'd never fly with a down chit. We agreed he would come back either to see me or a flight surgeon at HS-15's base in Jax to check his eyes after the cruise.

I could have belabored the points that I didn't think fatigue was causing his myopia, or that even if it **were**, fatigue is a basic staple of carrier aviation. He would be flying fatigued often, so even if that were the cause, we would have to correct for it. I figured he would be going to somebody else, in the hope that a "second opinion" would reach a different conclusion.

That night, I was invited to the Captain's "in-port" cabin for a "seance" after eight o'clocks. A "seance," I soon learned, was a euphemism for card game. The Admiral was there, too, and usually two other guys, at least one squadron CO, and either another department head or another squadron CO. Sometimes a sixth player would come. Although we played poker, we of course never gambled real money, just poker chips. This was heady stuff for me, just a doctor, playing with the big guys. They were real good at this. One suspected aviators played a lot of cards in their younger days. Fortunately, as I said, we did not play for cash, or I may have lost some real money. It was a time for the Admiral and the Captain to relax. It had been a long deployment. The banter and needling was truly expert, and riotous. I knew that these were smart people, but was impressed with how funny they could be too.

There were seances most nights at the end of the cruise, and I found myself invited for most of them, and to dinner beforehand a couple of times. One night, when I was really tired from a particularly long day, I was dealing a hand. The new SuppO, Bruce Bennett was playing that night too. The Captain and the Admiral never seemed to be too tired to have fun and be fascinating in conversation. It was infectious and yet it was clear that although aviators could play cards all night, I'd never be able to match that energy. I also wasn't as experienced as the Line Officers at cards. They had games like High-Low and Baseball. I'm just a Kansas City boy and we aren't good at card games, so when I dealt we had to play something simple like straight poker. Of course, we didn't bet money. Just poker chips, for keeping score. For some reason, a card came off the bottom of the deck while I was dealing. How it happened I still don't know to this day. My chubby little hands are not dexterous enough to do that kind of thing on purpose, and the card was something dumb like a three anyway. The Admiral quietly said, "No, I think you'll have to deal that one over, Doc. I don't want one from the bottom of the deck." Dealing off the bottom of the deck to an Admiral! Who could believe something like that is a mistake? It's not like stumbling on a loose carpet tack. He didn't lose stride or show any rancor, and he kept telling jokes, never repeating any punchlines. Snuffy somehow knew it was just awkward clumsiness, I guess, because he let it pass. First, only quick eyes would have noticed the gaffe. But then, only a person with an abiding trust and patience in others would be able to just let it go and not wonder when it would happen again.

The next morning, the 3M team flew aboard on the COD. Twelve or fifteen of them in the team, some wore coveralls, the others khaki. Because of the squinty, gnarly expressions, I figured that either they had been sucking persimmons for the last week, or they all had Tabasco sauce in their shorts. They gave us some speech about how they were here to help us, and then they dispersed to try to trip up as many FID sailors as they could. I went back to Medical and asked Rick to assemble the Corpsmen. Although I spoke to them most mornings at Quarters, I wanted to give them one last pep talk about the 3M inspection. I told them I thought they were ready and not to feel any pressures from the Inspection Team. Halfway through my little talk, Chief Hitzeman interrupted me to say I was being called up in the CIC, "Combat." One of the Small Boys in the Battle Group had a medical problem they were calling about.

Speaking to other ships about sick people called for judgment and tact. The young doctors or the IDC from the small boys only called because they needed help, not because they were looking for a lecture. Sometimes, there was enough information, and a confident IDC, that we could handle the problem over the radio. More often, the very fact of their calling was evidence that they couldn't handle that patient on that ship. So I was developing the attitude that if the other ship wanted to transfer a patient that meant that they needed to, regardless of what it sounded like on the radio. The Captain agreed with that approach. We insisted, however, on consultation first. We needed to warn them if we didn't think the patient could tolerate helo transfer, and we needed to be ready or to prepare for some patients.

I greeted Steve Wesselhoff, the CIC, or Combat Officer. Wesselhoff is a very intelligent guy with a clever wit, and an uncrackable stony expression. He and I had a running repartee, so we bantered for a few seconds as always, each of us sure we had outpointed the other (of course, impartial observers usually knew I had won). Redgie Gutshall was the TAO that day. "The Roberts has been calling, Doc. Their corpsman needs to talk to you." He handed me the headset from his chair so I could talk right across his desk.

All the ships communicating on the net could be heard, fragments of perhaps a dozen different discussions. The voices were all electronically scrambled so that other nations could not cipher the communication. American ships then unscrambled them, so the voices came out with an eerie metallic, machine-like timbre, whose only human quality was kind of nasal, whiny, and a little high pitched. You can't break in with "Breaker, breaker" like you can in a CB network on the highway. Only critical conversations are permitted on these overburdened nets, so presumably the ongoing discussions we all important. It would be unwise or at least bad manners to presume that one's own message is more important than the one on the air. I waited until there was a brief lull, then I broke in, "USS Roberts, USS Roberts. This is the Forrestal Senior Medical Officer standing by. Over."

A lag for the Roberts to receive, unscramble, and respond to my call. "***USS Forrestal***, this is ***Roberts***. We'll send for our Doc. Please stand by."

The "Doc" on the Small Boys, cruisers and destroyers, was an IDC, usually a First Class on a destroyer, and a Chief on a cruiser. The Sick Bay on their ship wouldn't be far from the CIC or com center. Still, I thought, since he knew I would be returning his call, he should have been standing by so I wouldn't have to wait around for him. However, it didn't bother me long because I enjoyed watching all the action in Combat, as the guys worked over all their various scopes and plotters. Because of all the sensitive scopes and scanners and plotters, CIC is usually dark. Table or desk lamps are confined to small pools of light wherever paper had to be read or produced. Conversations were held in moderately low tones, so that everyone could keep an ear available to monitor background conversations on the several radio nets or hear directions from the Combat Officer or TAO if they gave any. The stereotyped nasal robot-like voice was carrying on a discussion between two ships about some spare part, and between one other ship and some shore establishment regarding a port call. "Somebody wake the doctor up when the corpsman comes on in case he doesn't recognize where the medical conversation begins," Wesselhoff said.

"Good idea," I answered. "I wish you guys could let me know when Commander Wesselhoff wakes up too, but I don't think you could tell."

Somebody suggested that neither of us should jump into full time comedy work, and then the ***Roberts*** came in. "***USS Forrestal***, ***USS Forrestal***. This is the SMDR [senior medical department representative] from ***Roberts.*** I have a 23 year old white male with acute abdominal pain. Over."

As usual, the corpsman began with telling me the chief complaint and a little bit of the history of the present illness. In this situation, what we usually would want to hear next was the physical exam findings including the vital signs, then the course of the disease from the first symptoms. We found that on the red phone though the corpsmen, and young doctors alike, tended to focus on laboratory data, and medications. This caller did that. He told me about the white blood cell count last night and again this morning, the urine analysis, the blood sugar, and the EKG. "What about the abdomen," I had to ask. He answered that there had been no bowel movement. Finally, we determined that the patient's pain was very acute, but episodic. He had experienced some nausea and vomited once several hours ago. Perhaps the pain had radiated toward the scrotum once, but this was uncertain. The abdomen was tender, but not taut. Bowel sounds were either absent or not very active, but we weren't sure, because we couldn't tell if the corpsmen knew how to listen to the abdomen. There was no flatus. The urine was normal. They had no X-ray on the Roberts of course.

We had to suggest transferring the patient, and after he arrived, we learned he was suffering from renal colic, symptoms of a kidney stone.

That night, I went up to the bridge to tell the Captain that our transferred patient was doing well. I had already passed the word back to the ***Roberts***. The Captain invited me to a seance that night, but I told him I wouldn't be able to come. The next night was going to be the "Fo'c'sle Follies," so I wouldn't be able to work then, and I had a lot of work to catch up on. "OK, I'm sorry you won't be there, we may not be able to play for a while." I didn't know yet that the Captain was going to be busy with VIP visitors soon. "Look, I know you're going to be doing the flu shots soon. Don't forget what we discussed about medical waste and plastics. I don't want to go through what the Coral Sea did." He was really focused on that medical waste issue.

When I went back down to the Medical Department, we had a number of things to go over in meetings. I began by mentioning the Captain's concern about plastics and medical waste. We doctors chuckled about how the aviators pick up on funny little isolated topics to dwell on. Here we just transferred a guy from another ship who could have had a dissecting aorta or some terrible thing, and the Skipper was most interested in trash. Rick Combs was less amused. "I wouldn't brush off his concerns too quickly. The man has an uncanny instinct; that's how he got where he is." Rick also was plenty concerned about the medical waste and plastics. "Almost everything we have is plastic, Captain. We're not going to have room for all this stuff if we can't throw it over the side."

"You and I can go over that tomorrow, Rick. For now, it looks to me like we can fit everything in the Preventive Medicine office head."

Rick disputed that, he thought there would be too much for that one space, in fact, he suggested we should first use the Head from Ward Two, and spill over to the Prev Med head, actually the former shower stall, only as a back-up space. "And when do you think you're going to have time to walk around tomorrow? You said you want to be up on deck for the UnRep, the shots are starting, and the 3M inspection is going on." He was right, the next day was going to be very busy, but I told him I'd make the time for a planning tour for the two of us in the stash of trash, but I wasn't very enthusiastic.

We had a number of things to talk about. Although I was beginning to convince the department that we needed to get mandatory surveillance and preventive programs on a continuous cycle, the facts remained: it was the season for flu shots, and while everybody was still trapped on board it would be easier to "hit" everybody now than after the cruise was over and they dispersed, took leave, and so on. Rick, along with HM1 Rosenthal, and Senior Chief (HMCS) McGowan, had worked out schedules for getting everybody done. Since flight ops were over by now except for an occasional COD, we would be able to use the hangar bay, in three big lines. By taking two large departments, like AIMD or Supply, in a day, and smaller ones four per day, we could get all the shots done before the preparations of the last couple of days. Those last couple of days, the entire crew would be busy getting the ship super-pretty for arrival, and people would be getting so crazy that concentration would be wasted by then.

For some reason, only about half of the supply of flu vaccine was the right formulation for the transdermal jet-gun, so we would have to use syringes and needles for the shots for half the crew. The gun isn't entirely painless, but it hurts a little less than the needles. Also, some people develop troublesome blisters or other reactions from the jetgun, so the gun can't cover everybody. With those exceptions, however, we in the department favored the jetgun. Sterilization is a lot simpler, and so are supplies: no needles to deal with, to be pricked by or throw away, no plastic syringes. It's almost as easy as rubber-stamping correspondence. Step on the pedal. Next. Touch the gun to the arm. Step on the pedal. Next. The only time consumed is checking off the patient's shot record, on the left-hand side of his HR (Health Record). Too bad we could only use the jetgun on half of them. We decided to use it until we ran out of that form of vaccine and then shift over. We would ask every sailor if they would prefer to have the needle. Those who had trouble with the gun knew who they were. Everybody else would be amused by the question. What sane individual would prefer a needle? At any rate, we couldn't use the gun for more than half the flu shots. You will see later that adding an additional

2600 syringes for flu shots to the several thousand we already were using for TB tests mattered.

Finally, the marathon was all set. We would start in the morning. Rick had called all the DivOs together from all over the ship and explained the system to them. I had discussed it at eight o'clocks. Although I had an uneasy feeling about this big project, I told myself it was just because I hated the lines that would be involved. After all, we did need to get caught up, the crew did need to get the flu shots. We were going to do this right, and it was the right thing to do, so I resolved to quit worrying about it.

It was time to dismiss the meeting and let the medical officers and chiefs get back to work or for those who could, to relax for the evening. "Not yet, Captain, did you forget we have to talk about Womple?" Yes, I had forgotten. We had to talk about whether Womple could go home early on the COD. I had wrestled with whether just Rick, HMCS McGowan and I should discuss this, since it involved just one corpsman, or whether the other officers and chiefs should stay for the discussion. We wanted to keep discussions about individuals private, of course, which was an argument for the smallest group. On the other hand, sending one corpsman home early could have an impact on the thirty others who had to stay, and besides I was new and all the khaki[7] in the department knew HM3 Womple and could advise me.

"OK, Senior Chief, and LT Combs have to stay. We're going to talk about Petty Officer Womple. Everybody else is invited to stay, but you can leave if you want to." Nobody left.

The Senior Chief led off. "HM3 Womple's got family trouble again. We got a Red Cross message this afternoon. One of his kids is in trouble at school again and the Family Services Center suggested Womple should be there." One of the functions of the American Red Cross is communication with command about family emergencies. Arden Womple, in his mid thirties, was old for a third class petty officer. In fact, as the Navy was beginning in 1988 the first movements toward shrinking, Womple was facing potential dismissal for High Year Tenure, failure to progress in rank. He was more immediately facing dismissal for obesity, but that was a separate problem. He married a woman with several adolescents who seemed to be in trouble all the time with authorities at school or the Naval Station.

"Didn't he have to be flown back early at the end of our last deployment?" Doug asked.

"That's right," Rick added, "and halfway through REFTRA too."

"Captain, I think this is just more of his manipulative BS," somebody added.

Well, given Womple's general attitude and surliness, his motives might be suspect, but it was a real Red Cross request. We didn't question the Red Cross. They were on the scene at home. I said we had to accept the Red Cross authority.

There's no question about his going, guys. What we have to discuss is how to tell him, and how to deal with the rest of the corpsmen."

"No problem, Captain," said the Senior Chief. "I think that the other guys'll be glad to see him go, even though it'll leave more work."

It was true. Womple was a bully to the patients as well as the HNs and any of the other corpsmen he could bully. He was over 6', and as big and as round as a manatee. He had an impressive baritone voice with an authoritative diction that buffaloed even

---

[7] *Officers and Chiefs wear khaki uniforms, and everybody else wears dungarees or some other work uniform like coveralls. So the term "khaki" is often used to refer collectively to CPOs and officers.*

some of the corpsmen who outranked him. He was older and sounded so intelligent. If he hadn't been so sloppy, and had the grimiest uniform among the corpsmen, he would have been confused even more often than he was for a CPO.

Poor Womple had been counselled about his attitude, his appearance, and his demeanor toward patients a lot of times. He usually would sulk about it, but he had a remarkable record of seeming sincere and winning reprieves just before the worst possible things like Captain's Mast or Admin Separation. Still, his promotions were slower than Congress, which was why he might face High Year Tenure expulsion. With almost 16 years of service, he should have been a Chief, an E7, for a couple of years already, but instead he was still an E4 with no prospect of promotions. He dodged work, sulked around most of the time, just generally spread gloom. About three times, he had been processed for separation because of being fat, but it never quite went through.

The Navy had always had limits on obesity, but only enforced the limits sporadically and inconsistently until around 1980. With the gradual improvement in retention and pride in the 1980s, the Navy established body fat measurements. Above 22% body fat, members -- officer or enlisted both -- were placed on a mandatory weight loss program. Above 26%, a member couldn't be transferred or promoted and if he stayed above limits over a six month period, could be administratively separated -- fired. Two or three times, Arden Womple had been in the process of separation because of body fat. Once he lost down to 22%, and his prior command dropped the proceedings. A couple of years before, he was on his way out from the FID, when the ship's Legal Officer found some procedural omission, then Womple lost down to 24% again, and the process had to start over.

I too have been overweight most of my adult life, so I was probably ambivalent about Womple's obesity. Once I had complained to my father that the Navy focused too much on weight, and he pointed out, "It's for your own good. Besides, aren't the rules the same for everybody and didn't you know the rules when you joined?" If the rules applied to me, it was fair to apply them to Womple, I guess. However, I was worried that the weight might really just be a convenient scapegoat for dealing with a troublesome corpsman. Was it honest to get him out just for being fat? The real reason was he should just flat out be fired, but it's hard to fire people for that from the Navy just like it is from any big company.

We talked about this for a half hour or so, everybody having an unpleasant experience with Womple that they wanted to submit. Finally, though, everybody agreed with me that our own frustration with Womple could not stand in the way of his family's needs. I resolved to discuss the matter with the chaplain too, to make sure we gave Womple any support he needed. HMCS McGowan would make the arrangements with the ATO for Womple to leave on the COD as soon as possible.

THE FOLLIES

When the meeting was over I went up to the fo'c'sle for the "Fo'c'sle Follies" show, a tradition on all carriers. The Follies are put on by the Air Wing twice during the cruise. It's a long tradition for the "visitors" from the Wing to satirize their experiences and alleged abuse at the hands of the ship, and to lambaste whoever from the ship's company has attracted the most ire from the Wing. The first part of the program is for the Wing to recognize the best performers in various aspects of airmanship and safety, with competition among the squadrons for the best landing scores, best aircraft availability scores, and best safety records. This competition is richly and ingeniously mixed with humor, but not gently. The pilot or squadrons with the lowest landing scores are hooted and squirted by waterguns. Catcalls interrupt the proceedings frequently.

After the "formal" part of the proceedings, each of the squadrons in turn sing a song written for the occasion, usually bawdy, but always either boasting uproariously about themselves, or cutting one of the other squadrons -- or some unlucky target among the ship's company. This night, the "Bulls" of VA 37 had special T-shirts with the picture of NFO wings in a circle with a diagonal line through it, like a "no smoking" sign. The light attack squadrons, VA 105 and VA 37, who flew the only single seat airplanes left in the Wing, were proud of that, and missed no opportunity to malign the NFOs -- who were generally as numerous on the ship as the pilots. As the night wore on, a few of the "Bulls" were struck by eggs or whipped cream from unseen assailants. The "Bulls" song was accompanied by a trumpet and guitar duet, and had some clever puns and insults about the Mini-Boss.

The best song of the night was done by the "Thunderbolts." In a somewhat unusual departure, there was very little direct satire directed at specific individuals, except for an obligatory insult to how the MiniBoss slowed down flight ops by scolding pilots. Putting words about bombing missions to the music of "On the Street Where You Live," the "Thunderbolts" had the entire audience in laughter. It was certainly audience-specific humor, and would probably fall into the category of "politically incorrect" by now.

Then there were monologues by the CAG -- Pat "Martini" Hauert -- and Admiral Smith. Since the Follies are a production of the Wing, the CO of the ship is an honored guest but not truly a participant. The CAG was OK, but Snuffy definitely stole the show. Somehow, he squeezed in some inspiring words about the success of the cruise and the importance of teamwork, but his stage presence and stream of outrageous jokes were convulsive. Most of his jokes were about aviators and sailors, their families, the stresses and apprehensions about coming home. Some of the jokes had such crazy and baffling punchlines that any audience would have loved them, and yet even in that happy moment, more so later that night, everybody realized that the jokes were funny because they made fun of all the apprehensions and concerns that were gradually bubbling up as we were nearing home. It was sneaky. Every face was cracking and everyone was laughing, but Snuffy had slipped in a note about dealing with homecoming. He didn't dwell on it, but hid it in the merriment and let it linger there. Snuffy ended his conquering monologue and then the CAG introduced the skits.

For introduction the CAG said, "The only rules are there are no rules." That was certainly an understatement. Hilarious as they were, the skits, one performed by each of the squadrons, were merciless. First was a brief one about a discussion between Captain Pieno and Admiral Smith about alleged confusion on the bridge. Abruptly a couple of zingers about Captain Pieno's marital history -- he had been married a couple of times -- that were pretty disrespectful. I thought I saw the Captain's ears redden, but he being a dutiful aviator, would always just say, "no rules."

The A7 guys had a skit with faces stuck out of a sheet over boots, to look like short human puppets. These ridiculous looking characters were funny enough, but they parodied confusion in a two man A6 cockpit talking with confused Air Traffic Controllers on the FID. Even the Thunderbolts who flew the A6 laughed achingly, but still in revenge, they broke out their water pistols and shaving cream cans to pelt the other squadron.

Finally, near midnight the "Follies" ended. the show was as hilarious as I had always heard it would be, albeit more caustic even than its rough reputation. Some people may seethe a little about the jokes. Yet they knew that the rules were "There are no rules," and they themselves had attacked senior officers back when they had been J.O.s, junior officers. It was a ritual for the end of the cruise, a permissible way to express some of the tensions from this dangerous and confining life. Come on, it said, let's open up those wounds, laugh and heal one another. We are all brothers here and the cruise is over.

Still laughing as I filed out of the Fo'c'sle with the crowd, I mulled over the ingenious value of the "Follies." The culture of Naval Air depending on a complex blend of things. Dedicated loyalty and affection for the team. Imperative sharing and learning constantly. Pervasive optimism, and conviction that ours is the winning team. Most of all, maybe, fun. Six months at sea with only three port calls can strain the fabric. "Fo'c'sle Follies" wasn't just an hilarious show, it was I realized, an example of why this team keeps winning.

Before I went to bed that night, I stopped down at the Ward Room. In the lounge a number of guys were sitting around playing cards or chess, watching a movie on the big TV in the corner, unwinding themselves before going to bed. The informal dining room had a popcorn maker like the kind you see at carnivals or movie theaters, and there was popcorn available most nights. It was near midnight too, so "midrats," midnight rations, were available, usually just sandwiches and chips.

I saw Warren Lobs, the First Lieutenant, who was getting to be a pretty good friend. "Hey good show, huh?"

No response but a raised eyebrow. "Didn't you go down to the Follies?"

"Yeah, I was there for a while."

"Well, I'm still laughing. I guess you didn't think it was as funny as I did."

I expected Warren to make some Black Shoe comment about adolescent aviator behavior, but he had liked the Follies fine. He just had other things on his mind. "Gonna be busy the next few days, Doc."

We in Medical were going to be frenzied with catching up all the TB tests, HIVs and medical record reviews. We had agreed to do the annual body fat measurements at the same time, adding just one more notch to a hectic program. So I too had been thinking about how busy it was about to be. Thinking about HM3 Womple's problems, too, I had come down to the Ward Room before bed to unwind. Warren had some other things on his mind.

"Yeah, I guess the 3-M inspection is going to be a hassle, eh?"

"Oh, hell, I forgot about that! That's even worse!"

"There's something worse?" I was getting interested now. The festive final week was beginning to sound threatened.

"Right in the middle of the 3M inspection in a couple of days we have our last UnRep. I've got a broken PadEye that we have to fix before that, and then you know all the VIPs are going to start arriving tomorrow and they'll all be hanging around while all the activities going on."

I finished my popcorn in a hurry and went to bed. This was going to be a busier week than I had expected.

Early the next morning, the Corpsmen started getting set up for the flu shots, blood tests, and TB tests. We had special tables set up on both the aft mess decks and up in Hangar Bay I. Master Chief Morgan from the Supply Department had interceded on our behalf to use premium space on the mess decks. He said he owed us the favor because Doc Forbes had been so good for him. At the time I thought that Master Chief Morgan seemed awfully solicitous for some reason. Was his speech a little slurred, I asked myself? Senior Chief McGowan and Rick Combs had scheduled everything as carefully as they could. Right after morning sick call, we started the scheduled runs. People were to show up in their PT gear to make it easier to take the waist and neck measurements the Navy required for body fat determination, designated record keepers checked painstakingly assembled data bases to see what tests or immunizations the members needed. It worked remarkably well, but the whole department was involved. The medical department usual functions still had to go on, but we had pulled staff for the mass program, so the guys still in the department had to work a lot faster than usual, and everybody's work shift extended from 12 to 14 or 15 hours a day.

I have to admit I was kind of proud to see the process go so well. Hundreds of people filing into the lines and progressing as planned from one station to the next. Impressive and organized though it might have been, though, I vowed we would never be in this position again. It was a picture of military medicine we needed to get rid of. People should be able to sit in a private place and have private quiet conversations and treatment when their health was involved. We were going to get to that point on the Forrestal, I determined. As a representative of the command, furthermore, I had to feel that this wasted time. No matter how well we did it, making all these people queue and wait, even just fifteen minutes each, was very costly. Fifteen minutes times 5300 would be over 33 work-weeks tied up just by those standing in lines.

We were generating a huge mound of trash, too. Most of the squadrons in the Wing had done their TB skin tests on a different cycle, but still we were going to use more than 3000 tuberculin syringes just for the TB tests. Almost 4000 needle sets for the HIV tests.

Rick Combs went with me to check the storage of all the medical trash we were generating, down to the head in Ward II where we were stashing all the bags -- after they were first sterilized in the autoclave. It didn't look as though we would need more than the space in the Ward Two head, but if we needed to we could use the former shower stall in the space we used as the Preventive Medicine office. Looked as though we had it under control. I didn't know why medical waste had caught the Captain's attention so much. He sure had enough other things on his mind this week. Regardless of the reasons, Rick and I knew that medical waste and plastics disposal were more important now than they had ever been, so we were determined not only to keep it under control, but especially to reassure the Captain that it was.

BOSWELL IS A BOOK LOVER

It was a busy day, but they all were at sea. I had promised the doctors that we would review our medical library and order some new volumes. The department had a couple of journal subscriptions and about fifty books. All physicians are expected to own a few of their own favorite texts, but the department really needed a few new reference works.

We went around the room, letting every member suggest books that the whole department needed. Rock suggested a current volume on basic orthopedics. Doug wisely pointed out the large number of skin problems we saw and suggested a good picture atlas of dermatologic problems. Bruce Boswell, in his Tigger enthusiasm, jumped into the derm discussion.

"Have any of you seen this derm book?" he asked, pulling a small spiral-bound pocket book out of a beat up old canvas gym bag. "I used it in medical school, and I think it's just what we need here."

"You mean *osteopathic* school, don't you?" Rock threw in, in a manner everybody but Tigger thought was snide. Tigger didn't seem to notice. Some MDs are still a little contemptuous of osteopaths, DOs. In the military, we've mostly outgrown that. Some, however, like Rock, still do not consider DOs their true equals. Didn't bother me; Rock thought I wasn't his equal either.

"There doesn't seem to be much text and clinical guidance in that book, though," Bill Flynn said.

"It tells you just what you need," Bruce answered. "Look, there's a picture of each lesion and right beside it the name and the dose of meds for treatment. Just what you need."

That would be fine, Doug thought, but we still needed a good derm reference. He suggested one in addition to Bruce's spiral pocket book. Then Doug suggested we should consider a good text on Xrays of the extremities.

"This is just what we need," Tigger said, pulling another small spiral pocket book out of the old gym bag. "Great diagrams, easy to read, not a lot of useless text, you know?"

The group agreed his little pocket book was handy, but wasn't quite as detailed a reference as we needed sometimes when there was a tough film to study. We went around, bringing up books on four or five topics. For every one, Bruce had a little spiral bound pocket book that he pulled out of that bag. "Bruce, have you ever read an honest to god book? Do you know what a hard back **IS**!?" Doug asked him. Doug liked big difficult books. "Hey why bother," Bruce answered, as proud as if he had just solved America's illiteracy problem. "This is the kind of book you really need. May not impress anybody sitting on your bookshelf, but these babies fit right in the pocket of your white coat. You've always got 'em right where you need 'em."

Art observed, however, that none of us wore white coats on the ship, and besides, since Bruce had just shown us his entire medical library of nine spiral notebooks, a nine-pocket white coat was a critter he had never seen. I'm still not sure, but truthfully I really believe those may be the only nine books Bruce ever needed.

All that day, the lines kept coming and we moved people through. We kept up with Sick Call, and fortunately, it was not a busy week for any illnesses or injuries. So we kept up with normal work.

On the day of the last UnRep, Warren apprenticed me to BMCS Jones, the archetypal Bos'n's Mate. Senior Chief Jones had a craggy Victor McLaglen face that matched his sawmill voice. He showed me what the guys up on the Bridge had to be doing to steer us to our approach to the ***USS Milwaukee*** from whom we would take on fuel, mail, and supplies in ***un***derway ***rep***lenishment. Two ships can't just come alongside one another, shut down, and pass things back and forth. Dead in the water, ships can't control their positions, so the waves would knock them into each other and modern ships would flail one another to erector sets. The solution was to maintain steerage by steaming side by side close enough to stretch cables between the two ships. The warship was to make formation on the replenishment ship, whose job it was to maintain a straight course and a steady speed.

Conning alongside required keen seamanship, because if you got too far away, the cables and hoses stretched between the two ships would snap under high tension, and could cut a bos'n's mate in half as it whipsawed back. If you got too close, the Bernoulli effect would suck the two ships together, perhaps so strong that the rudder couldn't overcome it, or just as bad, that such a keen turn was needed that the aftercoming fantail on the carrier would still dash into the hull of the replenishment ship. Years before I had seen in the news that two Navy ships, completely alone in the vast Indian Ocean had collided. How could such a stupid thing happen, I had thought at the time. Big ocean; little ships. They had the whole Indian Ocean to themselves, why get in each others' way? Now I understood. It had to have been in an UnRep, and the Bernoulli effect sucked them together.

Down on the hangar bay with BMCS Jones and his crew, he talked one of the Gunner's Mates into letting me shoot the cat's paw over to the ***Milwaukee***. "On the ***Milwaukee,***" our loudspeaker announced, "stand by for shot lines fore, amidships, and aft!" With a shotgun, I fired the cat's paw, a ball of heavy cord, over to the other ship, trailing out line as it flew. Gunners forward and aft did the same. Bos'n's Mates on the ***Milwaukee*** scurried to catch the line and they tied rope to the ends of it. Then we pulled the rope back over to ***Forrestal***. Finally, using those guide ropes, we were able to attach cables and refueling hoses between the two ships. Since it was near the end of the cruise, we didn't need much more than fuel from the ***Milwaukee***, but we did take a couple of pallets of mail and some spare parts. It was dangerous work, with tons of equipment sliding over high tension cables, arrested and guided by Bos'n's mates pulling on ropes. Heavy leather gloves prevented most blisters, but careless movements could quickly sacrifice a finger. A number of the workers had to be tied to a capstan to be sure they wouldn't topple overboard if they slipped or fell.

The Milwaukee and most other replenishment ships carried a couple of CH46 SeaKnight helicopters. These twin rotor helos were used by the Marines to carry troops, but on these ships, they were cargo haulers. They had a big capacity, and their superior maneuverability was important for the adroit transfer of cargo from one ship to the other. When replenishment was done by air, it was called VertRep, for vertical replenishment. Most of the time VertRep and UnRep were done simultaneously.

The whole UnRep and VertRep today was over in less than two hours. The preparation and the clean up in this busy week added another couple of hours, though. Art Hawley had once described the process as a ballet, and he was right.

Normal work, and UnReps however, weren't all that the ***Forrestal*** did that week. The 3-M inspection team had been on board for several days and they were around everywhere. They were like the commie spies in J. Edgar Hoover comic books in the fifties -- they were everywhere. Anyplace there was a sailor trying to do work, there was a 3-M inspector asking him to demonstrate his preventive maintenance program. He had to faithfully go to the little instruction card kept in a special file place in the works space and then pick up *exactly* the *right* tools for the job at hand and then go back and log it in the three separate books or charts. Ed DeMartini or the XO, or their assistants tried to go around and see how well we were doing. All FID sailors knew that the 3M inspection was important, but we all especially knew that it was something you could put a score on, so it counted toward our winning the Battle E, the Carrier Championship as it were.

The 3M Inspection wasn't all of it by any means. The NAVOSH (Navy Occupational Safety and Health) team was on board too. Industrial hygienists, Environmental Health Officers, technicians, all came for the annual NAVOSH inspection. There are about two dozen screening and prevention programs on the ship that range from hearing conservation, heat stress prevention, asbestos surveillance, mercury and lead monitoring. So the NAVOSH inspectors were in every workspace, too. Sometimes sailors were confused about whether the inspector at hand was from the 3M team or the NAVOSH. The NAVOSH guy would arrive with his air sampling gadget, his chemical testing set, or his questionnaire, and the poor sailor would dutifully head off to the cabinet to get his preventive maintenance cards, only to realize he was responding to the wrong inspection. The food sanitation inspection team was on board from AIRLANT, too. Food sanitation was a target of stiflingly frequent inspections. For one thing, the Preventive Medicine techs in my own department inspected every gallery, scullery, bakery, and eating area on the ship several times weekly. The cooks and in fact the whole Supply Department hierarchy hated to see my guys coming. There is no acceptable level of mediocrity in dealing with cleanliness and sanitation. It just has to be done right, but that adds a level of frustration and tension sometimes to the cooks if the inspectors are not considerate or tactful. Indeed, I frequently had to warn HM2 Brian Haack that it was our job to promote sanitation, to help the Food Service do better, not just to punish and expose them for shortcomings. So, when the food sanitation inspectors came on board, it was to add not merely one more in the endless parade of inspections, but even one more irritant to S-2, the Supply division that ran food services.

The ship was crawling with inspectors of several kinds, but just the numbers and range of all these inspections wasn't enough to explain what a nuisance they were. Ships get inspected to exhaustion by themselves and outsiders all the time. Although this was more than usual, and irksome at the end of a cruise, what really made this klatch of inspections particularly irritating was that these were all especially picky inspections. The food guys crawl down on their bellies to find the little nitty microscopic grease smudges that even my sleuths had perhaps missed the week before (you see, the food sanitation inspections would affect and *reflect upon* not just S-2, but also Medical, the XO and of course the CO, too). The NAVOSH guys come and interrupt a busy forklift operator to ask him about work and rest cycles, earplugs, etc. The 3M inspectors more than once inadvertently asked one of the other inspectors to demonstrate some of their preventive maintenance procedures, provoking relieved pleasure from an onlooking crewmember but surprisingly little amusement from the other inspector. The crew was beginning to get more and more restive about coming home. The hangar deck was full of lines of people getting their shots and TB skin tests; everybody had to get at least one needle, so this was a further aggravation in the hectic activities. With all these strangers and all this activity, nerves among mere mortals would have begun to fray.

One additional little feature for us in Medical was that the food sanitation team and NAVOSH team were in fact composed in significant part with Medical Service Corps officers and some Chief corpsmen, the Environmental Health and Industrial Hygiene specialists. They would come down to our spaces in any spare moments, letting us feel like targets of opportunity. Inspectors, you get the feeling, are like IRS auditors. Once they get in the door, anything they find they feel to be fair game. One member of the Food Service team was LCDR John Perrault, a very intense, very precise fellow. Intense and precise are words that you like when you use them to describe a football coach or somebody who works for you. They're not happy words when they fit somebody who is inspecting you. Besides doing the food inspection, this prim, bookish fellow, who carried a thermometer in his pocket for measuring the temperature of cleaning water, had a personal interest in the new instructions about medical waste.

"I guess you got the CINCLANTFleet message about plastics and medical waste," he said, in what was disguised as a conversational tone, but I was convinced was a ploy of some sort. I thought at the time that his lips were pursed as he asked.

"Yeah, we got it," Rick answered him. "The Captain is right on board, too. Do you want to see where we're stashing the stuff?"

"Oh, no, I'm not here for that, I was just curious. Just wanted to know if you needed any help."

This was my first contact with John Perrault. Bruce Bennett, the new SuppO, had the same impression that I did, that Perrault was a snippy, inquisitive professional inspector. A couple of things didn't fit, though. Perrault was a former Marine, had a couple of tattoos on his forearms, and an impressive row of ribbons over his left pocket. These aren't things that often go with the kind of trouble-making inspector he seemed to be. Although I didn't think about it very much, I was troubled a little bit that I hadn't pegged John Perrault very clearly yet. Oh, well, after all these inspections, I'd never deal with him again.

TOO MUCH COMPANY

In detail after detail, the inspections and all their derivative activities complicated the trip home. But there was still more complicated outside interference. The VIPs.

There had been what I *thought* were VIP guests coming on board in our three port calls, local dignitaries and people who commanded the special attention of the Captain or the Admiral when they came to tour the ship. No, those weren't *real* VIPs. Real VIPs came on board in small numbers when we got underway from England, or flew on board from the COD everyday after we left. They all needed special tours of the ship, and staterooms of course. The ones who attracted the most attention were Senator Lawton Chiles and seven or eight of his staff. Senator Chiles, the senior senator from Florida -- the ship's home state -- had announced that he would be retiring from the Senate at the end of this term, within just a few months. So clearly this fact-finding trip was not a ploy to garner attention. No press accompanied him.

Well, maybe the press had not come just to accompany Senator Chiles, but they definitely had come nonetheless. They seemed to leave the Senator alone, I was told, but they wanted to see everything else. Human interest stories from the end of a six month cruise were maudlin, funny, provocative, a lot of things. The carrier is very photogenic, so the reporters, both TV and press, used their photographers a lot. Popular radio stations sent along one of the most popular disc jockeys who would record some shows from the ship to play on the air for a day or two before we would arrive.

So, the cruise is coming to an end, everybody is busy trying to maintain safety during the final few weeks. The XO and First Lieutenant are trying to get all possible cleaning and painting done before we get back to the States. The Air Boss and MiniBoss are trying to get the hangar clean, and the hangar and Flight Deck surfaces painted and for a good appearance for all of our families when we arrive in Mayport. The CAG and AIMD are trying to get all the airplanes in 100% ready condition for the fly-off, so all the planes can leave the ship a few days before we land. The 3M inspection, a source of discontent from the year before, and one of the most arduous and time-consuming inspections a ship must endure, is going on. A handful of other picky inspections are interrupting everybody's work. (We didn't have time to be grateful that INSURV and OPPE, the only two worse inspections for non-nuclear carriers, weren't happening) We were using thousands of syringes we had to sterilize and store on board to give everybody skin tests and flu shots, for which everybody was standing in long lines -- that I hated. Now on top of all that, we have to put on the happy face and escort all these VIPs around.

Captain Pieno seemed to thrive on all this activity. His daily 1MC talks to the crew made all the hassles sound like opportunities, and in fact, the crew seemed to take it that way too. Every time I stepped into the passageway, there was a tour going past with some of Senator Chiles' staff or a reporter, or an inspector measuring and recording some gauge or quizzing some crew member. The hangar was busier than it had been for the past three months. Like Lilliputians buzzing over Gulliver's body, mechanics and technicians covered and protruded from every airplane and engine, getting them ready for the fly-off. Dozens of others from the Supply and Air Departments were shifting loads back and forth to get ready for the end of the cruise and somehow touching up paint and the deck surfaces. All this extra turmoil was penetrated by the passage of various visitor groups getting their tours (all greeted with smiles and welcoming grace), and lines of people over in the corners getting their shots. Ozark, the XO, came around patting people on the back, and the Captain got around a lot.

Sam MacDonald was recovering well from his operation, and he was up and around. We knew he would require further specialist evaluation because of his cancer when we arrived home, and there were a couple of other guys who would require specialist consultations back in Jax. So Rick and HM1 Rosenthal arranged for an ambulance to meet us when we would arrive in Mayport. The Captain and the Admiral faithfully came down to see all the sailors on the ward every day. On the busiest days they never forgot to do this. Besides his genuine concern for the sailor, the Captain still had a special discomfort with the specter of a cancer lurking on his ship.

On the day we finished off all the shots and TB tests, I was out in the port passageway supervising the storage of bags of syringes, when the Captain sprang out of the Ward. "Well! Look's like the Doctor is in today! Missed your naptime today, Doc? Seems like every time I come by here you're out." I enjoyed his repartee, but the corpsmen enjoyed it even more.

"Doc, got a minute? I'd like to talk to you about one of your patients." Rich Gilboy, the Admin Officer, was with him. We went into my office.

"How's MacDonald doing?"

"Very well, Sir. He's eating all right and doesn't have much pain."

"He's not in any danger now?"

"No, Sir."

The Captain asked about flying him off the day before we arrived, to get him to the hospital as quickly as we could. I discussed that with Rock, who was adamantly against a catapult shot. I had to agree with him, but his staunch inflexibility and angry arrogance were insidiously making me lean toward arguing the opposite position, even though I knew we shouldn't put Sam on the COD. Besides we were now only four days or so out. Each day that passed, there was less and less difference between flight time and just waiting until we arrived.

Four days before we arrived, since it was the fall, the annual Combined Federal Campaign was in season. Time for the Annual FID TV marathon. The Captain hosted the show late at night while people offered up various prized personal possessions or stunts in return for bids on lottery tickets for the CFC. Somebody offered up a Hank Aaron baseball, somebody else an autograph of Jay Silverheels. I offered to swab and wax the decks in the Medical Department in return for a $300 donation, which my guys raised within twenty minutes. It took me over three hours to work it off, but for the whole three hours I was cheered and jeered on by no fewer than fifteen corpsmen.

Knowing we were going to be bringing Sam all the way with us, the Skipper didn't want that to be the subject of press attention or of panic among other families. He said he wanted a tasteful but honest notification to be sent ahead to the ombudsmen, not for general release, but so they could answer any questions if they were assaulted on the subject. I immediately went to the XO, to see if he could talk the Captain out of this. The ombudsmen weren't involved in this in any way, I told him. Can't you talk the Captain out of this? No, the message had to go. I went to Rich Gilboy, the Admin Officer. No, he said, he saw my point but the Captain was definite about it, and Rich himself did agree that the situation might be kept better under control if in a public panic the ombudsmen could know enough to help us keep calm in the community. I still thought nobody outside either the command or Sam's family needed to know anything, but I went along with Rich and helped draft the message.

I don't know how the Captain thought we would send the message he wanted without the word cancer in it. But when the message was released, the Captain was angry the other way. "Doc, of all people, you should know that cancer worries people! Why would you send a message like that!?" Rich and Ozark and I just looked at each other in befuddlement. He was our Captain and we loved him, but we agreed he was not always easy to please.

The arrival was coming close. Three days out we were within range of the jets. All but one F14 were "up." All the planes were cleaned, and had paint and trim touched up.

We all crowded up to Vultures row, Pri-fly, and any places up on the roof where it was legal to stand while the squadrons launched their airplanes. Last to launch were the F14s, the "Tomcatters," and the "Red Rippers." After they launched they circled back around and gave us a fly-by. They are beautiful in flight. With their wings swept back, they look like they're alive. The Rippers had posted a guy in Pri-fly who announced over the 5MC, "And Now, approaching from the east, gentlemen, the World Famous Red Rippers, Bullet Richardson commanding. The Red Rippers wish to thank you for the Cruise. God Bless America." The announcement was timed perfectly to be punctuated by the low pass of the squadron in a loud and tight formation.

The deck was clear now. The helos would leave the next day, then there would be no airplanes left. The hangar bay, cavernous without any customers, echoed in stark unemployment. The flight deck was empty. I had been looking forward to the fly-off, but now that they were gone I wondered why.

************* ******* **************

The morning of October the fifth was bright and sunny, about sixty degrees, perfect for Florida. We hit the St. John's buoy right on time at a little after 0900. From the inlet, you could see the crowds on the pier and a bunch of them standing all the way out on the breakwater. I went down to stand with John Gundlach and a few other senior officers on Sponson One, where the forward brow would go. There was a band playing, and a bunch of TV cameras all around. We searched the crowd for our wives. The deployment had been a lot longer for them than it had for us. We knew that, but we were a lot happier to see them, we figured, than they were to see us.

I found Ann down in the crowd and got her attention. How would I be able to describe any of this to her? Whether I ever could or not, the ***Forrestal*** was home now.

CHAPTER VI. BAD NEWS

The bulkheads, decks, and colors may all seem just about the same, but it isn't at all the same ship once the "yard monkeys" come onboard. The wear and tear on a ship from a six month deployment is unequaled by almost any other industrial plant. Even commercial vessels which may operate just as often have only a few percent of the crew density that a warship does. Also, modern capital ships are constantly fine-tuned and upgraded to remain literally up-to-date in critical technology. During "SRA," which stands for Ship's Restricted Availability, an intermediate level of overhaul is done. Electronics, tactics, aviation, all of the modern science of warfare evolves just as rapidly as space travel in this electronic age. Five thousand people live, walk, run, and pout in that vessel for 6 months. The sheer pace and density of work takes a heavy toll. Periods of renovation and repair must be interspersed with operating times just to keep the ship functioning. A 30-year-old ship such as the FID had undergone the cycle many times. Every year the ship would need more service to stay on the line.

While Mayport is not itself a shipyard, there is a genuine shipyard over in Jacksonville just ten miles away, with a couple of contractors. When one of the ships in Mayport needs an SRA-level overhaul, the contractors have branches out in Mayport, and they service our ships at our own pier. This is especially true for the aircraft carriers, which are simply too large to fit into the shipyard at Jacksonville Landing on the St. John's River downtown.

Shipyard workers are a unique breed of people. Just being a welder, for example, doesn't qualify by itself for being a yard worker. There is a culture associated with doing your welding, iron work, piping, sheet metal work, and all the other crafts on a ship. In fact, a high percentage of the shipyard workers are former sailors, largely hull techs and bos'n's mates. They sure don't look like sailors, though. Perhaps I saw two or three with hair no longer than their ears, but most of them had hair down at least to the neck, a few in pigtails. Stubble -- not beards -- was definitely de rigueur. The clothing selection kept always consonant with hair style. If some of the garments had been newer or more expensive, they would have qualified for Early Hells Angels or the mode of the Baltimore homeless. It was a studied, and definitely purposeful, design. The work was incredibly dirty, a lot of fumes, and there was a closeness among the yard workers. I figured the style was something of a work uniform. Perhaps they chose as diametrically contrasting a uniform as they could in order to tell them easily apart from the ship's crew. It worked. Nobody had any difficulty telling the sailors from the shipyard workers.

That actually had some dollar value because the contractor wanted to be absolutely certain that no jobs covered in his contract should be done or shortened by Naval labor. Whenever a sailor would be seen using a hacksaw, moving a pipe, or chipping any paint, the foreman was in the office of the Maintenance Officer within a nanosecond to complain. This particular shipyard was a nonunion shop, so there was an interesting tension involved. The workers themselves had no complaints at all; they were always happy whenever a sailor would do some of the work or take over a task. No problem, I'll just sit here while you do it. It mattered to the foremen and company reps, though. They kept a close protective watch on what work could be done (and billed) by them, and what could be done by sailors.

By the first evening in port, all the festivities had cleared out, families had completed the tours, and only the duty crew was left on the ship. Already the shipyard workers started invading the space. They had their big ventilation pipes, compressed air hoses, ventilating fans, and heavy-duty electrical cables running everywhere. Most impressive were the ventilation hoses. These were 10 to 12-inch diameter compressible vinyl tubes that had to run down into any space where ordinary ventilation would be cut off, or grinding would be done. There are spaces on a ship called voids that are purposefully designed to be left empty always. Voids needed to be painted, checked for rust, and inspected just the same as any other space. However, having been designed as voids, they had no intrinsic ventilation, so that air needed to be piped in and circulated if a person was going to be in there.

Since the sides and bottoms of voids are made of steel just like the rest of the ship, they consume oxygen. Even though painting retards oxidation, paint can wear out or, furthermore, even under the paint, there is still iron, and over years it still loves to oxidize, otherwise known as rusting. In a closed space, the oxygen can come from only one place, the air in the room. Eventually, the oxygen gets leached out so when the void is entered, it is not a vacuum, because all the other gasses, the nitrogen, carbon dioxide, and so forth, are still there, but no oxygen. The worker cannot "feel" the absence of oxygen, but he only needs to stay in the compartment just a few minutes before losing consciousness, and eventually dying. If the situation is intensified by physical activity in the space, like welding, or other work, he and his equipment suck up the remaining oxygen even faster. That's why these big pipes travel everywhere through the ship circulating air. They enter the ship mostly through the hangar bay, travel down through virtually every ladder well, and pass along all the passageways. The big 10 and 12-inch air pipes usually were tied up along the overhead. A passageway barely high enough to permit a person to walk now became compromised if two or three of those pipes were tied up with brown twine along the overhead. Sometimes a fourth or a fifth would be lying along the deck, or tied up along the bulkhead to allow room for feet. Then there were five or six small compressed air hoses to blow away dust, to operate pneumatic tubes, or for sandblasting. Skeins of thick, high-power electrical cable were mixed in there, too. There wasn't a normal passageway left on the ship. All of these various cylinders and cables ran through every passageway and obstructed anyplace you wanted to walk.

Further complicating travel around the ship were the canvas or naugahyde barriers put up everywhere. To protect against flying chips of metal or welding torches, or to hide work that was classified, many spaces had to be blocked, barricaded from ordinary traffic. So, in addition to the passageways already compromised by the tubes and hoses, the fabric barricades even completely closed down some that remained. Getting from one point to another during the SRA required relearning your way around the ship.

The simple fallout from all this construction work added a lot of litter and clutter to the ship. However, the simple construction fallout was only a minor element compared to the personal fallout from the shipyard workers. They were not allowed to smoke on the ship, but cigarette butts lay every couple of feet throughout the deck. Also, tobacco juice streaks and polka dots were beginning to appear on the bulkheads and decks. The contract said that the workers would always come in and clean up behind themselves, but they did it only when forced. Not only were the shape and form of the ship changed by the shipyard workers, but a dirty industrial ugliness was trying to squeeze out the sparkling crispness I had enjoyed so much.

The day after our arrival, I was alone in the Medical Department. I had given Doug some leave, and sent Rock to work at the hospital as surgeons always did when the ship came back to port. Sick call was relatively light. Most guys had other things to do that morning than to pay attention to minor illness. Phone lines having been installed as one of the first things that happens when the ship comes back to port, I telephoned my friend Commander Art Hawley, who was the SMO on the USS Saratoga, up in major overhaul in the shipyard at Norfolk, Virginia. Art went to the Saratoga at the same time I came to the Forrestal, but they had been in the yard the entire time, and were destined to stay there for another 6 months. I told Art that I had a lot of sympathy for him, as I was just now beginning to understand what a ship was like in the yard. Since an SRA was **much** less intense than a complete overhaul, I knew I was only seeing a fraction of what was happening to the Sara. Having been on the ship only about 3 months, I knew that we SMO's all had a kind of bond, so Art was one of the first people I wanted to call. "Did you hear about the SMO on the Coral Sea?" Art asked.

No, of course, I had not. We had kind of been out of the country for a while.

Well, the SMO on the Coral Sea had been fired the week before. It turns out some medical waste from the Coral Sea, not very much either, just a few syringes, had washed up on the beaches of North Carolina. I remembered Captain Pieno's pointed warning about medical waste, and remembered that Admiral Kelso at CINCLANTFleet was real agitated about the subject.

"Was that all, Art? Surely he did something else. The doctor himself wasn't the guy to throw the syringes off, was he? C'mon, they didn't fire him just for that! What else was there?" "No, that was it. Syringes on the beach, SMO's out of work. End of story."

Looked like the SMO on ***Coral Sea*** was going to pay the price. About one out of three SMOs get relieved. Art and I hoped this would be the only one for a while. Oh, the poor guy. He should have paid attention like we did. Now his career was ruined.

"Well, Art, that could happen to any of us easily enough. We just did HIV's and PPD's on 5,000 guys, you know. We've got a ton of medical waste, most of it plastic, that we are offloading just today. I can tell you it really crowded our department." Art and I commiserated about that for a while on the phone, and while we did I formulated a plan to try to stay ahead of this problem and maybe impress Captain Pieno with my forward thinking. It was not very busy that day in the Medical Department. One fellow came by with a tiny foreign body in his left eye at around 10:00 in the morning, and another sailor had a burned left index finger from mess duty, but otherwise it was pretty quiet.

I took advantage of the time to concentrate on the problems of waste coming out of the department, especially plastic, which was the major part of our trash. I knew that CINCLANTFleet and AIRLANT were both working on directives about medical waste, and we would have to respond to their guidance. For the present, however, just plan common sense may not be sufficient. Sometimes you just need to paint lamb's blood on your door to show you understand. We were going to take an aggressive direction not just to handle this right, but to let it show that the FID had the message.

There were really two problems with plastic. First of all, it can float forever. Secondly, it lasts forever. Most other soft trash would gradually disintegrate in the ocean or be eaten by fish. Metal would sink to the bottom and either be buried in the silt or eventually oxidize and dissolve. Plastic would float forever and last forever. It would be around to pollute the oceans for eons, but especially it could wash up on the beach like it did in North Carolina. The citizens, of course, had a right to be outraged. To me, though, that particular afternoon, the worst thing about medical waste on the beach was that SMOs could be fired.

I imagined for a moment what if I were in the shoes of the SMO from the Coral Sea? I did not have enough years of Naval service to get a pension if I got kicked out. Having left private practice, I really did not want to have to come back to a community and say, "I just got kicked out of the Navy. Can I open my office again?" My family would be dishonored. Maybe they could adjust to that, I don't know. But the being broke part... I knew that would be unpopular with my daughters.

As ugly as plastic or medical trash might look on the beach, it isn't really an infectious threat. Needles are ugly, of course, and people can be stuck or cut by them. Kids or bad guys might try to use beach needles for injections I guess. Mostly they get too sandy or dirty even for that though. The public outcry about medical hazards in the summer of 1988, obviously was about AIDS. Medically that was not a realistic concern. The HIV virus is very fragile despite its public image. As infectious agents go, the HIV is actually not very hardy. The infections that are transmitted by sex are the ones from mostly fragile agents that can only survive in moist, warm, and **living** environments. Sex organs, for example. If they are out on a counter top, or in sunlight, they perish. They can be passed from one person to another by means of exclusively moist warm "indoor" routes, like sex.

Ocean salt water is simply not a fertile place for germs. Neither the treponeme of syphilis, the cocci of gonorrhea, nor the HIV could survive in a syringe that floated in the ocean and then washed up on a beach. The problem was not biology. It was public anxiety and outrage. Irresponsible disposal of trash, pollution of public resources, and just the sheer ugliness of plastic medical stuff washing up on a public beach, all these were good reasons for public anger, sure enough. They shouldn't happen. Period. Still, what the public was mostly worked up about was AIDS, and that part was not a real issue.

Well, I knew this was important, and I was making a detailed plan to keep the FID out of trouble. We would account for every single syringe, from the day it came onboard the ship, until it was safely delivered to a responsible designated trash hauler. I refined our methods for storing plastics on the ship while we were underway. We would separate just plain plastic trash from plastic trash with any biological contact, like saliva, stomach fluid, stool, or pus. There would be provisions for sealing and double-bagging certain material. Anything that had biological fluids would be autoclaved after being bagged the first time and then would be bagged again so that sterilization was already guaranteed before we had to store it.

Of course, we had been doing most of these things already ever since that CINCLANTFleet message came out on 29 August. All of these schemes that I was working on this particular day were simply refinements of guidance given before, plus some new initiatives to make sure we stayed "ahead of the parade." I was partly just dressing up the bureaucratic trace. I drew nice flow diagrams, designed a series of log books that we would use for the sharp object disposal canisters. We would handle and sign for disposed syringes and such trash just like it was gold or documents. In the future, not only would I be able to show that we had a good process for all of our syringes and plastics and medical waste, but I would also have a set of log books that could trace every piece of plastic or sharp object from when it came to our department until when it left.

I was smugly satisfied with all of the plans and SOP's I had just devised and had neatly typed up. Next I designed a training program for the whole Medical Department. No university ever had a more clever curriculum for literature or science than the one I designed for our trash! Thorough and yet clear; sailor-proof, I told myself. And interwoven with such humor and cleverness in language that it even made me chuckle as I wrote it. We would make training mandatory but we would make it fun. Finally, I typed out a clever memo that was to be distributed and initialed by all members of the Medical Department. Keeping up what by now I thought was a rollicking background humor for emphasis, my memo unabashedly noted the recent firing of the SMO from the Coral Sea and warned that we did not want something like that to happen to the beloved SMO from the Forrestal, did we? I chuckled to myself as I read it. I thought the guys in the Department would kind of like the memo. It was one more example of the FID Medical Department being out in front. This had to be the most comprehensive plan ever for dealing with trash. After all, we were the Atlantic Fleet carrier that had been underway when the new instruction came out. We were the ones who had gone through the exercise of giving PPD's to 5,300 people, HIV drawings on that large number, flu shots to everybody on the crew, had maintained all of those plastic products on the ship. Yet we had carefully avoided throwing anything improperly overboard. We were the ones with firsthand experience, and successful at that.

Of course, if we implemented my new plan about doing shots and lab tests on a continuous weekly basis instead of just doing these mammoth catch-up exercises, there wouldn't have to be big amounts of plastic medical trash again. I never wanted to do it in that kind of mass again. Nonetheless, we were the first ones who had tackled this problem, and in keeping with our progressive and intelligent perspective, we were first on the block with a comprehensive plan -- staying ahead of the problem. Smug in victory, I chuckled again at the clever wording of the memo I had prepared for my guys, and at the irony that trash should get so much attention from a doctor.

I was interrupted from my amusement when Petty Officer Davis told me, "Captain, Commander Johnson is on the phone for you, and he says it's pretty important."

"Commander Johnson, who is Commander Johnson?" Davis didn't know.

It was "Grog" Johnson, the new Deputy CAG. He had replaced Commander Terry Hightower toward the end of the cruise, and I was just getting to know him. Since he was a member of the Air Wing and not ship's company, "Commander Johnson" wasn't a name I recognized quickly. Still, he and I had hit it off well, and I could tell I was going to like him. I didn't know why he called me at 2000 on a Tuesday night, but I figured that it might be to invite me to dinner or something.

"Did you hear about the syringes on the beach at Fernandina Beach?" What a coincidence. I had just spent the whole day on the subject of syringes on the beach.

"Where is Fernandina Beach?" I thought it must be something more about the ***Coral Sea***. That poor SMO. There was a foreboding itch in the back of my mind about this discussion already, though.

"Fernandina Beach. It's just 10 miles north of Mayport." This was my first week on the ship back in Mayport. Since I had only joined them in the North Arabian Sea, I wasn't yet familiar with the Jacksonville and Mayport area. "The news says that the syringes came from the ***Forrestal***."

"Don't worry, we didn't throw anything overboard, and we had real careful precautions to prevent it."

"Well, you'd better check into it, because the FID is being mentioned. I heard that CINCLANT was interested in this, and I think they had some trouble about it on the Coral Sea."

Trouble on the ***Coral Sea,*** indeed. The SMO got fired! "Thanks for calling, Grog, I'll look into it." I immediately went over to the Emergency Ward. We have a television in there up on a cabinet back in a kind of hole in the bulkhead out of the way. The Emergency Ward is one of a handful of places on the ship where CCTV always covers flight operations underway. If there were an accident on the flight deck, obviously we would need to know about it, so we keep a television for video monitoring of flight operations. In port, it might be different. If the television would be running all the time, the corpsmen on duty might spend more time watching TV than doing their work, so I had contemplated putting out some rules about when the TV could be on, and when it could not. For the moment, though, I was glad it was there. "Have you guys seen anything on the news?" Petty Officer Fields and Petty Officer Womple were watching MTV.

"No, but somebody said they heard something on the radio about syringes on the beaches."

This day had promises of turning bad.

I immediately went down to the XO's office. It was evening, and he was gone. I called the Command Duty Officer, the CDO, who acted as the CO's representative when the CO and XO were off the ship, to tell him what I had heard. He said he had heard some rumors along the same lines. Rumors are only rumors, but the more of them you begin to hear, you either suspect they may be true, or at least you recognize they can be repeated enough to become self-sustaining, like crabgrass. In any case, I was beginning to get worried. The CDO then told me that both the Captain and the XO were out of town for a few days. The Captain had gone to an annual convention of Naval Aviators called the Tail Hook Association. Ozark, the XO, was on leave visiting family in Arkansas. Captain Tuck, the CHENG, was the acting CO.

I went back to my office and called Rick Combs at his house. He, too, had heard some of the rumors. I asked him to stay on top of the news and to come in early the next morning. Then I called the CHENG at home. He had not heard about the rumors, so I told him that I had heard them from several sources.

"Doc, I thought you told me that we didn't throw anything overboard."

"Well, we didn't. There's no way those could be ***Forrestal*** syringes. We made damned sure that all of the corpsmen knew what we were supposed to do with the plastics and the syringes. There has got to be a mistake here. But I assure you we're looking into it."

"I'll be in early in the morning, Doc. We'd better try and stay on top of this."

The next morning at Quarters, Rick and I got all the corpsmen together, and I told them about the rumors I had heard about syringes washing up on Fernandina Beach. I asked if any of the corpsmen had heard any of the rumors and they had not. "How many of you guys remember when we talked to you about disposing of medical waste and plastics at sea back in September?" About half our corpsmen were on leave at this point, and some had duty the night before, so a few were not present. Of the 15 or so who were there now, only five or six raised their hands. "But I stood right here in front of you guys in September and mentioned this to you. Petty Officer Womple, don't you remember my mentioning this?"

"No, Captain, I really don't. Petty Officer Dunwoody did tell us that we had to be careful about plastics, though. I don't think we threw anything over the side after something like the first of September."

Two or three others remembered that I had come to talk to the corpsmen at Quarters, a few more than that remembered that Lieutenant Combs had discussed it with them. More than half of the guys assembled there realized that we had been stacking up bag after bag of medical waste back in a couple of our heads, but to my amazement four or five of the guys didn't even know that we had changed anything about trash disposal! Happily, none of those four or five guys had been involved in trash details over the last part of the cruise.

It was one of those lessons in communication. When only half of my department was still present, and even among them there were four or five who had no idea that we had a change in policy about throwing plastic trash over the side, that meant that if the <u>entire</u> department could be there, as many as ten wouldn't know about it. This, despite my coming to lecture the guys during Quarters, passing it on to all the petty officers, and the conspicuous stacking up of plastic and trash in two of our heads where guys couldn't use toilets any more! I was beginning to get uncomfortable again.

"Did anybody here throw any syringes or plastic over the side after the first of September, when we said not to do it anymore?"

Absolutely not.

"No."

"Nobody on the ship could have done it?."

"Well, it could have been some of the Air Wing corpsmen who aren't here anymore. Some of those guys seemed not to listen to instructions."

"Wait a minute. I felt we made it perfectly clear that the Air Wing corpsmen were integral members of this Department when we are underway. Lieutenant Combs and I talked to you at Quarters, too. We were all supposed to be one department. What do you mean 'Some of those guys'?"

Stifled expressions, shuffling feet. Another one of those gaps in communication. I thought we had solved the Air Wing/ship's company gap in the Medical Department. Maybe we had not.

I asked Rick to call over to talk to Bill Flynn over at Cecil Field, where some of the of the squadrons were. I called Grog Johnson to fill him in, and asked if he and Flynn would try to check with the corpsmen from the Air Wing. Grog had not heard anymore since the night before. We scoured the newspapers, and there were no comments.

I went down to see the CHENG, but since he was the Acting CO, he was hanging out up in the Captain's office on the O-3 deck. When I finally tracked him down, he was busy with all the other ship's activities. "Good morning, Doc, I hope your day started better than it ended last night." He was in a chipper mood and had no further bad information. I told him about my disturbing information at Quarters. Despite what I had thought was clear information to all the corpsmen, I was disappointed to find out some of them had not got the message.

"Welcome to the Navy, Doc. No message is sailor proof. You never tell them anything just four times, when you can tell them six or seven, and tell it in six or seven different ways, too."

Besides, it looked as though it might have been a false alarm. There was no substantiation about the reports that morning. We had been back in port 3 days, so if anything was going to come of it, we would have heard it by now. None of the guys in the Department had thrown any medical stuff over the side. Besides, I had seen all the plastics and all the trash being stored in the PMT room and in the head on Ward 2, so that I had firsthand knowledge that we had not thrown anything overboard, and we had a pretty good system in place. There were the nagging concerns that some guys seemed not to have got the message, and I did realize that we need to work on documentation of disposal, something I had only thought about yesterday, not while we were at sea. The attention to those new procedures was obviously necessary. We clearly needed to do some training so this would not come up again in the future.

MEET BILLY

Back in the Medical Department, there was a guy just checked in who had been beat up the night before. His name was Billy Dorsey, and he looked about 14 years old. A short fellow, around 5'6" tall, he had what would have been a cherubic face, if it had not been all pummeled, cut, and spattered with crusted blood. One front tooth had a diagonal chunk taken out, and his right eye was nearly closed. The left ear had a cut halfway down from the top. He had that characteristic melange of stale fruit and vinegar that is characteristic of last night's drunk. For some reason, only either cheap whiskey or cheap wine leaves just that exact smell. Beer can come close, but isn't quite sweet enough. And particularly among people who have been vomiting and haven't rinsed out their mouths or had anything to eat, the combined smell is not only characteristic, it's just downright repulsive. The smell is so bad you're inclined to feel sorry for anybody else who had to be in it with you, even the guy it came from, so I already had sympathy for poor Billy Dorsey because he had to put up with that smell, and longer than me. Dorsey didn't have much to say. He was obviously very tired, and looked like he still might be a little bit drunk.

Apparently, he and his buddies had been to some of the local bars last night. They started at "Big Jim's," and then they went over to "Cap'n Odie's." They told me that Dorsey started being belligerent with a couple of sailors from another ship, and had taken a punch at one guy who made quick work of him, but only left him with a black eye, apparently. According to his buddies, Dorsey just kept drinking although they told him he needed to get back to the ship, and he would fight with one guy after another. Not only is he little, but apparently Billy was not a very accomplished pugilist in those days, either. Finally, his buddies couldn't stand it anymore, but they couldn't get him back to the ship either, so they just came on back. Somehow me must have caught a cab and made it back himself.

Looking at him, you would never figure how anybody could want to punch such a cute little guy. An angelic looking creature, about the size of a leprechaun, he had a way of tilting his head to one side, and slanting his shoulders a little bit the opposite direction that called to mind either the Pillsbury Dough Boy or Winnie the Pooh. If he didn't smell so bad, I would have wanted to take him on my knee and ask him, "What would you like for Christmas, little boy." But he just smelled so bad.

After we looked him over, none of the cuts looked as though they needed sutures, and besides it was too long since his fights. We usually did not like to close cuts with sutures after several hours. After a few hours being exposed closing them up with sutures left too much risk of infection. I arranged for him to go over and be seen in Dental that morning because of the broken tooth and to see if there were any others broken. I phoned his DivO as we usually did for these young fellows who got too tanked up the night before. Alcohol was a major concern for us. Considering we had 5000 young guys, most of them away from home for the first time, we really didn't have as much trouble with alcohol as most groups of men that age. However, any were too many. We took those we had seriously. These young fellows needed some supervision and guidance. Besides talking to his DivO about his drinking and his injuries, Petty Officer Cedric Palmore called his LPO, to make sure that he had some senior enlisted supervision. Finally, whenever there was an "alcohol related incident," we made a referral to the CAAC, the Command Alcohol Abuse Counselor. Even a single isolated event related to alcohol had to be referred to the Counselor. It still is my opinion that even a single drunk incident means a problem with alcohol. The individual does not have to be an obvious drunk already. Even a single incident that leads to a driving accident or injury shows that the person has failed to control alcohol and could get worse in the future. Often what appears to be an isolated event is just really a sentinel, a herald. The first act of a new habit. The command owes it to him to begin tracking it, get him directed to treatment if necessary, and mobilize the resources that the Navy has. We have a long way to go on this problem, but at most commands we take it seriously, and we did on the Forrestal.

I tried to get Dorsey to talk with me about what happened to him, but I just did not seem to be able to engage him in any conversation. I tried to get him to talk to me about his drinking habits, what he had done the night before, whether he wanted to talk anything over. He just shrugged at me in a very engaging manner but did not want to talk.

That afternoon I went over to meet with the Officer In Charge of the clinic at Mayport. The clinic was supposed to back us up medically, and since we were in business just a few hundred yards apart, I wanted to make sure that we had met each other and taken every opportunity to work together. The clinic was a branch from NHJax, the Naval Hospital Jacksonville, which was more than an hour away. Mayport is about 20 miles east of the City of Jacksonville, and the Naval Air Station Jacksonville was about 10 to 12 miles southwest of the City of Jacksonville. Jacksonville traffic is almost as bad as it is in Boston, so it was approximately an hour drive between Mayport and the Navy Hospital, longer than that at rush hour. The branch clinic was not open after 1800 at night, and did not have a staffed emergency room. They did have a night watch, however, for "emergencies." I thought this was a little bit incongruous. Since all emergencies had to be sent elsewhere what was the staff for?. A bona fide emergency such as a heart attack would not be sent the one-hour drive all the way to NHJax, but over to the Beaches Hospital in Atlantic Beach, a place with marginal local reputation. Somebody with chest pain who seemed stable enough to last would be sent to either Mercy or Baptist Hospital. Those two were a little further than Beaches, but at least 20 to 40 minutes closer than the Navy Hospital. The **unstable** ones who couldn't travel would stay at Beaches. Too bad, maybe, because that might be the **worst** place for somebody who was very sick. Nonemergency, but hospital-requiring problems would be sent by ambulance to the Navy Hospital. With all this, although there were four ambulances parked outside the clinic, none of them were licensed as ACLS, "Advanced Cardiac Life Support" ambulances.

"You know you and your doctors have to stand watch over here at the clinic, don't you?"

"Well," I said, "with the Air Wing gone, our flight surgeons go back to the Naval Air Stations that the squadrons come from, and our surgeon has gone back to the hospital, so that the only medical officers left on the ship are myself, Lieutenant Doug Kempf, and CW03 Art Forbes. We stand the watch on the ship 24 hours a day, and we see patients 24 hours a day, which is more than the clinic." Also, it looked as though the clinic had six or seven doctors on their staff, so that they had a six or seven-section watch, whereas we had only a three-section watch on the ship. I told him I thought we would choose not to be in their watch rotation. "Well, there's a SOPA instruction that says you will," the OIC said.

"If you want, I can ask Captain Pieno or Admiral Smith to call SOPA to work it out." Since we planned to see all the ***Forrestal*** people right on the ship, though, it seemed best for the clinic to drop the subject. In the past, some of the carriers had closed down their Medical Departments at the end of the work day while they were port, so it made sense for their physicians to join in over at the clinic. I intended for the FID to keep up its medical services around the clock right on the ship. We did have better capability on the ship than the clinic did. We were our own hospital, a self-contained Medical Department for 6 months out of the year, so there was no reason in my mind that we should close it down when we were in port. The OIC liked that approach, although he told me that his doctors probably would not. I suggested they should all come on over and get a tour of the ship. It turns out none of his doctors had ever been to sea, although their clinic was in a home port that took care of about 15 ships, including two carriers, the FID and the Saratoga.

I had come over to visit the OIC at about 1440 that afternoon. He and I finished speaking somewhere around 1530, and he gave me a tour of the clinic. I asked if I could meet some of his doctors, but none of them were in the building. "They secure a little early, if there's nothing going on." Well, there it was about 1530, and none of the doctors were in the clinic.

I went back to the ship that day without as much comfort as I would have liked about our relationship with the clinic.

Formal dining in port was a real pleasure, but different than underway. For one thing, there were far fewer people who came to dinner. Not many officers or CPOs kept living on the ship in port. You could live on the ship without paying rent, of course. Some of us older people with families in other cities stayed on the ship, rather than pay for an apartment in town while supporting a household elsewhere. Single, young enlisted guys had better things to do with the small amount they earned as sailors than to pay for apartments, but almost everybody else lived in town. So the only people who came to formal dining were the duty crew and the handful of us who lived on the ship. That meant only about 15 officers in the Ward Room. At least one officer would have his family visit for dinner most nights on the ship.

The President of the Mess was, of course, the XO. In his absence, the senior officer present would usually preside at the formal dining. Being a Captain, I was always the senior officer. Yet, as a Staff Officer, I could never really be in charge of the ship. Since the CDO was the Captain's representative in the absence of the Skipper and XO, he would usually preside at dinner and sit in the XO's chair. In fact, with rare exceptions, at formal dining in port the head table usually seated everybody. We usually ate by candle light, although by the time the meal was over the lights would come on for coffee.

On this third night back in port, Mel Swartz, the OHO, Ordinance Handling Officer, was the CDO. Mel was an LDO, a Limited Duty Officer, the official term for what had been called a "Mustang" in the old days. Reported to be the most knowledgeable man in the fleet about aviation ordinance, Mel was responsible for all the magazines, inventory of any weapons on the ship, keeping all the weapons and their fusing in good condition, and overseeing the management of the day-by-day activities of the Weapons Department. He was basically the primary assistant to the Gun Boss. It was rumored that the OHO and the Gun Boss were not close.

He was a loud, outspoken fellow with a raspy voice and a ready laugh. A gregarious man with a bountiful inventory of anecdotes and jokes, his vocality and expressiveness put some people off. Nobody was indifferent about Mel Swartz. He also had a tendency to be a little bit of a needler, but he was willing to take a good joke, as well as dish one out.

Mel had an interesting characteristic. Many of us discover when we passed 40 that hair started growing on our ears, or eyebrows get bushy. Every couple of days the hair on the ears has to be cut off or embarrassing tufts start to grow out on earlobes or the tops. The OHO was similar but different. Mel was the only guy I knew who had such a tuft of hair growing out on the tip of his nose. He wasn't only different by having hair on his nose, but somehow by not noticing it either. He quite conspicuously did not shave it off. I figured he had to see himself in a mirror most days when he would shave. He did shave his cheeks and his chin, I know, because he never had any unsightly stubble on those parts. Yet the hair on his nose seemed to grow out close to an inch long. It was hard to look at Mel without looking at the tuft of hair on his nose. He didn't give any sign that he saw you looking at it, and never made any comments like, "I see you're looking at my nose. Does the hair bother you?" To the contrary, almost everybody who would talk to Mel just simply had to see that hair and had to be curious, as I was, about why he didn't cut it off.

It wasn't just a single hair like the hair that might grow out of the middle of a wart, it was a rich, full little tuffet. I had a little fantasy sometimes that maybe he was planning to braid it, or that he would comb it to one side when he got particularly dressed up. In fact, the OHO was one of the few people I knew who still wore hair tonic. He had dark hair, and when he combed it swept back somewhat, he used the exact style of Robert MacNamara, the old Secretary of Defense, or the characters from F. Scott Fitzgerald novels. Sometimes I wondered if he was hoping the hair on his nose would get long enough so that he could put pomade in it.

Everybody enjoyed formal dining when Mel was the CDO. Not everybody got a chance to speak because he rambled on so, but that didn't matter because Mel had good stories and good jokes, and we all secretly enjoyed looking at the hair on his nose and wondering about it. Interesting, though, nobody ever seemed to talk about it. I think we probably all wanted to, and we all knew that if we said anything to Mel about his nose hair, he wouldn't mind, we just never did. Maybe we thought it was bad manners. A lot of people seem to have hair that grows out from the inside of their nose, which was something you definitely would not talk about, but this was right out there on the tip.

Leaving the Ward Room that evening I ran into Master Chief Morgan, one of the most senior Chiefs in the Supply Department, the guy who had helped us get our tables set up on the mess decks for the shot-ex. He was always a kind of crusty fellow, but he seemed especially brusk tonight. When he returned my greeting, I thought his speech seemed a little slurred, something I had noticed a couple of times in the past few weeks. I reminded myself to speak with the SuppO about it. Master Chief Morgan might have a little drinking problem.

I went to bed that night generally content. I was adjusting to life in port, the routine was working out well, and other than all the pipes and disruption on the ship from the SRA, and all the noise, dust, and racket from the shipyard workers, things were going well. Admittedly I had been jarred about the needle and syringe rumors, but they seemed to have died out by now.

Next morning during sick call, the lines were a little longer than they had been the prior few days. More people were returning from short leave or liberty periods, and one of their first stops was back in sick call. It was getting to be winter, so we had a string of colds, and minor illnesses. Some of the guys had sprained their ankles or had other athletic injuries from their short times at home. Athletic injuries would start to be a bigger part of what we saw in sick call now that we were in port and guys could play basketball, softball, or other sports everyday now. Also, the automobile was back in our lives. Sore necks and facial injuries from automobile accidents were beginning to take some of our attention. When I finished in sick call that morning, there was a note on my desk to go see the Acting CO up in his office.

"Doc, we got a call from the PAO [Public Affairs Officer] over at NAS-Jax. They've started to have some syringes wash up on the beach down at Daytona. There was some stuff mixed in with the syringes that had the Forrestal name on it."

"But this is 5 days after we got into port. Besides, we didn't throw anything overboard."

"Here is the guy's number. Can you give him a call? He seems pretty sure that the name of the ship was on some of the stuff."

The PAO from Jax was not very cordial. "You guys are in some kind of trouble, and it's really causing us a problem here. You better go on down to Daytona and get a crew to clean up their beaches."

"Now wait a minute. We haven't even determined for sure that Forrestal was involved with this in the first place, and in the second place, I'm the Senior Medical Officer, not the trash detail."

"Instead of arguin' with me about this, you better get on down to Daytona and see what they're talking about. Whether you stay the Senior Medical Officer on that ship, or anyplace else in the Navy, might be an open question pretty soon."

I just hung up on him. I didn't like the direction that conversation was going. He had given me the phone number of the Beach Patrol in Daytona Beach, so I asked Petty Officer Cedric Palmore if he would give me a ride down there. It was a couple of hours' drive, and when we got to the Office of the Beach Patrol, sure enough, they had a red plastic bag just like the ones we used on the FID that had washed up on the beach. Inside the bags were some papers that clearly had the Forrestal name, and a handful of syringes. Fortunately, all the needles had been clipped off, but there it was, living proof of syringes and a plastic bag, with the name of the ship right on the bag. Oh, my God. The Beach Patrol Officer was a little bit sympathetic, but insistent. "There have been a bunch of syringes washing up on the beach, too. Every hundred or feet or so, we find a syringe or two washed up along here." I stayed and spoke to him for about another 20 or 30 minutes while we worked out a plan for me to get a bunch of FID sailors to walk the beaches and pick up any refuse we could find. My head was reeling. How could this happen? We had been so careful not to throw anything over the side. But there was the evidence, right in my hand.

HM3 Palmore and I drove back to the ship as fast as we could. I went up to the see the CHENG to tell him what we had found, and make sure we started dealing with it immediately. We had to get down there and pick up any possible scrap from the Forrestal, or any plastic that could in any way be attributed to the Forrestal, but most especially medical waste. While we spent the drive, Petty Officer Palmore and I, talking about how we would get the teams together, and get volunteers to deal with the pickup, spicules of fear about my own career poked into my mind periodically interrupting my train of thought. The Navy had just fired the SMO from the Coral Sea. He had not been kicked out of the Navy, apparently, but he had been transferred to some meaningless assignment in a small clinic somewhere at the end of the earth. At my Court Martial, I could just see the Judge or the Admiral saying, "And Captain Riley, your crime was all the worse because you had been warned by the Coral Sea."

Back at the ship, I immediately went to see Chuck Tuck, still Acting CO. Before I could give him my report, he showed me the morning newspaper. There it was right on page 3, reports of medical waste washing up over along a 12-mile stretch from Daytona Beach northward.

At Quarters that morning, we put out word all throughout the ship about the problem that had happened and called for volunteers. Chuck rented a bus for the next 3 days to take all the volunteers who would come with us down to the beaches to pick up syringes or any other medical waste. Only two volunteers from outside the Medical Department came. When we called the squadrons at Cecil Field and NAS-Jax, none of the corpsmen volunteered to come with us. More than a dozen of the corpsmen from the ship were willing to come. We spent most of the next 3 days walking up and down about 15 miles of beach looking for anything that could be from any Naval ship, and anything medical. Over that 3-day period, we picked up probably a thousand syringes, and five or six prescription bottles, two of them marked "***USS Forrestal***." Two other prescription bottles, however, were clearly marked "***USS America***." My heart leapt up. Could some of the syringes be from the ***America***? She has just been operating off the Florida Coast during workups.

A couple of the guys who helped us the most during this pickup were HM1 Dunwoody and HM1 Hugh Beaumont, our new orthopedic repairman. Beaumont, like Dunwoody, was older than most of the corpsmen. He was in his late 30's, a very intelligent guy, with a pleasant personality. He either was a college graduate, or had several years of college, and like myself was a Beach Boys fan. He had grown up in the Daytona area, and was very familiar with this neighborhood. He obviously felt bad about the syringes, and along with Dunwoody was one of the few corpsmen to realize that I was going to be fired because of this. That troubled him, and he tried to cheer me up the entire time. He made jokes, bantered with me about rock 'n roll trivia, and generally tried to make this into a fun exercise. After all, it was an opportunity for guys from the Department to get together and spend a little time on the beach. If it had been under other circumstances, we maybe even would have enjoyed it.

When we got back to the ship at the end of the third day, Captain Pieno was there, back from the Tail Hook Convention.

I learned that the Inspector General from AIRLANT had been making some calls down to our area. Oh, no, AIRLANT knew about it! Well, I learned, that was not the end of it. Not just AIRLANT, but also CINCLANTFleet and even the IG for the Department of the Navy up in Washington had heard about this.

I remembered what Myron Almond had told me about Captain Pieno being a screamer, and I remembered how angry the Captain had been with me about the Sam Macdonald case a month ago. I immediately went up to give him a full report. Might as well face the tempest head-on. To my surprise, he not only didn't yell at me, but his face wasn't even red. He asked me a few questions. He said, "You told me that you had this situation under control. Remember, you and I spoke about this back in August."

"Yes, Sir. Remember, I told you that we were saving all the medical material in the Department, and nothing was being thrown overboard. I can't explain how this happened, Sir. I thought we had it under control."

"Sometimes things happen just beyond your control, Doc." The Captain pointed out that with this level of public and Navy attention, we had to do an investigation to try to account for it. What he didn't say, and I knew, was that somebody was going to be punished, the Navy always had to have retribution. For one thing, the public insisted on it. But it was an old Navy tradition. This was very definitely in the Medical Department, so we all knew who would have to be held responsible. The SMO.

There are two books that govern investigations and justice in the Navy. One is the Judge Advocate General Manual, or "JAGMAN." The JAG Manual describes how investigations shall be done, sets standards for evidence, interviews, and documentation. Following an official JAGMAN investigation, the findings may lead to such proceedings as a Board of Inquiry, Captain's Mast, or finally Court Martial. The other important book is the Manual of Courts Martial. It seemed to me that we were going to wind up using both of those manuals before this was over.

The JAGMAN investigation was convened. The investigating officer was given the CINCLANT Fleet message of 29 August, with the explicit directions about handling medical waste and plastics at sea. I submitted a written report, not only accepting responsibility for the Medical Department, but clearly stating that Captain Pieno had instructed me on his concern about medical waste and plastics. If there needed to be such a thing as a noose for me, it was that the Captain had gone out of his way to warn me about medical waste. He had even told me that it was one of his priorities. It was a John Dean quality Smoking Gun. The investigating officer spoke to Rick Combs. After Doug Kempf returned from his leave, he was interviewed. Every corpsman on the ship was interviewed, some of them were called back from their leave early.

While the JAGMAN investigation was in its third day, the IG from AIRLANT, along with John Perreault, the Environmental Health Officer we met back in Chapter VI and considered a sourpuss already, flew down to Mayport to do an independent investigation. Although we had been out to all the beaches, scoured them and cleaned up the beaches for every piece of trash we could find (including non Naval trash such as plastic milk cartons), people who lived down there had found more. When the IG and LCDR Perreault came back from Daytona, they carried with them two boxes with some other syringes, and a bunch of other plastic trash, most of which was not even Navy. Since the FID was on the hook, though, nobody thought we should argue with the people who lived there. Any medical stuff found for months would be blamed on us, no matter what.

During one of their visits, John and the IG were accosted by news crews from two local televisions stations, and a protest group from one of the towns. John told me he suspected that the community group had been alerted by the news camera crews. When a camera was stuck in front of their faces, a reporter said, "When is the Navy finally going to take some action on this custom of polluting public beaches?" In the background, protestors were carrying signs about Navy pollution and the Navy being a poor neighbor. When the sound bite was played on local television that night, the two Naval officers were obviously caught off-guard, and could only say things like, "The investigation is still ongoing." But the chanting and bobbing signs of the protestors showed up well and looked like a multitude on a TV screen.

One editorial in the main Jacksonville newspaper the next morning argued that the Navy should be a more responsible neighbor. It mentioned the risk of AIDS and other terrible diseases that could be spread by medical waste on the beaches to injure harmless children. The paper said it hoped the Navy would not just have another coverup.

Two days later, I was called up to the Captain's cabin, to go over the findings of the investigations. Lieutenant Commander Mike Kunin was the Investigating Officer.

Here were the facts: By the rules that had applied up until the 29th of August, trash, including medical trash, could be thrown over the side as long as the ship was 50 miles or more offshore. Because of the place our plastic had washed up, the trash had to have been thrown out 3 days before we landed, hitting the current in just such a way that it would have washed to where it did. Had it been thrown out in the last couple of days, the trash would have gone to an entirely different area. So by the **former** rules, although what had happened was bad, it would not have been illegal. The investigating officers found that the Senior Medical Officer and the Division Officer, Lieutenant Combs, had set up proper procedures for handling the medical waste, and we had notified our department not to throw medical waste or plastic over the side any longer. Yet it appeared some corpsmen did not understand. Although the investigating officers were convinced that everyone in the Department *had been told*, they just somehow didn't fully understand or didn't remember. Therefore, it was the fault of leadership in the Department, failing to guarantee that everyone understood.

Despite that failure the investigation found that there was only a single incident of a corpsman from one of the squadrons who threw a single bag containing syringes and some other plastic medical containers over the side 3 days before we came into port. The individual had to be one of three corpsmen from the AirWing, but it was impossible to determine for certain who that might have been. Judging from the amount of refuse picked up on the beach, one single bag probably accounted for all that was found. When a single bag full of syringes came apart more than 100 miles offshore it scattered the little floating devils like seeds from a dandelion.

So there it was: the syringes and plastic were from the ***Forrestal***. CINCLANTFleet was furious about the matter, and the public was clearly outraged. The Commanding Officer of the ship had been mindful of the potential for medical waste being thrown over the side, and he had specifically directed the head of the Medical Department to insure such a thing could never happen. While the SMO and his principal assistant had taken steps to follow up on the Captain's guidance, a failure of leadership allowed a handful of corpsmen to not get the entire message, and on one occasion a bag of medical waste was thrown over the side in violation of directives. Since there were a handful of the corpsmen had not understood the directions, the corpsman, whoever he was, who threw the bag overboard could not be the one who was blamed. Of course, the officer responsible could and should be blamed, namely me.

Too many things had come together at the wrong time. The time of the year for flu shots, the end of the cruise, a new SMO who wanted to catch up on preventive medicine: all of this at the worst time there **had ever been** to have medical stuff wash up on a beach. Just after CINFLANTFleet announced this as incongruously one of the Navy's highest priorities, Forrestal got into the production of medical waste bigger than ever, raising the opportunity for this kind of misfortune and giving us a real good load of stuff to put into the hopper. Uncanny timing.

I didn't like the part where they included Rick Combs in the leadership problem. He worked for me, and I worried that he would get tarnished by the incident. He was only carrying out my directions at any point. Since I knew I was about to be fired, anyway, I told Captain Pieno the responsibility was mine, not Rick's and I apologized to the him for the embarrassment to the Forrestal, and to the IG for embarrassing the Navy.

The Captain said, "Thank you for a thorough investigation, Mike. You couldn't have reached any other conclusions. I will make a full report about this to CINCLANT Fleet and to Admiral Smith. Doc, I think your new instruction on this matter would prevent this from happening anymore. There isn't anything else you can do now. The Navy just has to stop throwing plastics over the side, and we all know that, but this policy was new. We wish it hadn't happened, but fortunately nobody was hurt, and really it was a kind of freak accident." The Captain asked me to stay while he dismissed the others.

I thought that he was going to privately tell me that he was going to send the case to a Board of Inquiry. I also expected him to express some anger or maybe hit me hard over the head with some heavy metal object. After all, something like this is an embarrassment to the whole ship (the whole Navy). It was going to cost the ***Forrestal*** the Battle E, and would probably hurt the skipper unless he was vigorous enough in my punishment before I was dismissed. I at least appreciated his doing what had to happen next in private.

It didn't happen that way.

The Captain told me he had confidence in me and the Medical Department. He told me had no choice but to issue a "Letter of Caution," a stern, official letter that serves notice or "caution" that the recipient better watch out and not mess up any more. While no officer wants to have something like that on his record, it's the sort of thing that if your performance is okay thereafter, needn't ruin a career. It's like probation. Under the circumstances, it was about the least punishment the Captain could have given me. By doing that, the Captain left himself in further jeopardy, though. If he had me Court Martialed or sent the case to a Board of Inquiry, that would have been the Pound of Flesh that tradition or the news media would have wanted. Somebody's career would have paid for the syringes, and the Captain would himself have been cleared by striking the swift blow for justice. By issuing me only a Letter of Caution, he could potentially be blamed for a "coverup" or for "going easy on the culprit." These were days when the public suspected coverups.

The Captain never said another word to me about that event, ever. He didn't raise his voice, he patted me on the back on the way out of the room, and he told me that he was further sorry that he had to give a Letter of Caution to Rick Combs, too. Apparently since there were two officers involved, each officer had to get a Letter. Once again, I told him it was my fault, not Rick's, and that I didn't want Rick to get tarnished by this. He told me not to worry, that if Rick's performance continued to be the way it always had been, by the time he left the ship the Letter of Caution would be forgotten.

Most commanding officers would have fired the SMO at that point, and both Captain Pieno and I knew it. Knowing how discouraged I was, Captain Pieno invited me over to dinner at his house that night. He never mentioned the syringes to me again, and never, never showed any lack of confidence.

The next week, Hugh Beaumont came to see me, somewhat sheepishly. He told me that he and a number of the other corpsmen knew who had thrown the syringes over the side, and that the person did it intentionally because he was angry at the Leading Petty Officer in the Department. It wasn't an accident, but was vengeful and done on purpose. Apparently, that was why Beaumont had been so solicitous the days we went down to pick up syringes, since he knew I was going to take the rap for somebody's angry stunt. He said it had been bothering him a lot the past few days, not only that it had happened, but that he and his shipmates had not come to tell me about it. He said that he had been worried that I might be fired, and that nobody had taken steps to try to protect me. He wouldn't tell me who the corpsman was who did it, though.

What good would it do for me to pass that on? It was over now.

CHAPTER VII. SRA AND INPORT

The SRA was going to continue for another 3 or 4 months. We would not start our "workups" for the next cruise until late February. It was all mapped out. The exact date for the first exercises and first movements of the ship were scheduled almost down to the minute. Usually, the carriers operated on an 18-month cycle. After a 6-month cruise, such as the one we just finished, there would be an SRA to do any repairs or updates, then workups stretched out over most of the next year. In our case, the cycle was being compressed from 18 months down to a year. We had arrived back in Mayport in the first week of October, and we were going to go out one year from then, so we had to squeeze all of our workups and any other things we were tasked with into just a year. It also meant once we started steaming in late February, we would be at sea or deployed at least half the time during the next six months, and then deployed for the next six. For the present, though, we were going to stay tied up at least the next 3 to 4 months, so I had to get used to operating my Medical Department with all those pipes and wires running through the passageways. Doing business was going to be a lot different tied up in Mayport than it had been while underway.

For one thing, my Department no longer had a monopoly in the medical business for FID sailors. They had options now, and several of them. A sailor could go to the Mayport Clinic. Even if he lived on the ship, he could simply walk off the bow, a mile and a half over to the clinic, and be seen in Military Sick Call over there in the morning instead of by one of us on the ship. It was 2 hours away to the Navy Hospital at JAX, but some of the sailors lived over on that side of town, anyway, where they may have been stationed before. For one reason or another, they or their family might prefer to be seen over at the hospital. It was common knowledge that the doctors at the hospital, also known as NHJax, or the doctors at the clinic were more apt to write a recommendation for "no duty" than the doctors on the ship. Although it is told to everybody in boot camp, many people in the Navy don't realize that a "no duty" chit signed by a doctor is merely a recommendation to the Command. Only the Commanding Officer and his delegated agents in the chain of command can excuse a person from work. The doctor only *recommends*. To be sure, a chief or officer disregards the advice of a doctor only at some risk. Still, the member given a "no duty" chit is supposed to either call his boss to let him know he won't be at work, and then turn in the chit when he returns, or bring the chit to the boss on the way home. Apparently, a number of the medical staff at the Mayport Clinic didn't realize this advisory relationship between physicians and command. Some of our sailors didn't recognize it, either, and some of them found it **convenient** to not recognize it. In the first few weeks, a much higher percentage than usual of our sailors were turning in "no duty" or "light duty" chits signed by doctors at the clinic and the hospital. A number of those chits recommended 7 to 10 days in bed, and then a mandatory follow-up with that particular doctor back at the clinic or the hospital, not with the ship's doctor.

I had spent a lot of time with the corpsmen telling them that I intended our Department to be the primary medical contact for all FID sailors, that I wanted us to be the "family doctor," not only for the sailors but for their families. This would entail a helpful attitude, and an eagerness to assume responsibility for their care, though. Several times I would walk by the ER on the way to my office and overhear a corpsman telling a patient, "You'll have to come by tomorrow morning in Sick Call for that." That was exactly the kind of comment I had tried to fight the entire time we were underway. It always amazed me how the guys expected the rules would change as soon as we came into port. Whenever I heard it, I would intervene, and find out what was bothering the sailor, walk right into the ER with the sailor and make the corpsman help me with the treatment.

After the patient would leave, usually with some minor problem, I would ask the corpsman why they didn't go ahead and treat the patient at that time. "Well, I thought that's what Sick Call was for."

"But you weren't doing anything now. It would be different if you were busy. You're just sitting there reading a book."

"Well, we always just tell them to come back the next morning."

No, we did *not* tell them to *come back the next morning*! If you are treating somebody else or if there is some emergency going on, that is one thing. Sure, we schedule Sick Call so that people can bring their routine problems in the morning. If he is here right with you now and alive, why not treat him right then if you have time. That way he won't **have** to come back in the morning. It's another way to cut down on lines in Sick Call. I tried to impress on the corpsman that there was some reason the guy would come in whenever he would come in. Maybe his injury was hurting him, maybe he was worried, maybe he had trouble getting off the next morning. Trying to get across the service aspect of medical care was a constant effort. Not just doctors, but anybody who works in a medical setting, so often thinks that people should have to conform to the system. No wonder, if sailors got turned away on the ship, that they would go to a clinic. Our corpsmen all understood this, and they too believed in giving service. Sometimes, though, when people are accustomed to routine, it's hard to break out of it.

One day, I was writing out some charts and realized I hadn't spoken to the SuppO about my concerns that Master Chief Morgan might have a drinking problem. It's only about fifty feet down to the Supply Dept office, so I went down to discuss it with Bruce.

"I appreciate your calling it to my attention, Doc. We'll look out for it. Did you actually **smell** alcohol on him?"

"No, just the speech. Now that I think of it he's been kind of grouchy lately too, and don't you think he's been looking real tired?"

"Yeah, but we're busy as Hell. He's a pretty good Chief, Doc, but I know you can't always tell. He doesn't have any past history of alcohol trouble."

Just then, I felt a little embarrassed and a little guilty. As a neurologist, there should have been a lot of things I would think of in a guy with slurred speech. Was I starting to confine my diagnostic thinking to just automatic lines? I'd have to talk to Art Forbes about this. I knew he had been seeing Master Chief Morgan for something.

Back in the office I returned to the paperwork and left the door open. I heard a sailor come in and complain about a cough and a sore throat while HM3 Arden Womple was on duty. In his basso-profundo voice and typical condescending attitude, Womple said, "Well, there's nothing I can do about it now. You can either wait until Sick Call tomorrow, or if I were you, I would go on over to the clinic over on the base." That kind of comment tripped my fuse. I immediately jumped over to the ER.

As usual, Womple had a soup-stained shirt, had not even got out of his chair when the sailor came into the ER. He had a magazine opened up on the desk, and had not taken the sailor's pulse, temperature, or blood pressure.

"What's the problem, sailor?" I asked.

The guy had been feeling ill for a couple of days and had a fever. He had been coughing and had a headache. I spent about a half-hour taking his history and treating him. We gave him something for his cough, and I called up his DivO to ask for him to have the rest of the day in the rack and to stop by to see me tomorrow morning to see whether he could go back to work then. Then I closed the door. Womple looked surly, but did not seem to understand what he had done. I reiterated for him my effort to treat people on the ship rather than send them over to the clinic, and asked him if he understood me.

"Yeah, but what are we supposed to do if somebody comes in sick in the afternoon? We can't treat them here."

"Who said we can't treat them here? I'm a doctor, there are 20 corpsmen around here at work. we've been treating them here for the last six months. What in the Hell are we in business for?"

Arden didn't even want to work hard enough to even look back at me stupidly. He just shrugged and began reading his magazine again.

"Hey, did you just decide this conversation is over?"

"Well, I thought you were through."

"HM3 Womple, I never did expect you to agree with everything I said, but try to think of this as though I'm the employer and you work here. If we looked at it that way, would you be anymore likely to be interested in what I have to say?"

Womple just shrugged again.

"Look, Petty Officer Womple, I certainly can't threaten you, and you are too old to scold. EMI is not something I like to use for anybody, especially not somebody who has been around as long as you have. I am trying to get you to understand that we are here to provide a service, and we are going to function just like a real clinic around here. If you don't give me some sign that you understand that, I'll try to get you assigned somewhere that you do understand the boss."

"Yes, Sir." He made a half-assed gesture to stand up, but that was the first time I heard him say the "Yes, Sir" word in that entire discussion. When I left there, I didn't feel any better about what Womple was going to do.

A couple of days later, still worried about that interaction, I met with HMCS McGowan and Rick Combs to see if Arden was having more personal problems, as he had during the deployment. McGowan checked with Arden and with the Family Services Center. Arden told him to "bug off," and the counsellor said the family problems weren't too severe. In fact the Center had been surprised that Womple had been allowed to come home early from the deployment.

When we had been back in Mayport about a week, Commander Kit Henessy, the Skipper from HS-15, the Red Lions, called to follow up on the eyeglasses we discussed at the end of the cruise. He wanted to repeat his visual testing when he wasn't tired. I knew it was still going to show that he needed eyeglasses, but if he was going to feel better about it, why not? When we repeated his refraction he still needed a little correction for astigmatism and about a -1.25 correction for myopia, nearsightedness. When we dialed that up on the phoropter, he recognized that his vision was much better.

Since we had first raised the subject during the cruise, he thought it over and was willing to go ahead with the glasses. Frankly, I think the reason he wanted to wait was simply that when the cruise was over he would be living at home, not among his fellow aviators, so wearing glasses wouldn't be quite as visible. He would, of course, wear his glasses when he was flying. No aviators wanted to wear glasses or to admit that they needed them, but modern aviators also wouldn't expose themselves or others to hazard by leaving them off. With their visors down, other people couldn't see them wearing the glasses most of the time, anyway. Still aviators are aviators. They would wear them if they had to, but just as soon not talk about it.

Although he was the first one, Kit wasn't the last of my patients from the cruise that I heard from that week. In the mail I received a summary from Oliver Leen's treatment at the Navy Hospital Naples. The course of his pyelonephritis was detailed, and his response to intravenous ampicillin had been able to cure the infection. Once the infection was under control, a small adjustment in his regular insulin dosing got the diabetes under control, also.

Once his pyelonephritis was repaired and the insulin dose adjusted, Leen was back to appearing pretty healthy. He convinced the internist at the hospital how well he felt, and how much the Staff needed him. The internist knew that we had a robust Medical Department on the ship, and saw that with just 2 1/2 weeks of hospitalization the patient's blood sugar was back in normal range. By simply taking his insulin, which Oliver showed the doctor he knew how to do, they agreed that he should be able to return to the ship. Of course the young internist had never been to sea, so he didn't realize limitations in our Medical Department. Most especially he did not realize that Oliver had hidden his illness at a time when he was very sick all alone in his stateroom. If he had become comatose, and if his fellow officers had not gone to look for him, he might have died. The regulations, and furthermore just plain common sense, in my opinion, called for a "Medical Board," a process and a medical document that establishes an individual's diagnosis and limits his duties and his assignments. In this case, dependence on insulin prohibits an individual from going to sea.

With Oliver's prodding, the internist simply wrote a discharge summary that allowed him to return to the United States, and in the recommendation at the bottom of the summary recommended that he return to his duty at sea with the Staff.

I was frustrated by the results, and angry at what I considered manipulation of the system. Probably I took it too much as a personal affront, when I should have confined the whole focus to only the matters of Leen's health and effects on the command, and should have overlooked the technicalities. His health **was** important to me, though, especially on the ship. I was afraid that the next time, particularly if he hid his illness again, the outcome might be worse. I telephoned Oliver Leen and told him that I thought there had been a misunderstanding. "No, there was no misunderstanding, the doctor at Naples thought I should return to full duty without any problem."

I told him I had no choice but to discuss it with the Admiral, and to refer the case back to another internal medicine consultation at NH-JAX. Leen obviously did not like that advice.

When I went to see Admiral Smith he had already spoken to CDR Leen. Always loyal and concerned about his officers, the admiral wanted to be sure that Leen's career was not damaged. As long as he took his insulin, wouldn't he be the same as anybody else?

The last thing I wanted to do was be the adversary of a Naval Officer. I was supposed to help guys like Leen fill out their careers and stay healthy, not punish them. I told the Admiral that, and assured him that it was Oliver's safety I was most concerned about. None of us wanted to find Oliver Leen dead in his rack some morning. I had carried this discussion as far as it needed to go. Snuffy Smith didn't need my elementary sermons on things he understood very well. Furthermore I knew that he was every bit as concerned about Oliver's health as I was. He just wanted to protect the man's career too if he could.

I recommended that the admiral let me refer the case to the Chief of Internal Medicine over at NH-JAX, Captain John Seibel, and that we just have him review the matter.

The Commander went to see Dr. Seibel, even though he didn't want to. As I expected, John agreed that with the amount of insulin CDR Leen took he should not be on sea duty, and that was what he recommended in the Medical Board. Finally, it was settled. CDR Oliver Leen was officially not fit for sea duty. I felt somehow guilty, like I always did when I had to tell an aviator he couldn't fly anymore, but I was relieved that Oliver Leen wouldn't be in that dangerous position at sea again.

MAYPORT

The first 3 to 4 weeks I worked just as many hours as we had while underway. Doug and Art took some leave, so I was the only doctor on the ship. I was still getting to learn things about the ship, and the crew, so by the time I finished seeing patients and writing up my notes it was usually pretty late in the day. Gradually, however, I was able to get a little spare time. When Doug and Art returned from leave, I did not have to see all the patients myself. I was getting a little faster working with the ship's bureaucracy and records systems. I began to have time for jogging again and seeing a little bit of the town.

The Mayport and Jacksonville area are way up at the northern part of Florida, so they are not entirely unscathed by winter. It never got really cold, though. Most days we stayed up in the 50's or better, and only very rarely dabbled down to the 30's. Maybe because of the coastal winds or something, we had a lot of bright days. I explored jogging from Charlie pier down to the main road on the base which was called "Maine Road." There was a large lagoon in the middle of the base right across from the Base Exchange area, with a sign that said, "No swimming. Beware of alligators." These were earnest signs in northern Florida. The kids who hung around the pond saw the alligator occasionally. He apparently was only about 6 feet long, but we all took him pretty seriously. More of a hazard than the alligator, however, was the flock of geese who hung around the northern edge of the lagoon right by the day care center. Geese are not only confident animals, they are pretty aggressive. More than a pack of barking dogs, a sensible jogger would be hesitant whenever he came by those geese, because they would run up and nip at your ankles. Sometimes I imagined being in the headlines the next morning listed as "Navy Doctor Mauled to Death by Pack of Wild Geese."

Just a quarter mile past the geese was the beach. The beaches in this part of Florida were flat, had very find sand, and stretched for miles and miles uninterrupted. To be sure, there was a big chain link fence all the way around the Navy Base, and it extended right down to the beach, halfway between the high tide and low tide lines. A guard was stationed there to be certain that unauthorized strangers wouldn't just walk onto the base.

On the very north end of the beach at the Naval Station, right at the inlet, was a complex of buildings called the Fleet Training Center. Here a conglomerate of training activities were carried on, both for people who were assigned to ships and would come to the FTC for refresher training, and for people on route to assignments at sea. For example, the fire fighting school was here. It was just like the fire fighting school at San Diego and Norfolk. Some of the people who had come to the Forrestal would have intermediate orders to the FTC for a couple of weeks for fire fighting if they did not have that training elsewhere first. Every Tuesday and Wednesday around midday, a big black cloud would rise up from the FTC while they suffered through the exercises on fighting a big oil fire on the simulated deck.

There was an 18-hole golf course, always busy, winding through the base. It ran from over near the housing area on the beach, all the way back to Maine Road, and then crossed the road over toward the Naval Air Station, just inland and along the southeast side of the main Naval Station.

The Air Station was primarily there for the LAMPS helicopters on the "small boys," the destroyers and cruisers. The H2 helo, now almost 30 years old, had been developed for the antisubmarine mission primarily off the back of destroyers and cruisers. It fulfilled a number of other functions for the small ships, of course, but its main mission was to hunt submarines just as the H3 was on the carrier. A small but very capable aircraft, the H2 had a crew of three, the two pilots and the sonar operator/crew man in the back. All Navy helos had two pilots.

One of the places I liked to run the most was out the back gate from the Navy Station to a perimeter road around the runway. The perimeter road ran out to the right and bordered up against the old fishing village of Mayport, a rustic little settlement along the St. John's Inlet. There were no openings in the chain link fence around the Air Station, but of course you could see through to the old village. Some of the people kept chicken coops, with very funny looking chickens. They were both scrawny but sinewy-looking with high red topknots and real long pointy spurs. Kept in different cages from the kind you usually saw for egglayers or roasters, we figured those were fighting cocks. The houses were an eclectic collection of shacks and old Gulf style southern houses. The road turned down along the main runway and ran past a mile or more of marshes mixed between long expanses of green, lawnlike grass. All the away around the runway you would double back and run north again on the other side. Turning right would divert the run back to the golf course, a circuit of around 5 1/2 miles. If instead you went all the way around the main road and back up to the beach, the trip was a little over 8 miles.

Only one road led into the Naval Station and Naval Air Station at Mayport, appropriately enough named "Mayport Avenue." Stretching 3 1/2 miles without a bend, curve, or even flicker, Mayport Ave. seemed a lot longer than it was. There were only a few kinds of businesses on that route: honky-tonk bars, tire stores, used car lots, and pawn shops. Well, that's not exactly true. There was one small shopping center, the first Food Lion store I ever saw, and a couple of tatoo parlors. Mayport Ave had two very different identities. During the day, especially at rush hour, it was a 3 1/2 mile parking lot for the unfortunate souls who were squeezed into the home of two dozen ships and 12 helicopter squadrons on a single road. By night it was North Florida's Times Square.

A few of the night spots on the Great Honky-Tonk Way were known as the Flamingo Lounge, Cap'n Odie's, and Big Jim's Gold Coast (or just "Big Jim's" to the insiders). Down at the corner where Atlantic Boulevard, the main east-west road, intersected Mayport Ave., there was a fake-adobe liquor store and bar combo that had a semi-pseudo western motif and a big, brown horse shoe painted on one wall. It didn't have a name, at least not where you could see it. I never went into Capt'n Odie's, the Flamingo Lounge, or Big Jim's, but of those three, Big Jim's scared me the most. I fancied myself a pretty rough hombre in my younger years (no doubt a laughable self-delusion), but I freely confess that there was no time in my life when I would have been brave enough to go into Big Jim's. It had the kind of look to the outside, and the intimidating impression of the parking lot, that anybody who had not killed five or six men with his bare hands didn't have a chance in that place.

However, the toughest looking of them all was that semi-pseudo western place down at the corner of Mayport and Atlantic Ave. I called it "The Corral" because that just kind of seemed like what it should be named. Occasionally, somebody would roll out one of those illuminated trailer signs in front of the Corral to advertise country music or something. There was always at least one misspelled word or missing letter. The sign might say, "L_dies nite Wesday nite." The place looked rough. I was told that the reason they had a western motif wasn't so much that the people there were especially devoted to western music, or any other music for that matter. It was just that they hoped the western music would drive black guys away. It was so rough looking I sometimes felt nervous just driving past it. I never remember seeing any cars in front of the place, but it never went broke in all the months that I drove past there.

The sailors mostly stayed away from Big Jim's. Even sailors as young and feisty as they can be, especially with a snootful of booze, recognized that Big Jim's was a good place to avoid. So it wasn't a place too many went to very often. The worst beatings I had to take care of in the emergency ward seemed to come from Big Jim's. One night, a sailor had a deep knife cut almost from ear to ear across his neck from an attempted throat-slitting. Somehow the attacker had just not pushed hard enough. I admit this particular guy had a fleshy double chin, but the attacker seemed to miss all the major vessels and never even cut into the windpipe. Most guys who got beat up at Big Jim's had a piece at least two inches bitten out of one ear or the other, it seems like the right ear a little more often than the left. Their noses were almost always broken.

Another interesting thing about Big Jim's was that no Forrestal sailors seemed to lose a fair fight in there. From what my patients told me, there was some dirty fighter who always seemed to sneak up from behind and hit my guys. For any of the sailors who were sober enough to talk, it was always "He sucker punched me." This mystery puncher wouldn't have touched my guys in a fair fight. They never saw the guy who hit them. He always seemed to jump out from behind them and punch them for no good reason. The Forrestal sailors were "just standing there, minding my own business," or "talking to this girl," when they were mysteriously attacked without provocation. How he was able to keep punching them for so long and so accurately, and also to bite out a piece of their ear, was always a mystery to me.

By contrast, the beatings from Capt'n Odie's weren't near as bad. To be sure, the guys from Capt'n Odie's had a lot of black eyes, an occasional broken tooth, and less often a cut from a knife. But the guys who went to Capt'n Odie's always claimed to have won their fights. As opposed to Big Jim's, where they only lost because of the dirty sucker puncher, at Capt'n Odie's I always should have seen the other guy.

If the bruised and bloody face in front of me had just come from Capt'n Odie's, the sailor always reassured me that he had eventually finished off the other guy. About a third of the time, the beaten sailor had a buddy standing behind him who would silently shake his head, smile, and look down at the floor. The buddy would discreetly signal me that the FID sailor had lost. However, I prefer to believe that all the guys at Capt'n Odie's won their fights, and the FID sailors at Big Jim's were all sucker punched.

One tragi-comic irony from Capt'n Odie's seemed to never register with the FID sailors. The main reasons for going to Capt'n Odie's were that the music was good, and that there were a lot of very friendly women. Now, no FID sailor in history ever had to pay for a date, so I know that these women danced and spent time with our sailors just because they liked them, and because they wanted to spend time with young men. It was said, though, that some of the good looking and friendly young women at Capt'n Odie's were married to sailors from other ships. Indeed, when we returned from our deployment, a few FID sailors found that their wives had taken up with other men, some from Mayport. How many of those had met their new loves in Capt'n Odie's I don't know.

Petty Officer Brian Haack was very fond of Capt'n Odie's. He was also fond of falling in love. It seems like the first night we got back into Mayport Brian had to make it over to Capt'n Odie's. By the time we had been there about a week, he brought his new girlfriend in to show her around the Department, and as the guys often did, he brought her by my office to meet me. It was around 1900, and as usual I was finishing up my paperwork for the day. The corpsmen liked to bring in their girlfriends, as a teenager would bring them by to meet their parents. "Captain Riley, this is my girlfriend Linda." She was a very clean-cut, outgoing and charming young woman. She stuck out her hand with a lot of confidence and did not have the kind of shy frivolity that a lot of the young women who came around the Medical Department did. Brian was around 22, and I guessed that this young woman was somewhere between 26 and 28.

"Where are you two off to tonight?" I asked.

"We don't know yet," Linda said. "We both like to go dancing." Unsaid, I guessed they were probably going to Capt'n Odie's. About a week later I learned that Brian was planning to get married. This was the modern age, so I guess they weren't in a big **hurry** to get married, but Brian seemed to spend a lot of time at her house. I tried not to get into the private lives of my corpsmen, or to give out too much advice. I knew that advice was usually not welcome even with your own children, and so you had to be very careful how you used it with others. I told Brian, however, that moving into somebody's house wasn't like in the movies. It carried more commitments than you might realize, and probably a young man in his position should be just as careful about that as he would be about getting married. You could tell my advice amused him by its old-fashionedness. It was as though he thought it was cute for me to be concerned, but quaint and outdated just the same.

Art Forbes popped into my office one afternoon. "Skipper, I need your help with a patient, or I guess with his boss." Art and I both knew I was no skipper, but he called me that, I suspect because he knew I liked it. What a craftsman. He had won me over, though. Art worked harder than I had even realized at first, and despite his deceptively spicy exterior he never stopped thinking about his patients. "It's Master Chief Morgan, Skipper. He refuses to take his damn blood pressure medicine and he keeps smokin'. He knows he's s'posed to be in here to let me check his pressure every week until we get in under control, but I just can't get him in here. He keeps givin' me excuses. Can you talk to the SuppO?"

"Sure I can. What's his pressure been running, Art?"

"Last few times its been around 105-115."

I knew Art was referring to the diastolic, so I asked, "What about the systolic?"

"That's been as high as 180-190. But that's been almost a month ago. I can't get him in here. When I go down to his spaces, he always seems to be someplace else."

As bad as those pressures were, considering they were in a guy only in his forties, who was on treatment, the meaning of the pressures might be worse than just the numerical values. I called the SuppO immediately. Guiltily it crossed my mind that the speech problem I had noticed might not have a thing to do with alcohol. High blood pressure causes disease in the small arteries in the brain: that can affect speech. Medications can slur speech. Hypertension can damage the heart, and diminished cardiac output can affect the brain. His blood pressure was out of control.

"He's on leave, Doc," Bruce told me.

We called Master Chief Morgan's leave phone number. Disconnected. He would be back in less than a week. Art would bring him in so that I could go over the case with them.

"One last thing, Art. Does the Master Chief have a drinking problem?"

"Used to. Don't think he does anymore... but you know, I've wondered whether that has anything to do with the pressure getting out of control. Seems like it got worse about the time the cruise ended." Art and I worried about the Master Chief the rest of that week.

One day around that time, my morning started off bad. The OOD called me from the Quarterdeck to tell me my bicycle had been crushed. There was a bike rack tied to the brow on the pier. I do have to admit I sometimes thought it a little strange that nobody but me seemed to use that rack. It seems that overnight, the tides had been a lot worse than usual and the metal frame from the brow shifted quite a bit more than usual, in the process smashing the bike rack and my ten-speed into an eight foot paper clip. I was still stewing about that when HM1 Tom Dunwoody came to my office to tell me that Petty Officer Hugh Beaumont was on the phone. Beaumont was the biomedical repairman who joined us late on the cruise, and who had been so supportive during the high stress over the needles. He had also been mysteriously hinted about some foul play around the event.

"Hey, where is he, by the way? I didn't see him this morning. Did I forget he was on leave or something?"

"No, Captain, that's why he's on the phone," Tom explained. "He didn't come in this morning, and he's calling in now."

Beaumont impressed me as a little older, a little more mature than the others. Even as a First Class Petty Officer... he seemed to belong higher, like a Chief. We had a trusting approach to our guys as much as we could, so we wanted to work with guys like Hugh if he had a problem that kept him away from the ship one day.

"Sorry, Captain, having a little personal problems at home. Can I get leave for today?"

I said we'd try to help if he needed it, what was the problem?

"Well, the wife and I are having some problems, you know after the cruise and all. Guess we just need to get the trust thing back, you know?"

Ah, the famous 'Trust Thing.' It means so many things and such different ones to everybody. Certainly I knew that my simply coming back to the Navy, and being so far away from the family was a strain on trust in our house. Sure, I worried about it too, but it maybe meant something different to Hugh. "What about trust, Hugh."

"Oh, you know, what she's thinking, what other people are thinking. You know it can all run together when people think or talk about you."

I didn't get it. "When people talk about you, Petty Officer Beaumont?"

"You probably can understand what I mean. I know it's been hard for you, too, Captain. I mean, I know there are people who would like to see you hurt around here. And I think that's too bad. It's that same trust thing. Loyalty. You know that's what's wrong in this country, trust and loyalty. It's like back with McCarthy, you know?

"Oh, I'm so tired, I'm not making any sense," he realized.

"Not really, Petty Officer Beaumont. I don't follow you. Have you been up all night?" He had. "Have you been drinking or taking medications?"

"No!" he said quite angrily. "I told you once that I don't have any substance problems anymore." As a teenager he drank too much for a few years. "Substances are part of the problem in this country."

I told him to get some sleep and come to see me in the morning. Immediately I asked HM1Dunwoody and Chief Hitzeman to come into my office. "You guys been seeing anything funny about HM1 Beaumont?"

No.

"If I wanted to check with some of his buddies, who would I ask?"

"He's kind of a loner, actually, Dr.Riley," The Chief told me. Neither of them had noticed any wandering speech, or anything else strange. I asked them to pay attention and resolve to be sure to check up on Beaumont the next morning.

We were interrupted just then, when Billy Dorsey was brought in his DivO. Once again, he had a big cut over his eyebrow, and his mouth and cheeks were swollen. He had some scrapes on his hands and elbows. He had obviously been beat up again the night before. He was walking a little crooked, bent over slightly to the right. As I examined him, I pressed over the midaxillary line on his right rib cage, and he jumped about eighteen inches instantly. I was a little afraid he might have a broken rib.

"What happened last night, Billy?"

"Nothin'." Funny, while it was nothing that happened to him, he still had that coquettish little grin. It kind of made you want him to be your little boy. On the one hand, I wanted to scold him, but on the other hand, I thought I should find a rocking chair someplace and sit down and cuddle with him a little bit. His tousled red hair had the character you used to see in the Buster Brown ads, like somebody purposefully laid it at those angles. Only if you got within two feet and had the smell of that stale, semi-rotten alcohol from the night before pierce the cuteness, it reminded you that poor Billy's life was beginning to be a mess.

"Billy, we asked you to go see the alcohol counselor the last time. What did he say?" I knew what he said. The note back from the alcohol counselor had said that Airman Dorsey was an immature fellow who had been introduced to his first alcohol contacts, and he would need a lot of watching. The CAAC had recommended that Billy be directed to attend AA meetings for several weeks. We had an AA group on the ship that was very vigorous and met every day, twice a day while we were underway. His DivO had not followed through on that, however. I had phoned his DivO twice in the interim, but had found only indifference. "Boys will be boys." Now, here was Billy again, beat up for the second time in a short period. I filled out another CAAC report and resolved that I had to talk to the Air Boss about him directly.

To check out the possibility of a rib fracture, I requested a chest X-ray. The HN who was on duty shuffled his feet, mumbled something that might have been a little bit like "Yes, Sir." and then left the room. AN Dorsey and I were alone then, and he looked at me sheepishly like a little boy whose daddy might not take him fishing that day because he had been naughty. In a few minutes, HM1 Dunwoody who was supervising that day came in to take Dorsey for his X-ray. I figured HM3 Hastings was back warming up the X-ray unit, or putting film in the cassette.

While they went off to get the X-ray, I looked after another patient who had a fish hook in his finger. Just outside of the Charlie pier where we were tied up, there was a long, rock breakwater that stretched out beside the St. John's Inlet. When guys were off duty, they would frequently go out and fish off that rock pier. Anglers know that it is common for people to get fish hooks stuck in their earlobes and fingers, but only people who work in emergency rooms know **how** common it is. There are little barbs at the end of fish hooks, so they can't be just pulled out the way they come in. The hook needs to be pushed all the way through if it is not already, and the eyelet cut off so that the hook can be curled right back out, by the pointy end. This is usually pretty easy to do on fingers and earlobes, but sometimes a little tougher on cheeks or chins. The thing we were most concerned about was the possibility of an infection. Fish, fish hooks, and worms can bring a perplexing panoply of bacteria, and cause serious cellulitis. I usually did not like to give "prophylactic antibiotics" but after removing the fish hook, I usually required the individual to soak the affected hand in a disinfecting soap solution for about 30 minutes or so. That's what we were doing with this patient after I took the fish hook out when a very sheepish HN Rodriguez walked in.

CORPSMEN TOO

Rodriguez was a new corpsman, a very quiet fellow, and always eager to help. He walked into the ER, sidled over in front of the desk where I was writing a few notes, and just stood there with his hands behind his back, looking down at the deck. He could see that there wasn't anything more to be done with the patient who was just sitting down and soaking his hand, and obviously I didn't need any help writing the note. Still, Rod stood there shifting his weight from first the left then the right foot, then back again, staring at the deck, saying nothing. Now and then his foot would kick at the corner of one of the tiles.

I finished writing the note about the fish hook patient, and was still waiting for Billy Dorsey to come back from his X-ray, and I looked up at Rodriguez, who still had nothing to say, just shifting back and forth from one foot to the other.

"What's up, HN Rodriguez? Do you need me for something?"

"Yes, Sir. Well, Sir. I guess I need to talk to you. Senior Chief said I should ask to see you in your office." He said all that without making real good eye contact, still mostly concentrating on the deck tiles. I didn't need all my powers of marvelous insight to recognize this was a bad sign. "Well, it looks like you've got some kind of trouble. It will be a little while before they get back with those X-rays. Why don't we go into my office and find out what's the trouble."

Getting HN Rodriguez to tell me what was the problem was harder than opening a box of corn flakes. Every time I thought I could get him to come to the point, he figured some other way not to open up. It seems that he had just bought a new pick-up a couple of days after finishing the cruise. The vehicle had needed some new tires, but he couldn't get the kind he wanted in Mayport. To get the right kind of tires, he had gone down to Neptune Beach, then over to the outskirts of Jacksonville. Nobody had what he wanted. So he decided to get them someplace else, and he finally did. Then last night he had gone out to eat with some buddies, and one of the friends needed to be dropped off at the Post Office. Then HN Rodriguez had to call his mother, then it was getting too late. Then his buddy had to go over to somebody else's house. Then there was...

"Enough! Will you please tell me what the problem was?! Did it have something to do with the car?"

"Well, Sir, I'm not sure they could really make it stick."

"Make what stick?" It turns out that, finally, after that round-about story, HN Rodriguez and some buddies had gone to Capt'n Odie's for a few drinks. When he came back on the base, in his new pickup truck (Why did a single 19-year-old kid who lived on ship need a pickup truck?), he had been stopped for driving while intoxicated.

"Why did they stop you if you weren't doing anything wrong? How did they know you had been drinking?"

The answer to that is the old standby familiar to all doctors. "I just don't know. I only had two beers." Any drunk person you ever see in an emergency room, especially if they have just been stopped while driving, or if they just got beat up, always consumed "just two beers."

Rodriguez had not really sought me out because he wanted my advice or because of his conscience. DWI was a major offense in the Navy, and a major offense to Captain Pieno. Being stopped for DWI on a military base causes an entire cascade of unpleasant things to happen. There is an official notification to the command, which Rod knew was already in the works. Unless there was some remarkably unusual extenuating circumstances, and there never were, the member's driver's license would be suspended on all military bases for at least one year.

Captain Pieno, like most CO's, took DWI seriously and insisted that being caught for DWI was a ticket to Captain's Mast. It was a way for him to personally keep track of guys who had alcohol trouble and demonstrating the Skipper's personal concern about it. Although my experience at Captain's Mast had shown that Captain Pieno's reputation at NJP, the legal term for Mast, was grossly exaggerated, the sailors didn't know that. Most of them would much prefer to stand in front of any hanging judge, or perhaps to be flogged or keelhauled, rather than stand before Captain Pieno for Captain's Mast for anything, much less DWI. So, Rodriguez had not come to me as a conscience-troubled supplicant. He knew very well that he was in a whole bunch of trouble, and that I was going to find out before too long anyway. I had spent so much time talking about drinking and driving with the corpsmen that HN Rodriguez knew very well where I stood on the subject. We had talked about recreation and sports the guys could do when off duty. We worked on departmental group activities without alcohol. We had buddy systems. And on top of all that we also gave warnings about consequences. Furthermore, I was tied up with Billy Dorsey, and one other patient who was now waiting out in the passageway. I was beginning to wonder why it was taking so long to get Dorsey's' X-ray. Truthfully, my frustration with Dorsey's drinking had already tightened my spring about young guy's alcohol problems. HN Rodriguez was also 19, just like Dorsey. There was a more than additive effect having both of them there with me at once.

"HN Rodriguez, I'm so mad at you I can't talk about this right now. If you expect me to give you some sympathy under these circumstances, you can forget about it. Do you remember the four or five times at Quarters before the end of the cruise when I stood in front of you and all the other corpsmen and asked you to be very careful about drinking and driving when we returned?"

Rodriguez's response to that was the same as his round-about circumlocution a few minutes before. He threw his arms up, and started to talk, he babbled on about how he really didn't think he had too much to drink. Teenage excuses. I knew that the security force on the base were experienced. They knew all the signs. If they said a 19-year-old guy was driving under the influence, it was probably because he had been zigzagging, had avoided apprehension, or had run a red light. If they said a guy had been drinking, he had been. Rodriguez started to interrupt me.

"Never mind. I think you'd better see Senior Chief McGowan, then make sure you get hooked up with the CAAC, and then you'd better go down to see Master Chief Shulman to see if there is anything we can do to save your career. I want to talk to you this afternoon. I <u>hate</u> it when any of my guys have to go Captain's Mast. I swore that nobody in this Department was going to go to Captain's Mast. You let me down and the whole Department, now get out of here!" Master Chief Shulman was the Command Master Chief. He was the Senior Enlisted on the ship. He maintained a kind of paternal oversight on the enlisted guys, keeping all the chief and master chiefs organized, and bestowing the right attitude as much as possible among the troops. He also was the sailor's advocate if the sailor needed an advocate with his own department head or the skipper.

I liked Rodriguez, so why was I getting this upset, I asked myself. Isn't this one of those predictable leadership situations? Slowly it came to me. It was, I realized, more of a **parenting** situation. One of the reasons I felt so close to Rod and a couple of the others was that they were exactly the age of my children. I was feeling guilty these weeks about not being with my daughters now and when I saw guys like Rod needing a parent it struck me that this day, my daughters were missing a father because I was down here. The situation was real enough by itself -- I was worried about the kid! In my guts, though, I was mad at myself as though I were letting something somehow like this happen to my Mary or Abby by not being with them. They were the two older ones, the teenagers.

Having already been worked up by all these thoughts, I was now starting to fester about why I didn't have Dorsey's X-ray back yet.

When I stepped across the passageway to the view box, Petty Officer Lopez had brought three chest X-rays back. One of them was so overpenetrated it was just a black shadow with the faintest evidence that there was a heart someplace in the middle. Another one had pretty black/white contrast, but it completely cut off the top of the lung. A third one was an attempt at a rib view. To look at ribs specifically requires angling the chest in a certain manner so that the profile of the ribs at a certain level are up against the film in a way that gives the best resolution of detail. Rib detail was not entirely clear here, but good enough that I could see in the tender point there did not seem to be a fracture. The fact that HM3 Lopez had to bring the films, but especially the fact that the films were so poor told me that HM3 Hastings had not done them.

Petty Officer Eddie Hastings was often sullen, not an inspired genius, and usually pretty listless. He took excellent X-rays, though. These were not the work of Petty Officer Hastings. "How come Hastings didn't take these films?"

"Well, Sir, maybe you should talk to HM1 Rosenthal." HM3 Donovan Lopez was real hard to understand. He was born in the United States, but raised by his Haitian parents and married to a Haitian woman, so that he spoke creole exclusively except when he was on the ship. He was nearing completion of his baccalaureate degree, and he was probably one of our brightest corpsmen. It was just hard to understand him. He could sense my frustration about this situation, and it was quite apparent that he was quite frustrated about his own difficulty with the films. One of Donovan's traits was that he never liked to be the bearer of bad news. It was becoming clear that had something to do with Eddie Hastings. There I was already angry, so out I go looking for Rosenthal. Rosenthal wasn't in the Admin. Office, and he wasn't over in Medical Supply. Finally, I found him over in Medical Records. I didn't even have to ask him the question. "Eddie is UA, Cap'n." Unexcused Absence, or UA, is the Navy term for AWOL.

"Where is he?"

"Don't know, Sir, but I think we can guess. This has happened once or twice before. In port, Eddie sometimes takes a room over at the Quality Inn and drinks all night. He usually gets up okay the next morning, but once last year he overslept, and he probably did it this time, too." We sent one of the corpsmen out to find him, and sure enough, he was hibernating in a drunken funk on the second deck of the Quality Inn a half-mile outside the gate.

By the time they brought Eddie back to the ship, Petty Officers Lopez and Brannom worked together to finally get a good set of chest and rib X-rays on Billy Dorsey. Nothing broken and no pulmonary contusion evident. He apparently just had a bad bruise. I had spoken to his DivO, as well as the alcohol counselor. We could not legally confine him to the ship without Captain's Mast, but his DivO told him he couldn't leave the ship for the next 2 days, and we were going to check up on his attendance at AA meetings. After he had a thorough evaluation with the alcohol counselor, we would decide whether he had to be in Level 2 treatment, or whether just putting him on buddy care and making him go to AA for a while would be adequate.

Two and a half hours later, Eddie Hastings came into the Medical Department. He had bags under his eyes, and looked a little blood shot, but he had a clean set of dungarees on and was cleanly shaven. Oh my, he looked so ashamed, so dejected, and so contrite. His demeanor contrasted starkly with HN Rodriguez. For one thing, Eddie was somewhere in his mid to late 30's. Whereas, Rodriguez was full of excuses and wanted to tell me all about how the situation wasn't as bad as it looked, Glaze was so sorry, and so embarrassed. Here was my third major alcohol flap of the day, a guy who had been UA, a pretty serious offense, and he had jeopardized adequate medical care. All that made me pretty angry. There was more, though. I was frustrated because of the alcohol in those two younger guys, but in retrospect I think I was angriest because of my frustration with the Medical Department. Although we have only one fully trained X-ray tech assigned to the Department, there is supposed to be adequate cross training that good X-rays can be taken by several, if not most, corpsmen even if the X-ray tech is away for some reason. In Eddie's absence, it had been a classical goat rope to try to provide a simple chest X-ray and rib films. It wasn't just Eddie's fault that he had not been there so that we had to call on the other corpsmen. It was also his fault, (but especially my fault), that the others were not adequately trained to take good films. Training the other corpsmen in X-ray techniques was one of the main functions of the fulltime X-ray tech. Obviously that had been woefully neglected in the entire crew we had on duty that morning.

Having said all that, I was surprised to find that instead of anger, I was worried about Eddie.

"Petty Officer Hastings, I need to know if there is something wrong."

No answer from him. He just sat there looking at the deck. I decided to give him some time to talk, maybe if he were not pressured he could tell me more. It seemed like we waited there for most of the day, although I guess it was probably only 5 minutes or so.

He shuffled in his chair a little bit, looked up at me as though about to speak, but then it dropped out. He put his hands together and looked back at the deck again, and we started another long silent interval.

Finally I couldn't stand it anymore and I was about to talk when Eddie decided to say something. "I'm sorry. I know that doesn't help, but I've just had a lot on my mind." Again, I let him be in control as much as he wanted to be, so I didn't say anything more. A few more minutes went by. "Sorry I was late this morning. I didn't do it on purpose." We waited silently again.

"Petty Officer Hastings, do we need to talk about what's wrong?"

"No, Sir, I can handle it myself." Another one of those painful long silences. I was beginning to wonder if this was going to make me miss my next couple of meals. Finally, when he still didn't say anything, I had to. "Petty Officer Hastings, I'm not going to put you on report. You know I prefer that we handle problems within our Department. However, you are a Petty Officer. The more junior guys look up to you. Try to help me out here. They know that UA is a fairly serious offense, and a Petty Officer would usually lose a stripe for that. We didn't turn you in, and you're back on the ship now, so UA is out of the question. I'm not interested in giving you a hard time about this, because it's clear there's something bothering you. But I can't help you if you don't tell me."

Still more silence, still looking at the deck.

"Well, you sure have a right to not want to talk just to me. I really think it looks like you need to talk to somebody, though. Maybe you should think about talking to Petty Officer Brannom or one of the chiefs. In the meantime, you know I have to turn you over to the CAAC. Have you ever had trouble with alcohol before?"

"Yeah." No further comment. Later, I found out that Eddie had been to Level 2 treatment before. He had been recommended for Level 3, the inpatient program, twice at prior commands, but always transferred right around the time that he was supposed to go in. That should not happen. For a sailor who needs Level 3 program, or has unresolved alcohol difficulties, they are not really eligible for transfer. If a command doesn't help a drinking sailor enough with his problem, they can't transfer him. In other words, one command cannot just ignore a fellow's problem and dump it on the unsuspecting next command. It is an added safeguard that works most of the time, but a few guys slip through the pages occasionally... and the sailor himself sometimes participates in the slip-up.

Eddie Hastings had exasperated the senior petty officers in the medical department, and Doug Kempf who had been there for two years had no confidence in him. Well into his thirties, Hastings would be facing high year tenure within a couple of years if he didn't get promoted, and it was hard to imagine that with his attitude and performance he had any chance of promotion. Art Forbes and Senior Chief McGowan determined to spend more time with him, encourage him, see what other help he needed, and be sure we got him back with the CAAC.

It turns out that Eddie had for a while been an active participant in the AA meetings, but had only been going sporadically, if at all, for the past several months. I also asked the CAAC to help us decide whether HM3 Hastings should get into Level 3 treatment. "We need to have a course of Level 2 first, Captain."

I pointed out he already had Level 2. "Well, not here on the FID, and he never really finished it." Level 2 was a kind of intense day treatment program that involved both class room, group meetings and a little individual counselling. It had a good track record in some cases, but on people who were on a brink more or less, not really hooked as it were. The Level 3 inpatient program was reserved mostly for Level 2 failures.

"How about Antabuse, Doctor Riley?" the CAAC suggested. Antabuse, or disulfiram, is a drug often used in alcohol treatment programs. There's some controversy about its role, and even about whether it helps at all. The patient takes the pill once a day, usually in the morning when well motivated. If a person with Antabuse in them consumes any alcohol, they get violently sick. Knowing that, presumably they won't take or won't tolerate alcohol in a moment of weakness later. Antabuse is surely not for everybody. Whatever merits it may or may not have, I always felt it had no role at all if the subject wasn't the one who wanted it. So the CAAC and I decided we would talk it over with Petty Officer Hastings depending on how things went during Level 2 and his AA meetings.

The next day I went to see the XO about HN Rodriguez. "I know you got the report chit about Rodriguez' DWI. He's a great corpsman, though, and I really gave him Hell yesterday. He's got the max number of hours of EMI I could assign, the Base Security took away his drivers' license, so he won't be driving his new pick up for at least six months. XO, is there any way you could just keep this down at XOI, and not make him go to Mast? Honestly, he's had plenty of punishment about this, and I'm sure we've got it under control."

"Doc, you know how strongly the Captain feels about DWI."

"Yeah, but if he knew how hard I've already come down on this guy..."

The XO said he would do what he could. I even called up to talk to Lonnie Pizza, the Ship's Secretary. I told him what I had told the XO, and asked if he could look out for the chit and maybe avoid Mast on this one case. If at all possible, I wanted to keep our problems inside the department; I never wanted one of my guys to go to Mast.

It didn't work.

Three days later, HN Rodriguez had to stand before the Commanding Officer at Captain's Mast. Underway, Mast was usually held in Aux Con so the Captain could stay near the Bridge. In port, Mast was held on the Fo'c'sle.

The Captain stood behind a lectern. The offender, in dress uniform, marched smartly to attention in front of the lectern, then respectfully removed his cover. The Command Master Chief and the Chief Master at Arms stood on either side of the CO, and the witnesses, in this case Rick Combs, HMCS McGowan, and me, stood to the Captain's left of HN Rodriguez. Although conducted a little bit like a trial, Captain's Mast is **not** a procedure to determine innocence or guilt. If you weren't guilty, you wouldn't **be** there. That's why its real name is **N**on**J**udicial **P**unishment.

Captain Pieno started off easy and reassured me from my first visit at Mast that his frightening reputation was exaggerated. I had come this morning to stand by my sailor. Usually only the DivO, Combs, and the CPO would accompany the offender. I was concerned about Rod, though, and wanted both him and the Captain to know that. I guess I hoped my being there would make it easier on him. The Captain in a normal voice said, "You are accused of operating a vehicle while under the influence of alcohol, and further more of doing that on a military reservation. That is violation of UCMJ code ____. Is that true?"

Oh no. Rod lifted his arms in that expression way he used with me and started to ramble on with an explanation. He was supposed to stay at attention. Captain Pieno did not like BSers.

Senior Chief Shulman, the Command Master Chief, intervened. "Just say 'Yes Sir' or 'No Sir' and stay at attention."

"Yes Sir"

Fortunately, the Captain didn't show any irritation. "Captain Riley, do you have anything to say?"

"Sir, HN Rodriguez is an excellent corpsman, and until this matter a squared away sailor. We've given him a very stern punishment in the department, he's going to AA meetings, and I really think we can trust him to go back to the standards he knows we expect. With the Captain's permission, I think he has learned his lesson." I hoped that would be persuasive.

"Son," he said to Rod, being I thought paternalistic, rather than intimidating, "How long have you been in the Navy?"

"Two years, Sir," Rodriguez said, remembering to stay at attention -- and obviously being even more relieved than I was that the Captain was going to counsel him rather than devour him.

Continuing on just as quietly, the Captain asked, "How long have you been a Bum?"

Rod was puzzled. He angled his head to the left like a confused puppy.

"Stay at attention when I'm talking to you!"

Rodriguez started to gesture again as though to speak. Master Chief Shulman didn't bother to step in this time. It was too late. The Captain was roaring as he cut him off.

"I'm tired of writing letters to mothers about dead sons! I'm tired of answering the police about innocent people killed by drunken bums who are too dumb to stop drinking or too damned unconcerned not to drive! Which one of those are you?!"

"...I," Rod started, unwisely, to answer...

"Don't interrupt me when I'm talking! What are you staring at me for!"

This was the Captain's Mast I had heard so much about. Captain Pieno's neck and temple veins bulged out. His head tipped to the right and left as he excoriated Rodriguez. Standing at least ten or twelve feet away, even I was a little frightened.

Finally, Rod was fined about $500, restricted to the ship for about a month, and given a suspended loss of one paygrade. That meant he wasn't busted one rank yet, but he would be with any slip ups at all. Most emphatic of all, though, was that Rod and the rest of us were trembling.

BAD NEWS JUST WON'T GO AWAY

The syringe matter was not quite over yet. One day, Captain Pieno was interviewed on the evening news in Jacksonville. Fortunately he had a lot of poise. It looked like he had probably been on television before. The interview began benignly enough. A very young reporter, somewhere between her first assignment in a very small town and her hopeful next assignment in a bigger market, was conducting the interview up on the flight deck. It was kind of a cloudy day, so the picturesque opportunities of the shipyard were suppressed by the gray background. In fact, the gray sky, the gray day, all the gray hulls around the basin behind us set a tone that was far from upbeat.

The interview began with reporter saying something about the Navy was a longtime, well-known neighbor in Jacksonville (she didn't say the term "good neighbor," though). Then she described the aircraft carrier as a floating city, and spoke about the remarkable responsibility of the Captain "for any tragedies or crimes" on the ship.

Obviously the Captain had some experience with the press because he took charge of the interview with his personality and open answers. It was a sparring match, though, with the reporter trying to stay on the offense, but the Captain answering all her questions like a friendly neighbor.

Her eyebrow rose ominously, and she said, "But the only medical waste on Florida beaches this year was from the ***Forrestal.***"

"That's not really true, you know. There were a number of items of trash from a British vessel down in the Key West area, and a number of containers for various medical supplies down in the Canaveral area that had the names of some of the commercial vessels, too. But that's not the point, Gloria. What happened a couple of weeks ago was inexcusable. We on the Forrestal, and in the Navy, feel very badly about it, and we are going to redouble our efforts to prevent this sort of thing happening again."

She then asked if anybody would be made to pay for the mistake, a question that I of course took rather personally. I was kind of afraid the Captain was going to mention my name. He said, "Remember, I am the Captain, so I am ultimately responsible for this kind of thing. If anybody should be punished, I guess it should be me. However, to answer your question, yes, there was disciplinary action taken against the department head involved."

The reporter asked, "Do you mean the Medical Department?" But the Captain just said he thought that was as far as he should go. On that, at least the televised portion of the interview, ended.

That same night, the Captain had me over to his house for dinner again. He had done that the night after the first investigation, too. We didn't even talk about the syringes or anything about the investigation.

Your Captain is your Captain, whether you're playing racquet ball with him or having dinner at his house. Away from the ship, he didn't think of **himself** as the skipper, just as John, and he invited a friendly cordiality. He and Carolyn were good hosts. He was a friend, but of course he would have to be The Captain to me. They had a lot of books in their house and enjoyed history, Stephen King, and long probing discussions about human nature, so I enjoyed visiting at their house and conversation with both of them.

Captain Pieno had begun his career as a navigator on transport air craft, I think. During the Viet Nam War, there was a great need for A-6 BN's... because so many of them were being shot down. Captain Pieno loved the go-fast side of aviation, so the A-6 appealed to him. A lot of people, especially A-6 BN's, will tell you that the person who is really in charge of the A-6 is the BN, not the pilot. (Of course, A-6 pilots, of which Tim Thomassy, the next Captain of the Forrestal was an example, had a somewhat different view.) Well, Pieno apparently became one of the most decorated aviators in Viet Nam, and he had thousands of hours in the A-6. He had a very successful career after that, too. Nobody seemed indifferent about John Pieno. Some people in the A-6 community just didn't like him at all. They would say that he was pushy and aggressive. The others, about equal in number to the first group, either had worked for him and said they would follow him any time, any place and under any circumstances. Or they had not worked for him, but they admired the way he fought for his squadron and fought for getting good things for his squadron.

While he was a squadron commanding officer, and maybe a few years before that, there was a reservist named John Lehman, who was also an A-6 BN. Lehman apparently had never been on sustained active duty, but had served all of his Navy time exclusively in the Reserves. His fulltime job was in and out of government, with various jobs in the Department of Defense. At a certain time, though, in his very early 40's he became the Secretary of the Navy. While in that job, he continued his Reserve obligations, including his annual 2 weeks of active duty. John Pieno was known to have been a friend. Lehman spent at least one of his active duty times serving in the squadron Pieno commanded. Once when asked what it was like having SECNAV be a lieutenant in his squadron, Pieno was quoted as saying, "It's no problem. I treat him just like I'd treat **any** Secretary of the Navy."

The competition is keen to become a squadron commanding officer. The competition for ship commands is even tighter, being chosen only from among the very top-rated squadron CO's. So at each cutoff point, there are plenty of opportunities for jealous also-rans to complain about those who win the jobs. There were rumors that Captain Pieno only won command of the "RAG" (Replacement Air Group, an advanced tactical training squadron) because of his connection with Secretary Lehman. The same rumors would say that's how he was selected for command of a carrier too. Captain Pieno knew those rumors. He didn't ever comment on them in my presence, and I'm sure he didn't to anybody else either. Being friends with the Secretary of the Navy would not explain why his first squadron and the RAG were both fabulously successful, nor would it explain why he got the Battle E as CO of the ***Savannah***, his requisite "deep draft" command before taking over a carrier.

Therefore, it seemed to me that if there were any advantages to being a friend of the Secretary of the Navy, they were indirect. Also, Pieno was no "yes man" so I was convinced that his success was deserved. His time on the ***Forrestal*** was drawing short, and he would be up for Admiral in about a year. Years ago, he had decided that if he did not make Admiral, he was not going to "hang around." Being a Navy Captain is something a lot of people aspire to, not what I would call "hanging around." He had been on the fast track his entire career, though. I knew what he meant. Although he and I did not discuss it, I was more than a little worried about whether this flap with the syringes would spoil his shot. We would find out in a couple of months when the Battle E would be announced. If Forrestal could get the Battle E, I figured it would not leave any lasting scars on the Captain. I found myself among those who would work for Captain Pieno anytime.

************************* *************************

As the autumn wore on, Art and the SuppO forced Master Chief Morgan to let us monitor his blood pressure. Sure enough, the medicine Art had been giving him worked... when he took it. No particular side effects that bothered him, he just didn't like to take medicine. Also, the Master Chief's wife, the SuppO, and Art all told me he didn't have slurred speech at all. That's the way he had always talked. Must have been my imagination. I did worry now, though, whether the blood pressure could have done it. As a neurologist, I knew a lot of people had subtle cerebral or pontine effects from their hypertension that unsuspecting observers do not easily recognize. While we couldn't convince him to give up the cigarettes, he did take the medicine, and his pressure stayed around 135-145/95-100.

These were the last days that Ozark would be with us. I spent as much time as I could hanging around his office. That wasn't much with the schedule we were keeping, but in our short friendship he had been good to me and he was a fountain of necessary wit and humor. On his office bulkhead there was a painting of a squinty-eyed, gnarled up cowboy with his tobacco stained teeth gritted and his stubbled chin in a sneer. A caption at the bottom of the painting said, "There was a helluva lot of things they didn't tell me when I signed on with this outfit." I used to like to come and sit in his office and bask in the wisdom of the painting.

THE NEW XO

One day, I flounced in looking for his reassuring optimism and humor, but I was suddenly struck dumb. There was a strange Commander sitting with him, wearing a leather flight jacket without a Forrestal patch.

"Hey, Doc, I'd like you to meet my relief, Mitchell Vaughan!" Mitchell Vaughan had just come by to begin an orientation. He wouldn't be checking in until later. A year or two younger than I was, he had a friendly handshake, an open smile, and a great reputation. With a quick excuse about needing to go save lives or something, I ducked out of the office. The nerve of that guy; taking Ozark's place! We would get acquainted later, I knew.

One late October evening we were finishing coffee after dinner, when Lt Steve Tobia, who was the JOOD, got a call on his brick. A young sailor from the Air Department who was UA from work that morning was reportedly holding his wife at gunpoint in their mobile home and refusing to let her in or anyone else out. Steve excused himself to find out the details, but the story pretty much took the pleasure out of after dinner conversation, so the crowd dispersed. I followed Steve out to the phone in the lounge and sat around while he got the story.

"Well, guess there's no firearm. That part was incorrect. Domestic dispute, apparently no violence, just a lot of shouting. He refuses to come out. Apparently his wife is still there, but he's not keeping her."

"You going to call him?"

"They don't have a phone, just use the phone booth at the trailer park."

There were several mobile home parks out on Mayport road, ranging from pretty nice to o.k. None of them were really awful, although a couple did adjoin auto salvage dealers or honky tonks.

"I think I'll have to go out there and investigate," Steve said.

"Lieutenant, I don't think that's a very good idea. First of all, investigating is the Police's job. Secondly, there was a report of a firearm..."

"We know that was incorrect, though."

"How! You only have the same quality of information refuting it that you had reporting it! Domestic disputes are some of the most dangerous things that even professional experienced officers deal with. People get blown away by husbands with guns. Why don't you ask the base police to go check it out first?"

Lt Tobia was willing to try that, so he called the base police. They had no jurisdiction out in town, they told him.

"Well, you'll have to call the local police."

That was a less popular idea.

"Doc, we don't even know that there's anything illegal yet. If we get the local police involved, it really escalates everything a lot further than we want it to go. I'll have to go out there and check it out."

There was no talking him out of it, so I went along.

We drove out the gate down Mayport Ave and I noticed the trailer parks more than I had before. The first couple of parks closest to the gate looked pretty rough. One on the left side was out behind an auto parts and salvage lot. In fact, it wasn't so much behind as it was merged into the gravel-surfaced lanes of the park. The aluminum and powdery faded paint of the frayed small trailers blended imperceptibly with the car carcasses and hub caps scattered around. One expected chickens to run out from under the scattered machinery parts. A little further down, there was a park with the big seventy-footers, many of them with siderooms sticking out. None of these were frayed. The lanes were paved, and there were small well-kept yards around each trailer.

Finally, we came to the one we were looking for. This one had only rental mobile homes. It was out behind a laundromat and a small half-occupied shopping row. It was a hot evening, and all the hinged windows on the trailers were open -- which meant these weren't airconditioned. Here and there folks sat on the little steps up to their front doors sipping from an RC or beer bottle.

Two Naval Officers in uniform, one carrying a brick, are pretty obvious in a trailer park, even in Mayport. "That's the one you're looking for. Over there," shouted one of the porch-sitters, a guy in bib overalls and no shirt. The brown trailer he pointed to was one of the few with all the windows closed, but at least the door was open.

I insisted we call to the trailer from behind a tree. LT Tobia was embarrassed by this, but went along anyway. "Jones," he called, "This is LT Tobia from the ship! Doctor Riley is here with me. Can we talk to you?"

No answer.

He called a couple of times without answers. I was getting a little nervous. Could this be the behavior of a dangerous young man. Or could he have killed himself and his wife?

The neighbors had been watching this for a while, but the guy in the overalls spoke up again. "Ain't nobody in there anymore. They been gone a half hour or so."

Timidly, we walked up to the trailer and peaked in. No bodies. There was a .45 automatic pistol on a table in the living room. So much for the "It's safe, there's no weapon" philosophy. Back at the door, a little boy on a bicycle said, "They're down at the phone," and pointed over to the laudromat. Over there was a young couple, one of them just hanging up the phone, the other staring toward us. When they saw us looking at them, they started walking our direction.

The young woman didn't look disturbed at all, but the sailor was obviously very tired. He was disheveled. His eyes were boggy and dark. His clothes were rumpled. "He's OK," the woman said. "He's calmed down now."

"You ready to go back to the ship, AN Jones?" the lieutenant asked.

The sailor said he would, but he wanted to get some things out of the trailer. I talked him out of that because of the gun. Lt Tobia took the Airman back to the ship when one of the chaplains arrived.

It seems that Airman Jones was 18 and Mrs. Jones was 16. They had been married only shortly before the deployment, neither of them had been out of Tennessee before. They couldn't afford a car. She had not been able to get a job. The only way they could afford the rent of this trailer was to take in a couple of subletters to rent bedrooms. When Mrs. Jones and one of the renters told Jones the day before that they were having a child, AN Jones expressed his great disapproval of that plan. The other guy left in a hurry, but Jones kept his wife in the trailer all day fretting about the gun. They had just been on the phone with her parents, trying to get enough money for her to return to Tennessee.

We brought Jones back to the ship. A skinny, morose fellow who looked a little older than his 18 years, he didn't want to talk much. Later that night, we arranged to admit him to the psychiatry unit at NHJax, because I was worried about his injuring himself. The Chaplains and ombudsmen tried to help Mrs. Jones get back to Tennessee, but she needed a couple of days to get her things together.

I sat down late that night trying to figure how to write up the report for the Captain.

CHAPTER VIII. CHANGE OF COMMAND

Gradually, the autumn gave way to winter, as much as Florida can. The SRA remained intense. With the needle guns clanging away all night to resurface the hangar bay above my stateroom, I had to shift up to the Gator's cabin on the O-3 level for a few weeks. My admiration for Doug and Art grew weekly. Their work days began before 0700 every morning, and many days ended late in the evening. On rare occasions they were able to finish up and go home by 1600. Years ago when I worked at Bethesda, I scorned medical folks who went home that early. I used to think it was more evidence that the guys on the ships didn't work as hard as us hospital doctors. I knew better now. Their average work day, even in port, was more than 10 hours, sometimes stretching well past 16. Even that tally overlooked the fact that sometimes they would go to work in October and not get home until April. Whenever they could find an eight or even a six hour work day, they were welcome to it. Despite Art's crusty attitude, and Doug's stern Prussian personality, they were both very good clinicians, the kind of people I would like to have for a family doctor.

Turnover in the ship's company was high at this time. The Personnel Department on the ship, along with BUPERS up in Washington, tried to concentrate the turnover to homeport periods. So, we were seeing probably more than 200 new people every month. Also, the Reagan buildup years were conspicuously drawing to a close. Not everybody who left the ship was going to be replaced. All the parts of the ship still had to function, but we would be doing it with fewer people. The fact was that the services were shrinking. Little did we recognize how much they would be shrinking in the next 5 to 10 years, as events would prove later.

One of the new people was the XO. Shortly after he relieved Ozark, he summoned me down to his office to brief him on the Medical Department and the health of the ship. Mitchell Vaughan had a reputation of being one of the hardest working and brightest people in the HS community, the people who fly the H3. In the first few minutes with him, it was obvious that he deserved the reputation. Showing him a few tables and lists of our personnel and our inventories, I started a prepared brief to describe the department. "Our main functions can be described as preventive medicine, occupational health, medical treatment ..."

"In preventive medicine, do you distribute condoms?" he interrupted.

Caught off guard a little, I said, "Well, yes and no." The issue of condoms was really more complicated than it seemed on first blush. Yes, we did have condoms in the department, and whenever a sailor came to ask for one, we gave him at least two -- opportunities to need them sometimes can be more than once a night. Condoms were for sale in the ship's store, where sailors could easily get them. Furthermore, by tradition and regulation certain self care hygienic items like sunburn lotion, insect repellant, and condoms are Class VI items, self care supplies, not medical. It had been demonstrated over the years that sailors who had enough foresight to come down to the medical department for their condom would be just as likely go to the ship's store and buy one. It wasn't the **price** of condoms that kept sailors from using them, it was **thinking** about them in advance. The fortunes of youth sometimes place young people in an opportunity they had not foreseen. It's not being *free* that makes condoms be popular, but being *thought about.*

"Do you make them available when guys leave the ship on liberty?"

We were getting into details here, when I thought we were going to be going over the department in general. Only thirty minutes were scheduled, then the SuppO was coming to brief him. Were we going to spend the whole time on condoms, I wondered?

"Not on the quarterdeck..."

"Why not?" the new XO interrupted, "I think we ought to be ***proactive*** on this, don't you? I mean, you're the doctor."

I tried to explain that use of condoms wasn't simply related to ease of acquisition. He didn't agree with that. Then I reminded him of the complications of wives' opinions and public relations considerations in giving out condoms as sailors depart the ship, and the XO said, "We'll do it smart, though, we won't just do it without thinking."

The XO conducted the rest of the brief asking questions. He was well-informed and knew the most important areas related to health on the ship. I didn't always get a chance to fully answer his questions before he brought up a new one, but I was impressed by his depth of information and his energy level. Beyond the information we exchanged, though, this interview just kind of clarified for the record something that was already clear enough for me. I already knew without being told who was in charge. But if I'd had any doubts, today's talk demonstrated who was the XO and who was the Doc.

The drudgery of the SRA was wearing on everybody. Although the yard workers had been cheerful at first, the incidence of minor skirmishes between the yard workers and crew members were increasing. Cigarette butts lay about the deck in corners here and there. Workers usually did not clean up at the end of a shift unless they were forced to. That caused friction because the crew, even the youngest and newest members, thought of the ship as something more than just home. The ship, kind of like Jonah's whale, was alive to us, part of our family. To the yard workers, it was just a dirty place where they had to come to work. That difference in attitude, taken together with the crew's restlessness, set a little bit more distance between the yard workers and us. We never had any major outward problems with them, but the everyday friction built up gradually. The yard workers with their black, grimy Harley-Davidson tee shirts, scraggly hair poking out from under their hard hats, occasionally dropping a cigarette butt on the deck... These guys shared the tight passageways and work spaces with well scrubbed young men in dungarees or khakis, who were proud of doing well on inspections, and looked on the environment as a kind of parent.

The yard workers, non-union mostly in this shop, periodically complained about the "great deal" the military members had with various benefits packages. For their part, all the military people realized that their ragged looking counterparts had incomes double or triple a Navy salary.

The SRA just seemed to go on and on. We had reached a point where the big round pipes and myriad cables seemed to be just regular parts of the ship. The nuisance was so ingrained we almost forgot to wish for it to go away. We saw shipmates moving on, had to adjust to new coworkers and new bosses, and somewhere in the back of our minds, knew we had to get ready for the deployment with a long series of workups yet to come.

As January wore on, we began to think about Captain Pieno's relief. He had been in a command a little bit more than a year and a half, his time had to be coming to an end. The Battle E would not be announced until sometime in late March. We all wanted to win it, as much for the Captain as for ourselves, and we wanted him to be there when we got it. The crew would miss him.

In the Department Head meetings, we were already missing the old XO. Things were different. Where Ozark used to ask for advice and invite interchange, Mitchell said how he wanted things done. He was a bright officer and had a lot of experience, of which he was very confident. He didn't seem to need our advice or experience as much as his predecessor. The new AIMD Officer, CDR Kevin Myette, a feisty shortstop of a guy, joined me and "Clark" in trying to needle the XO whenever we could. It didn't make much difference, though. The new proliferation of memos and instructions kept growing, and the XO never let up on his constant attention to detail.

Captain Pieno had inherited a good ship's crew from his predecessor, Tim Wright. The ship had just completed a major renovation before Pieno took over. With his own version of "tough love," occasional detonations at Captain's Mast, but his obvious affection for the crew, he would be missed.

Since the SRA began, there had been a 15 to 20 percent turnover in the ship's company. Of the 85 percent who had been there a while, none were indifferent about Captain Pieno. About 10 percent were deadly afraid of him. They had either seen him at Captain's Mast or reprimanding somebody, or they had heard the legends. Another 5 or 10 percent disliked him, or stronger. These might include officers or chiefs he had chewed out. I still considered myself a little bruised from the episode after Portsmouth, for example. Some didn't like his cowboy reputation, his old-fashioned Hell-bent-for-leather aviator attitude. Some people, mostly aviators, were simply jealous of his success, I suppose.

Nobody was indifferent to Captain Pieno. Everybody else thought he was one of the best leaders in the Navy, and were devoted to him. I was among this group. I admired the way that both he and Snuffy came down to the Ward everyday on the cruise to see our patients, each of them coming alone and not drawing attention to themselves when they did it. The positive attitude among the young sailors on the ship, the exuberance of everybody who was a member of the team, all these were the responsibility of the Captain. Most of all, though, was the way he had stood behind me after the syringes. I would always wonder whether that event and the notoriety around it was what kept him from making admiral. He must have wondered about it, too. He never showed me any rancor or resentment, though. In my lowest days, he just invited me over to play racquet ball. Of course, I was one of the few guys he could always beat in racquet ball, but I think he may have invited me even if I could beat him.

The new CO had been identified, an A6 pilot named Louis Thomassy. We began hearing one thing or another about him in January. He had mostly been a West Coast sailor. The OHO, Mel Swartz, had worked with him when Captain Thomassy was the CAG on the ***Midway***. He liked him, and said that he had a particularly good touch with the crew. The XO warned he was known as a "religious zealot," and implied there would be a puritanical change in the way things were done on the ***Forrestal.***

Captain Thomassy was apparently a Chief of Staff in a Surface Group up in Norfolk. The first week in February, he came to visit the ship for a few hours. We heard him bonged aboard, but nobody saw him. He and Captain Pieno visited for a couple of hours, then we heard him bonged off again. That kind of surprised me, because if it took 7 days for John Bigbee and me to turn over just in the Medical Department, I figured it would take at least 10 days to 2 weeks for the commanding officers go over everything about this behemoth.

The SRA continued, the passageways were dingy and dusty. The noise continued to be awful. However, the week after Captain Thomassy came to visit, we had a going-away party for Captain Pieno and Carolyn. It was held down at a fancy Saw Grass Hotel in Ponta Vedra, south of Mayport. We had some roasting speeches to say good-bye to Captain Pieno. We all had an opportunity to give him some gifts as mementos. From the Medical Department, we gave him a fish hook that Doug Kempf had been saving for over a year, and I recounted the story behind it. During the last workup cycle before the deployment, the FID was operating in the Caribbean. In the middle of one critical tactical operation the radio beamed up an emergency call from a fishing trawler. Someone on the trawler had reportedly traumatically amputated his arm and was bleeding to death. Captain Pieno terminated the tactical operation and turned the ship around, traveling about 20 miles to be within helicopter range of the trawler.

They launched an H3 from the Red Lions, to save the fisherman's life. It turns out that instead of an amputation of his forearm, he had a fish hook through one of his fingers. When brought to the ship, he was crying out and thrashing about, but Doug Kempf had simply removed the fish hook, soaked his finger, and the man returned with only a minor puncture wound. In order to "save" this life, the super carrier had terminated an entire day of tactical operation, hundreds of air flights, and an awful lot of DFM. I was able to embellish the story a little bit when I told it, but Captain Pieno was pleased to have the fish hook as a memento. Then at the end of my speech I said, "I'm sorry that's all we have to give you, Captain. We in the Medical Department also bought you a very expensive gift, but in a moment of carelessness I just threw it over the side." Everybody in the audience knew what throwing things over the side meant to us that year, so the remark brought the house down.

The week after the dinner, all of the trailers and wagons were finally removed from Hangar Bay One, and the doors between Bay One and Bay Two were closed. The deck up in Bay One was painted nicely, and all the pad eyes were painted white. Banners and flags hung from the overheads, and a dias was up in the forward end of the hangar. Clearly, plans were being made for the Change of Command Ceremony. It was announced that Captain Thomassy would relieve Captain Pieno on the 25th of February.

Preparations for the Change of Command told us a little more about the new XO. Meetings with him were not exchanges or dialogues, but soliloquies. These often came with his pointing out that some department or another had not taken some action that he wanted. "But how was I to know you wanted that?" the department head might ask.

"Didn't you read the 5050?" That is the serial number for administrative notices about conferences or meetings. The XO and his new Ad-Min Officer, Max Small, liked to put things in writing. There was a proliferation of 5050's on a bewildering variety of subjects. They had become so numerous, they sometimes got all clogged up in the memo production line, a memo logjam. Like too much paper in the commode, their bulk hampered their own flow. The 5050s sometimes did not arrive until the deadline listed in a memo had passed. So, at various meetings the XO found himself berating somebody for not complying with a memo he hadn't received yet.

For the Change of Command, Rear Admiral Dunleavy, Commander of Naval Air Forces Atlantic Fleet (COMNAVAIRLANT or just AIRLANT), would be the guest speaker. Admiral Dunleavy was about the first NFO to reach flag rank, and probably the first NFO who had commanded an air craft carrier. He was an A6 BN, just like Captain Pieno, and the only flag officer I ever saw with a Boston accent. According to rumor, Admiral Dunleavy and Captain Pieno did not get along, and apparently it went back a number of years. Some speculated that it was because of Captain Pieno's close relationship with John Lehman, others said it was because Pieno's squadron had showed up Admiral Dunleavy professionally some years before. Yet others noticed a difference in their personalities and suggested Admiral Dunleavy may have disliked or envied Captain Pieno's flamboyant style.

Since Admiral Dunleavy, as Commander of AIRLANT had the main vote in awarding the Battle E, many doubted that we would have a shot at it as long as Captain Pieno was in command. I, of course, fretted that the ship's otherwise flawless record would be blemished by our syringes. They had, after all, received a lot of press at the end of the deployment.

The week before the Change of Command, Captain Thomassy came to the Forrestal for two days of meetings with all of his department heads. The XO lined us all up and requested that we rehearse our briefs with him before we spoke to the new boss. He suggested I change a number of the things I was going to say, and gave me some guidance on words and sentence structure in my brief. From the grumbling that afternoon in the Ward Room, I suspected the XO had given other department heads similar explicit guidance in how to brief the new skipper.

When the time came for my brief, Tod Graef and I discovered that the XO had scheduled us in a combined brief as though Medical and Dental were part of the same department. Walking down the passageway to the office he was using for interviews, we encountered a tall thin man with frosty grey-white hair and recruiting-poster posture, his shoulders squared back. He was wearing his leather flight jacket with a squadron patch on one side and a Midway patch on the other. Tod whispered to me that "He looks like he's been sent from Central Casting." I knew what he meant. The new skipper had a bearing a little bit like Jeff Chandler. With his shoulders squared back and his crest of white hair, I remembered what I had been told about his being a religious zealot, and I braced myself for a strict introduction.

As soon as he spoke, though, my apprehensions disappeared. A very cordial, and friendly personality, Tim Thomassy had a folksy manner about him, and actually a kind of country accent. He was from western Pennsylvania, but his manner of speech was midwestern, almost Missouri. Before he heard anything about our departments, he wanted to learn about us personally. He told us a little bit about his own background and his family, and he said, "Look, I can't learn everything about your department in 2 weeks, much less a half an hour. I just wanted to meet you guys now and see if there is anything you need me to work on immediately. We'll get into detail gradually as we get to know each other." Neither of us had emergent problems. We were both so fond of Captain Pieno that we were apprehensive about whoever would take his place, and we probably expected some kind of ogre that day. We were so relieved by how pleasant he was that we were almost speechless.

There were a number of interesting contrasts between Captain Pieno and Captain Thomassy. By his own description, Captain Pieno had been a borderline juvenile delinquent in his youth, and he used to say that he spent a major part of his teenage years on probation. He had one of those hand-made tatoos with the word "John" on his left shoulder. He would like you to infer it was put there by a rebellious teenager on his first night in jail. If you suspected there was still just a touch of the outlaw lurking under the skin, Captain Pieno would not intentionally dissuade you. Captain Thomassy was a scholar athlete who went to the Naval Academy. After the Academy, Thomassy was married to his high school sweetheart for over 25 years. Pieno's second wife Carolyn, was almost 20 years his junior. He drove a bright burgundy Porsche, Thomassy a small, tan pickup truck. Except in his flashes of fire, Pieno had an urbane, smooth way about him. Captain Thomassy, by contrast, had an open, almost "aw shucks" ingenuousness. While they both came from A6s, Thomassy was a pilot, Pieno was a bombardier-navigator.

Yet, they had much in common, too. After all they were both from Intruders. After thousands of hours flying in that airplane, a camaraderie exists among people who have to do it together. There is an attitude about counting on another guy in that airplane, about sharing, about an entire philosophy of flight that extends into your general being. Both of them operated at a very personal level. Their styles were to give trust and to be trusted. They demanded a lot of their people, but gave instant and permanent loyalty to those who lived up. They were both very accomplished officers, after all they had both achieved command of an air craft carrier. Ambition is the driving force among a lot of naval officers. These were two men who cared more about their crew and more about accomplishing the mission than they did about their own careers. That was one of the most striking features about each of their personalities, and something that became evident within the first day of knowing them.

There were a number of Changes of Command that winter. Just a week or two before I had been to the Change of Command for the VA-37 Bulls in which "Shaky" Jacobson took over from "Jet" O'Hora. The bigger the organization, the better the Ceremony. Change of Command on an air craft carrier is a rousing experience! In a different time of year with a better weather guarantee, a ceremony could be held up on the flight deck. In winter we had to settle for the hangar bay as a reasonable second. It is as tall, as wide, and much longer than a big city auditorium. Over in one corner the band plays a medley of marches, mostly Marine and Navy songs. The ship's divisions stand at parade rest in formation in their sparkling uniforms. Then the music stops, the XO over in another corner reads off the names of the dignitaries. By Naval custom, a Bos'n's Mate rings the ship's bell to introduce flag officers or other commanding officers.

Just like watching a Shakespearian play or a familiar opera, anticipation only enhanced the excitement. Knowing what was coming next only intensifies the pageantry

Bong, bong... "Commander Carrier Air Wing 6 arriving." Pat Martini Hauert, the CAG, entered. Bong,bong... "Captain Louis E. Thomassy, U.S. Navy, Arriving." The bell again and then, "***Forrestal***, arriving,"to introduce Captain Pieno. The Commanding Officer is never introduced by name, just by the name of his command.

Then came the flag officers. Navy and Marine Corps bands always try to do outdo one another in the jaunty, snappy, almost jazzy quality of Ruffles and Flourishes. It has such a spunky, sassy swagger that it announces to any audience, "We may be admirals here, but don't forget we're sailors." Admirals get more bongs than Captains. First, came our new Battle Group Commander, Admiral Richard C. Allen. His call sign was "Sweet Pea," but it was going to take a while for me to figure out why they ever called him that. The first few times I saw him, he had such a stern almost frowning appearance that I expected him to be a grouch. I wouldn't know Admiral Allen as well as I did Admiral Smith or my captains, but I came to realize he was a man with a good sense of humor, and a warm personality. Finally, came the star of the day, Commander Naval Air Forces Atlantic Fleet, Rear Admiral (two stars) Dunleavy.

For true believers, these ceremonies are almost intoxicating. The music, the coordination, the celebration of pride and dedication, all convey an overpowering and pervasive sense of community, of family, of belonging.

The Chaplain said a brief prayer, in the ecumenical all-encompassing style that Navy chaplains use. Then Admiral Dunleavy gave his speech.

There was a rumbling of anticipation as to whether he would announce the Battle E, but we knew that it was not due for another month or so. It just would have been a nice touch if he could tell us that day. Dunleavy had a way of pacing semi-informally on the platform when he spoke. It would have been a distracting habit for some speakers, but it just seemed natural with him, and conveyed his sense of comfort and conversation with the audience. He spoke of these being uncertain times, of these being years of change, he said the only thing certain about our future was uncertainty, and that the face of national defense would have to change, that America would always need the kind of people we had on Forrestal to represent American values. Familiar ideas shared sincerely among friends are not mere platitudes. Besides, he told us things we liked hearing, so we were all pretty well pumped up.

Then at the end of his speech he said, "I know you're all wanting to hear about the Battle E. It's not due for another 6 weeks.

"... But the Forrestal is the E! Here, John [speaking to Pieno], you know you won it, or rather your crew won it in spite of you. Congratulations, men of ***Forrestal.***" We were all on our feet cheering one another and the Captain, and not a few of us were choked up. Then the Admiral turned to give Captain Pieno the Legion of Merit.

On the starboard side of the hangar, a gray and white blur flickered in my peripheral vision, and I heard a tub-like "thunk." Four sailors in the formation suddenly slouched down on one knee to look at something on the deck, and an arm waved in my direction. I ran over there, and saw a six-foot tall, black bos'n's mate face down on the deck. There was a little blood over by his left shoulder. He slammed over like a tree right in formation staying at attention all the way down to the deck. Military formations not uncommonly have somebody black out, a little bit more often in a hot environment. It was a little warm on the hangar bay that day, but not hot. Nonetheless, standing at attention, immobile for about 45 minutes, the blood pools in a young man's lower extremities, and he can faint. Usually his buddies will grab his elbows, may think they're helping by propping him up, but by doing this they deprive him of the horizontal position that would allow blood to go back to his head. In this case he fell straight forward just like there were hinges on his toes and he were a straight oaken door.

Well, that was the end of the Change of Command ceremony for me. Seaman Crowell had a through and through laceration on his chin, an abrasion on his nose, and one broken tooth. Fainting was what made him fall, but he hit the deck so hard that he sustained a concussion also. We had to take him down by litter to the Medical Department to scrub up his abrasions and sew his chin back together. About the time I finished sewing the seaman back up, I heard on the 1MC the dignitaries departing the ship to go over for their formal luncheon. After the admirals were bonged off, I heard Captain Pieno being piped over the side by name for the first (and last) time, "Captain John A. Pieno, U.S. Navy, departing." And then almost incongruously, Bong, Bong, "Forrestal, departing." That, of course, was Thomassy. The Change of Command was complete. We had a new skipper.

After the guy who fainted on the hangar deck, it was quiet most of the rest of that day. It occurred to me a few times that could be a harbinger of how things would go with our new easy-going Captain. The SRA was drawing to a close, and we knew that workups would begin pretty soon.

Late that night, after finishing up some paper work in the office, I trudged out toward my stateroom and I bumped into HM1 Hugh Beaumont in the passageway. He had duty the night before, I thought, why was he here tonight?

"Tell you the truth, Captain, my wife and I are having some problems, so I'm staying on the ship for a while."

"Sorry to hear that, HM1. Seemed like things have been going better for you." When he came to see me after our last talk, a couple of nights' sleep had made him a lot better. The rambling, peculiar talk had disappeared, and I dismissed it as due to fatigue.

Beaumont's work and records had been slipping a little lately, though. The chiefs and I had discussed it just the day before.

"Anything I can do, Hugh? Want to talk for a while"

"No, she's just tired of me, that's all. I'm just not enough anymore. She's just a bitch, that's all." And he walked away downcast. My Dad always warned me not to get involved in people's marriages or romances.

I went to bed that night around 2000 and started reading the new Larry McMurtry book ***Texasville,*** which I enjoyed until I fell asleep about an hour later. At 2300 one of the corpsmen had to come down and bang on my door. "Captain, we need you down in the Emergency Room." It was Master Chief Morgan, the guy Art had brought to us about the blood pressure. He was having trouble breathing. His wife was there, too, and she was pretty anxious. Although they lived only ten minutes from the Navy Hospital, an hour's drive away from us, they never liked it much at the Navy Hospital, so they came all the way here to the ship, where despite Art's scolding, the Master Chief trusted the medical care. Probably not the best choice that particular night. He was plenty sick.

"He can't breathe," his wife said. "He says he can't get a deep breath. We just got home today, and he's been like this the whole time. I had to talk him into coming in."

"You having any pain, Master Chief?"

He didn't want to talk much, like he had to spare his breathe. "No..." quick inhale, "just hard to breathe."

I listened to his lungs while one of the corpsmen took his blood pressure. His heartbeat was over 100. His lungs had the wet rales throughout that meant pulmonary edema... severe congestive failure. His blood pressure was around 220/150. He was restless, couldn't sit still, characteristic of pulmonary edema.

"Let's get some oxygen started right now. Master Chief, have you been taking your medicine?"

He nodded yes.

"No he hasn't!" His wife interjected. "Yesterday, I noticed most of the pills were still in the bottle, so I got on him about it."

I gave him some furosemide, a diuretic, intravenously, and we took an EKG. It only showed what we call a strain pattern, but the rhythm, except for being fast, was normal.

Going to the phone to call the Mayport Clinic for an ambulance, I told the guys to take a chest Xray right away while we waited for the ambulance.

"You'll have to wait while we call the ACLS ambulance from town. We can't send a cardiac patient in our ambulances," the corpsman from the clinic told me.

"OK, but this guy isn't having an MI or an arrest. He's got malignant hypertension and pulmonary edema. What he needs isn't ACLS. It's to get to the hospital in a hurry."

The chest Xray confirmed the pulmonary edema and the Master Chief was doing a little better after the diuretic and on the oxygen. Ten minutes went by and no word about the ambulance. I called the clinic back.

"One of Liberty's ACLS ambulances is down and the other one is on a call. We had to call another one from town. They should be over there in about half an hour."

"No way! This guy needs to go to the hospital. You people have four ambulances over there, why don't you send one over here like I asked?"

"Sir, I told you we can't send a BLS ambulance for a cardiac patient."

"But what this guy needs is rapid transport, not defibrillators. Do you have a physician on duty?"

"Yes, sir, I'll have Dr. White call you."

We gave the Master Chief some nifedipine, that got his pressure down a little.

Two or three minutes later, Dr. White called. "Hello, Doctor White speaking. I'm a family physician."

I explained the case again and asked for help in transporting the patient as soon as we could over to the hospital.

"Well, what if something happened en route?" He asked.

"What if something happens by not sending him? He's not having an arrest, he needs to get to the hospital for treatment. What are those ambulances for?"

"All right, but you'll have to take responsibility..."

Take responsibility! "You son of a bitch, that's what I ***do*** for a living. Just send us the ambulance please." I called the Emergency Room over at the hospital -- where I was wishing Mrs. Morgan would have brought the Master Chief in the first place -- to pass on all his details and to tell them he was coming.

Our ER was busy that night, and I sent one of our best corpsmen over in the ambulance with the Master Chief.

Thirty minutes later, I was finishing up with a fellow who had sprained an ankle when the ER from NHJax called.

"Is this *Captain* Riley?" When they wanted to show contempt for you, they called you by rank rather than "Doctor."

"Yes, are you calling about Master Chief Morgan? Thanks for getting back to us so soon."

"Yes. Well. Did you know that Mr. Morgan is in pulmonary edema." Funny what goes through your mind sometimes. A Master Chief Petty Officer hates to be called "Mr." His name is "Master Chief."

"Of course, that's why we sent him to you..."

"Well, for a life-threatening disease, don't you think you should tell us before transporting someone like this? I mean I'm going to go ahead and take care of your patient, but we don't have to accept a patient in transfer without prior consultation."

In fact, it had been a different doctor I spoke to forty minutes ago. "But I did. Didn't Dr. Holt tell you the patient was coming?"

"No. The first we knew of the patient was when he arrived on our door."

I explained that I had discussed the entire case with Dr. Holt, including past history, EKG findings, course and treatment here, the whole works. Dr. Holt's shift ended after that and he had not passed the information along to this angry doctor.

"I find that hard to believe," the new doctor told me. "That doesn't sound like Dr. Holt. We have the patient here now. They can sort out the rest of the problem in the morning."

Master Chief Morgan was admitted to the ICU that night, and his breathing improved a little as the night went on.

Early the next morning I called to find out about his progress, and as usual the nurse in the unit said, "I'm sorry, we can't discuss patients on the telephone."

"May I speak to the Master Chief's doctor, please?"

The staff doctor was too busy to talk to me all day, but I was at last able to talk to one of the interns on his case, who explained that it was hard to get his blood pressure down still, but "I guess you know Mr. Morgan was pretty sick. They really botched up his care over on the ship. He's lucky to be alive. They didn't call to say he was coming over or anything. Just sent him over in a BLS ambulance. Lucky he didn't have an arrest on the way over here."

Yeah, lucky.

About an hour after that I got a call from the CO of the hospital, who had been called by Dr. White from the clinic. "What the hell's going on over there!"

I yelled back a little and he backed off. Later, though, I found out that Dr. White and the second ER doctor had filed a Quality Assurance complaint about me at the hospital.

The most important thing was that the Master Chief's blood pressure got the treatment he needed. A couple of months later, though, we learned he was transferred to one of the universities for further treatment and finally had to leave the Navy on disability.

That was a busy week in the department. We had a lot of patients besides looking after the paperwork that seemed to be growing as we filled out more and more reports in the advancing workup cycle. We were still readjusting the department for the new XO and the new Skipper, too. This week, the XO wanted to talk about "no shave chits." He decided that we had been too lax in issuing no shave chits and he wanted to "tighten up" the system.

Navy uniform regulations require a clean-shaven face. Sailors can wear moustaches, but have not been allowed beards for a decade or more.[8] Whiskery stubble, however, has never been allowed. Well... except for the "no shave chit." With a medical excuse, a sailor would usually be permitted to avoid shaving. Sounds simple, doesn't it? It is simple for the individual healing from a transient problem, like eczema, or a cut. He grows a little stubble for a few days until the lesion heals and then he resumes shaving. The chit from the doctor shows the boss that he's under treatment. The problem is something called *pseudofolliculitis barbi.*

The term means a condition of the beard ("barbi") that imitates folliculitis, infection of the hair follicles. It brings tears to all ships doctors in the U.S. Navy. A saga of our time, there is pain in the PFB story for everybody. It is a legalistic bureaucratic mire-pit, a recalcitrant medical problem, a military principle, a turf battle, and in the bargain a racial symbol too.

Curly or kinky hair is shaped the way it is because it grows out of its follicles real flat and it loops around the way package ribbon would if you pushed it out from a slit. A long curly hair with a natural rounded tip merely circles itself around and around making loops. When a flat hair is cut, though, its own tip turns into a sharp little flat edge. As it grows, each sharp little hair kinks back around, and likes to dig back into skin or into an adjacent follicle. For white guys, this may cause an occasional "ingrown hair," a form of bothersome pimple. Black men, though, have more curly kinky hairs than straight ones. They can have dozens, hundreds, of these back-bending little stabbers. They can create lots of bumps on the skin, some of them developing abscesses or cysts -- PFB. We aren't real good at treating this. The best way is just to not shave.

What about regulations?

Uniform and personnel regulations say that if a person has a condition that makes it impossible for him to comply with the uniform, he's unfit for Naval Service and must be Administratively Separated. Remember 1910.2? Can't shave, can't be in the Navy.

While most commands consider it a "medical problem," (it's a skin rash, isn't it?) most medical guys say it's only a medical condition if you shave skin than shouldn't be shaved.

To black sailors, shaving rules and no shave chits are a form of racial harassment. PFB is not just something **confined** to black men, it is **very** common among them. It's not a disease, but a trait of being black. If they have it, they have to show their no shave chit to go on liberty if they have stubble.

When I arrived at the Forrestal, Doug was handling most skin problems, and he usually gave out six month no shave chits. By promoting a six month interval, Doug had cut the PFB visits quite a bit. Recently, though, we had this new influx of CPOs and officers, all of whom had accumulated years of their own local expectations about how

---

[8] *Beards had been permitted briefly during the 1970s as one of the "Zumwalt" initiatives. The novelty probably irritated more people than it pleased, though. I don't think we'll ever see them back again.*

long no shave chits should last -- none of those expectations bearing any reality to the situation. Foremost among them was the XO.

"Doc, I saw a guy with an actual beard last week. He had a six month no shave chit. I thought no shave chits had to be renewed every two weeks," the XO told me once.

Showing him one of Doug's chits, I emphasized that the note said it was a "medical recommendation" to the sailor's supervisor. The note recommended that the sailor should be allowed to trim his stubble down to 1/8 of an inch or less because of his condition. "Doesn't sound like a beard to me, XO."

"Doc, I want you to change our policy about this. I want all no shave chits to be renewed every two weeks, and no beards."

If every one of the hundreds of FID sailors with occasional PFB would need a doctor's note, that would increase our attendance at Sick Call significantly. We would have to deal with this later.

Later that week, Petty Officer Del Rosario brought in a Health Record and a special request chit to release the Health record over to the clinic. The sailor involved had a follow-up appointment over at the clinic.

"What's the problem? Why can't we see him?"

Del Rosario just shrugged, so I asked him to bring me the patient. The twenty year Seaman looked tired, but not terribly sick. He had seen Dr. Darrow over in Sick Call at the Mayport Clinic a few days before. She filled out a "Bed Rest" chit, told him not to work for a few days and come back to her for follow-up, but bring his Health Record.

He lived on the ship, I noticed. "Was there a problem getting into our Sick Call?"

"No sir," he didn't make eye contact,"it's just..."

"Have we offended you somehow here?"

"No, sir, it's just I really have been feeling bad and I thought if you were really sick you should go to a real clinic. When I went over to the clinic, that's what they said too."

Who knows who "they" were, maybe the receptionist, maybe Dr. White. Going through the history, the seaman had been sick for a little over a week, mostly fatigue, headache, sore throat. Dr. Darrow, who seemed to be one of the better doctors over at the clinic, thought he might have mononucleosis, and she took some blood tests that she was going to follow up that morning. I examined him myself, felt some big lymph nodes, and the tip of an enlarged spleen and found myself agreeing with her diagnosis.

We sent him over for his follow-up with Dr. Darrow, and I called to talk with her about his case, to compliment her on her management and ask her to send the FID sailors who found their way over to the clinic back to our Sick Call so we could look after them. She agreed to "release him as soon as he's stable."

Dr. Darrow was the nicest doctor over there. I thanked her and bit my tongue.

No sooner did we hang up than the XO was on the phone. "Doc, can you come down here right now?"

Chuck Johnston, CO of the MARDET, the Marine Detachment, and his First Sergeant were down at the XO's office already when I got there. A young Marine, a 20 year old Lance Corporal, had shot himself in the head with a .44Magnum in his bathtub. His wife found him when she came home from work around noon.

There had been no clues. He was a good Marine, no recent problems, no drinking or drug history. No suicide note. No signs of background mental illness or new crises.

Despite our efforts, the threat and specter of suicide would prove to be a growing menace in the Navy.

CHAPTER IX. SPRINGTIME AND WORKUPS

Finally, we were about to do what ships were supposed to do. Our long SRA period was over. It took only about a day to get all the fladderap out of the passageways, all of the tubes and hoses and pipes. They had been gradually moving one or another of them out over a couple of weeks. Once we got them out, we had to have a pretty busy "field day" to get the entire place cleaned up, but the crew was so glad to get rid of it that it wasn't hard to get all hands to turn to.

We were entering the cycle of "workups," underway periods that would grow progressively longer and more difficult while preparing for the next deployment. Over the year between the recent deployment and the beginning of the next one, almost half the crew would change, so a lot of people had to learn their jobs, learn about flight operations, all the complicated things that an aircraft carrier does. They had to absorb all the subtleties of dealing with one another, and all the traditions. Classes and reading could teach us all a lot, but the only training that really counted was underway. "You fight like you train."

There would be a sequence to the workups. First, just the ship's company, we would begin by moving the ship, practice driving it, just making the ship work, no airplanes. Then we would practice, we and the Air Wing together, landing airplanes and shooting them off the pointy end. Then we would get into fancier driving of the ship and flying of airplanes. We would even let some other squadrons come in to practice landing on our flight deck, do the "carrier quals" that all squadrons needed to do. At a certain level in its readiness cycle, every carrier had to take its turn doing the carrier quals for the East Coast. Later, the Captain and his war fighters, once the ship and the Air Wing were trained in all their fundamental movements, had to practice all the complex interactions of battle techniques and tactics. There would be some exercises of tactical maneuvering, and during these times we would test out some of the new equipment that the operators had put on board during the SRA.

Inspections! Throughout the entire process, various oversight agencies would come by and test and inspect us as we did some of these things. Every department on the ship would have progressively harder and harder things to do. This included the Medical Department, right along with the Air Operations, Engineering, Weapons, and everybody else.

Finally, we would go through a Rite of Passage called REFTRA, for "Refresher Training." REFTRA was a legendary "Hell week" experience that all ships of the line had to go through at a near-graduation point in their workup cycle. The term "Training" in REFTRA had been a ludicrous misnomer for perhaps more than a generation. It wasn't training, it was harassment and (to whatever degree there was anything legitimate about it all) it was a testing, a kind of certification that the Navy used to let you move on to advanced phases of workups.

On the East Coast, the organization responsible for REFTRA was down in Guantanamo Bay, Cuba, known as "GITMO." So, a synonym for REFTRA was "GITMO Training." The Small Boys, destroyers, frigates, and cruisers, would actually go down to GITMO for 10 days or 2 weeks, pull into the pier there, do some of their testing while they were tied up, and then do their operating in the Caribbean. Aircraft carriers had to do the whole exercise underway down in the Caribbean.

There would be five or six underway periods before REFTRA, something you could pass or fail. Well, you couldn't really fail it, because you just kept doing it over and over again until you finally pass, even if the ship were to stay another two or three weeks. REFTRA was more about safety and basic shipboard stuff than it was about being able to fight, or do tactics. Surely, the war fighting stuff was included, but the ship would have to go through that during "advanced phase" and then finally, during "battle group phase." Those two cycles carried progressively more difficult tactical and strategic work and gradually more coordination with other ships. Especially in the battle group phase the important goals were coordination with other ships in the battle group. This included coming alongside for underway replenishment with the auxiliary ships, coordinating antisubmarine warfare (ASW) with the destroyers and our helo squadrons, coordinating anti-air warfare (AAW) between Aegis cruisers, our E-2 aircraft, and our fighters.

The first step in workups was called "Fast Cruise." It's an oxymoron. Nothing fast about it. Nothing cruise about it either. You don't even sail. Fast Cruise is a one-day dress rehearsal for getting underway. All the cables and connections to the pier are shut down. Everybody on the ship goes through their particular procedures for putting the ship in action. A sea and anchor detail is assembled on the fo'c'sle, and the entire team including the Quarter Masters on the bridge practice getting underway. Communications go down to DC Central and the entire Engineering Department. We exercise moving the deck edge elevators up and down. Internal communications is tested. The ship makes its own electricity, meals are prepared. In other words, we practice as though we were being underway, but with the safety of really not going anywhere. The ship stays tied up.

For all of the not going anyplace, Fast Cruise can still be a very trying experience. With all the new people onboard, it isn't just the sailors who are new, but department heads and division officers. In the past few weeks only one major department head had changed, the First Lieutenant. Ed De Martini, who had been the Assistance Maintenance Officer and the rescuer of our 3-M program, was now the First Lieutenant. Warren Lobs had gone on to the staff of a reserve center in New York.

Bob Montgomery, the Ops Officer, would soon be relieved by Steve Wesselhoff, who had been his assistant as the "Combat Officer." Rookie Word, who had been the Skipper of the "Thunderbolts" would become the new Combat Officer, and like Wesselhoff, Rookie would fleet up to OpsO in a year. Larry Osborn, after almost two years as the Mini-Boss, finally fleeted up to AirBoss when Ray Laturno left.

Rookie, Steve, and the new Boss invited me to join their bridge group. When all our work was done at night while were underway, starting around 2300 or midnight, we'd play bridge for a couple of hours and unwind. We were all about the same age, the parents of teenagers, and we chatted and joked while we played. Rookie and I were stuck with one another as partners, though, because both the Boss and Wesselhoff got cranky, especially at these late hours, if you lost count or opened a bid wrong.

It was becoming evident to everyone that over the next 6 to 9 months the pace was going to accelerate, and we would be getting underway more and more. Those prospects mean different things to different sailors, adventure to some, unspeakable apprehension to others, but stress in one form or another to everybody. Even if you didn't know the ship's schedule, and didn't know all the extra time the Chiefs and DivOs were spending with their guys, you could review the logs of the Chaplain's visits or the roster of cases at Captain's Mast and know that something was stirring in the crew. Romantic problems with girlfriends, drinking and brawling in town, disciplinary problems in departments, all these were showing up in those two places.

Hugh Beaumont had been looking rumpled and worn out, so I asked him to sit with me late one afternoon. "I think we have to talk. Things aren't going well for you these days, Petty Officer Beaumont."

He stretched his elbows out on the desk, bent his head forward. I was glad he felt he could open up. "Can I just tell you a few things, Captain?" I nodded. "Well, you know I told you a while ago I wasn't good enough for her. Well... she got a job as a ***cocktail waitress***! Isn't that perfect?"

"Well, Hugh, what's wrong with that."

"Captain, she's a school teacher!"

"I heard teaching jobs are hard to get around here. She might make more waitressing, anyway."

"Sure and with all the work on the side... probably even some of my shipmates!

"She's tryin' to take everything else, too. She's gonna get the car, the furniture, the kids, everything!"

"You mean a divorce?"

He nodded, started to tear, wiped his eyes. They had been married about thirteen years.

"Has she filed already?"

"Not yet. She will, though. Bitch."

I asked if they had been to a counsellor, chaplain, family services. No, she refused to go.

"How about if I call her?" He agreed to that, but reluctantly, but he knew she was going to say no, he told me.

When I called Mrs. Beaumont the next morning, she was very guarded and cold. "I won't talk to you now. Are you on the ship?" Of course. "Then I'll call you back."

Immediately she rang back. "Oh, good, it **is** you, Captain Riley. He's been so strange, I wasn't sure."

Hugh had been going to watch the house at night, accusing her of carrying on with other men. She hadn't been dating, she told me. "He imagines all kinds of things. I'm worried!"

We arranged for the couple to go over to Family Services. I don't know what I must have expected, but somehow less than what happened. In a couple of days, the counsellor and Mrs. Beaumont came to see me together, and we talked of Hugh's forays into her workplace where he had been arguing with her in front of customers, accusing her of promiscuity, hanging around in the neighborhood when he wasn't at work.

"Has he hurt you?"

"Oh, no. Nothing like that. Hugh is **not** violent at all. It just frightens me."

So I notified the XO, we had to give Hugh official orders to stay away from the family and the neighborhood for a while. Most important I arranged for him to see the psychologist over at the Mayport Clinic the next day.

Besides the family and romance stresses that reflected what was happening to the lives among the crew, the case mix in Sick Call was different too. Bob Dylan might be right about not needing a weather man; we could tell the wind was changing (or there was some bizarre new virus in the air) just by the sign-in list. We were beginning to see people with a new cluster of maladies. Flat feet, sleep walking, and bedwetting for example, things doctors usually see a lot less than sore joints, coughs, and headaches, had become actual outbreaks. Whether their feet had ever hurt them before, it wasn't until now in the late winter, just before we were going to start getting underway, that they reached that point that they needed to see the doc.

We had a handful of guys who suddenly began wetting the bed or walking the decks in their sleep, but far fewer than the flat feet. These three conditions are old standbys before a ship starts getting underway, but the mix varies from one crew to another, perhaps with the local "grapevine." Homer Moore, the SMO on the ***USS Enterprise,*** told me that they didn't have too many flat feet but a lot of sleep walkers on his ship. Now, sleep walking and bedwetting are well-known signs of anxiety. Maybe they should reasonably be anticipated among young people about to go to sea. Proper medical evaluation, reassurance, sympathetic attention to a young man's concerns are warranted for transient sleep disturbances like these in general. And yet the form that these conditions take just before ships movements tend to be distinct. The sleep walking always occurs where a crowd is gathered, and several witnesses wide awake. Miraculously, these patients never seem to fall down any of the ladders or trip on hatch covers. Their hands are always stretched out horizontal, like in the movie images of ghosts. Bedwetting, which most people would like to hide, gets quickly reported -- announced in fact -- by the patients to everyone in the berthing compartment. In the confined spaces of those compartments the prospect of a recurring urine smell throughout a deployment agitates the shipmates, so they become vigorous witnesses. People who suddenly discover their bedwetting just before a deployment celebrate it unabashedly when they bring it to our attention during workups.

This year though, the most common new condition in sick call was the outbreak of flat feet. Years ago, it seemed intuitively obvious to physicians, as well as the lay public, that if God gave most of us an arch in the bottom of our feet, those who did not have such an arch must have some kind of disorder. I guess we have thought that way about a lot of physical things. Left-handed people were considered to be somehow disadvantaged, and other people with anatomical variations are often considered to have a "disorder." In the last 20 to 30 years, though, evidence began to suggest that biological variety is not necessarily disease, being left handed or having flat feet for example.[9] Even among soldiers who do a lot of marching, it turns out that if God put less of an arch in your foot than he did in somebody else, that's not a disease. While doing a lot of marching or working on your feet on a steel deck may make your feet sore, it happens to people *with* arches just the same, no less and no more, as it does to people with flat feet.

Some guys didn't come for treatment or for our examination at all, but just to bring us a letter from the private physician or the family doctor from back home, saying that the flat feet or the allergies disqualified them from sea duty. "Doc, my family doctor said that I'm going to have to leave the Navy because of these flat feet. He said to give you this letter."

All of these complaints had to be considered and examined. A number of things have to be considered in each history and sometimes X-rays or lab tests have to be done.

So Sick Call was growing busier and taking longer every day.

"SN Jones, I'm glad to tell you that you don't have a major problem here," we might start up our summary after all the testing -- carefully avoiding a comment that would imply "nothing is wrong," because experience proved that would anger them. We tried to be reassuring, and lay out a plan for helping with, say, the flat feet. It never worked, though. A veil came down over their face, the eyes kind of glazed over. When a sailor wanted off the ship and considered himself ill, no medical explanation would work...

---

[9]*Truthfully, there are a couple of diseases that cause laxity in ligaments and tendons and cause foot pain among other symptoms. Conditions that do this only to the feet and no other part of the body are exceedingly rare. When real diseases of the muscles or joints cause flat feet, other parts of the body are invariably affected too.*

"I want to see a specialist!" was usually expressed in the tone reserved for ,"I'm not talking until I see my lawyer!" In fact, two sailors on different occasions presented me with letters from their lawyers on the subject of flat feet.

A consultation to see the specialist was a dilemma. When a specialist was not necessary because we could fully handle the problem on the ship, we didn't want to overburden the specialty clinics. There was already a three week wait in the orthopedics clinic -- adding unnecessary consultations only stressed out the oversubscribed doctors further. I also thought we should let the ship know we were confident in our diagnoses when we were. The crew might get the idea that if we always needed a specialist back-up on everything, how reliable could we be? During the three to five weeks a sailor might be tied up with visits to the specialty clinic, he could be lost to his department, and with our sailing soon, that was a concern. Such an absence was sometimes necessary to take care of our sailors, but for an *unnecessary* consultation, it would be wasteful. On the other hand, we in the Medical Department wanted to be as certain as we could be; some days we would have liked to have a specialist go over every case.

There were other causes for more business, too. It wasn't only the new outbreaks. The number of minor accidents, corneal abrasions, lacerated scalp, cuts on fingers, were also accelerating. The number of sprained ankles and other athletic injuries didn't increase, but now they were a little more trouble and they healed slower. More guys were observing when they came to Sick Call, "You know, Doc, I don't think I can work with this," or, "Can I have a no duty chit?"

There were other kinds of chits besides the "no-duty" ones that were causing us problems: the no-shave chits again. The XO had insisted that the fuzzy stubble and every-third-day distant shave that we advised for PFB would be acceptable, but only if the sailor got a renewed note from the doctor every two weeks. Not a note from a corpsman, not a form letter.

There were a couple of hundred black guys on the ship who had this problem. If they all had to come in every two weeks, that just added a whole flock of people who didn't need real treatment.

"Doc, this is the way it's done everywhere in the Navy. Why do you have to be different?"

"XO, for one thing, it's done differently at just about every command. For another, for some of these guys, **MOST** of them, once we have tried antibiotics, or retin-A, or hydrocortisone, if they still get it, they're always going to be vulnerable!"

Mitchell Vaughan was not so much a hard-headed man, it was just that I usually couldn't persuade him to listen to me. That day, I just got lucky, I guess. I showed him the parts of the Personnel Manual about suitability for service. "Look XO, it's not really a **MEDICAL** problem at all, it's a personnel or uniform issue. You can either separate these guys from the Navy because of their condition, or you can let them adapt to these shaving practices ... but it's permanent. They aren't going to quit being black just because of my medicine."

"OK, Doc, I've got work to do, for heaven sake! You win." Finally. The XO agreed. We in medical would first try to treat a guy for a transient condition. We had a three step several week protocol for that. If he still had shave bumps, we could send a note to his boss to either separate him from the Navy according to 1910.2 (which we knew they would never do) or his **BOSS** -- not the Medical Department -- would permit modified shaving. So finally, from now on, our only shave chits would be for the few guys with transient or first-time problems.

FINALLY GETTING UNDERWAY

The week finally came for our first ISE. It was only going to be about 2 days underway. We would leave about midday, giving us an opportunity to take everything very slowly in the departure to try to avoid the mistakes of hurry, and to have as few accidents as possible. All the other departments, just like mine, welcomed the chance to spend the morning tying up the inevitable loose ends before the first underway period. Indeed, we had plenty of loose ends, and some of them smelled a lot like alcohol.

We had to have Sick Call just like we did every other day, of course. Not surprisingly, about twice the usual number showed up. By now, we had made Sick Call more efficient and diminished the lines quite a lot. Sick people or people who said they were sick went to the front of the line. Then, sailors who were just finishing the night shift work were next. Everybody else was asked to return 30 minutes later at 0800. The longest anybody waited before seeing a doctor or corpsman was ten minutes.

I had been able by now to enforce the rule that our corpsmen did not turn people away. If a person felt he needed to be seen at 0630, he didn't have to wait around for Sick Call to open at 0730. He came to the Emergency Room, and he was seen. There were minor exceptions, such as with HM3 Womple, who still would turn people away even if they were vomiting or bleeding on the deck. We tried not to assign Womple to ER duty. For the most part the corpsmen knew that whenever somebody showed up, he would be treated.

Well, on this morning, the line started forming around 0630 in spite of our new system, and there had been a steady stream of people outside the Emergency Ward from about midnight onward. Since we were going to be getting underway, Big Jim's and Capt'n Odie's had a lot more business than usual that night.

When Sick Call hours were over, a little later than usual that morning at around 0930 I had a handful of sailors I needed to call the hospital about. Two guys had fractures, one a "boxer's fracture" of his right fifth metacarpal, a typical fracture from punching something hard. Occasionally it can happen from punching a particularly rigid jaw, but among sailors nowadays that particular fracture is usually the result of angrily punching something even more rigid than somebody's face, such as a concrete wall. That's what it was in this case. A young bos'n's mate punched a wall. They do that for different reasons: taking dares, showing off, temper tantrums. Another member had a fractured forearm from falling off his bicycle.

We couldn't keep guys with casts on the ship. Of course, if we were deployed, days away from any port, then we could put casts <u>on</u> people, but we didn't like sailors with casts to stay on the ship. A fracture, with or without a cast, limits a person's mobility. Imagine if the ship ever went down, or the individual were blown over the side into the water. Either a fracture or a plaster cast would compromise swimming and water survival. Admittedly, this was a pretty small possibility, and to people who didn't have to think about it a lot, it could seem like a silly concern, a well casted fracture in a healthy young man. It was peace time, why should you expect an aircraft carrier to sink? Well, in the short time I had been on the ship, we already had one guy who was blown over the side. What if his survival at sea had been compromised by a cast on his arm? It would be worse yet on the leg. Even getting up and down the ladders on the ship became hazardous if you had a cast on an extremity.

The orthopedists at the hospital usually seemed pretty unsympathetic with this, and even their surgical director did at times, also. When I would call about these problems, they would say, "What's wrong with the cast?" I would explain the problem, and they would say something like, "Well that's not my problem. If you're going to worry about things like that," [implying anybody who would ask such a stupid question must not have enough *important* things to think about] "you have to take it up with somebody else." Finally I would wind up calling the XO of the hospital who would speak to the orthopedist, and eventually the patient would go over to the hospital.

There should have been a way for us on the ship to make arrangements to berth a sailor with a cast someplace on the shore while we were at sea. As it was, we were forced to get an orthopedic surgeon to take responsibility for the patient from that point forward. Surely, the orthopedists were right, that a minor fracture that was adequately casted shouldn't have to tie up an orthopedic appointment when people were already waiting too long for orthopedic appointments. Regardless, I couldn't take them with us to sea and our only choice at the time was the hospital.

I wish it had just stopped at ankles and wrists. We had another guy with a broken face. He had been punched a number of times at Big Jim's, had a broken nose, and by our sinus films looked as though he had a fracture with a fluid level in his maxillary sinus. I had to call the ENT doctor about him, a phone call I always dreaded. When I phoned the Otolaryngology Department, I was put on hold, where I lingered for about 5 or 10 minutes. Finally, a corpsman came. Suddenly there was a dial tone. Somebody at the hospital must have pushed a button accidentally. Surely, they would not hang up on us on purpose.

I called again, was put on hold again for 5 minutes, and once again the same corpsman came to the telephone. "Good morning, this is Dr. Riley again. I was waiting for Dr. Eilers." "Oh, he's tied up in the OR and won't be able to come to the phone for a couple of hours."

"Well, we're about to get underway here, can I talk to one of the other ENT doctors?"

"No. Dr. Simons is on leave, so it's only Dr. Eilers."

"Well, what can we do? We're about to get underway, and I need to ask Dr. Eilers consultation about a patient."

"I don't think there's anything you can do. Maybe you can write out a consultation, and Dr. Eilers will call you back."

"But I won't be here in a few hours."

The corpsman didn't say good-bye, jump off a bridge, or anything, he just put me on hold. I waited about another 5 minutes.

"This is Dr. Eilers. What do you need?"

Dr. Eilers and I had spoken together in the past. I had tried at various times being normal, submissive, aggressive, angry, or supplicant with Dr. Eilers in the past, and it never seemed to work, so I just described the patient leaving any emotion out of my description.

"Well, that's no problem, just bandage him up and put him on an antibiotic, I'd recommend Keflex, or ampicillin. Then just make a routine appointment and I'll see him in a couple of weeks."

"Well, we're going to be underway here, and this guy works in the engine spaces where it's pretty hot. He looks pretty bad, and I'm a little concerned about his going up and down the ladders in all that heat. Do you think you could help us by putting him in medical hold[10] so he can stay behind?"

"No, he really doesn't need that, you can just put him on light duty there on the ship, and I'll get to him in a couple of weeks."

---

[10] *Medical Hold was a status over at the hospital. We couldn't do that in Mayport yet at that time. Since it was a status of hospitalization technically, only one of the hospital doctors could arrange it.*

"But I don't have the option of just putting him on light duty here on the ship. He needs to stay behind while we're underway."

"Well, what would you do if you were on a deployment?"

I tried to explain to him that we were not on deployment. It just isn't the right thing to take a guy to sea on a 2-day exercise when you don't really need to.

"Well just assign him to the Beach Det." The Beach Detachment is a small group of the ship's company, mostly from the Supply, Admin, and Security Departments who stay behind looking after certain ship's business while the ship is underway.

"That's not what the Beach Det is for. I'm not allowed to put patients there. This is what the Medical Hold is for, though, isn't it?"

Finally, we got to the bottom line, "Well, putting a guy on Medical Hold requires a lot of paperwork. I just don't have the time for that. I'm a lot busier than you are. You'll have to figure something else out." Dial tone. He had hung up.

This was already taking a lot of time, and I had a few other patients I had to deal with. We were going to be getting underway in a little over an hour.

After all these months, I had looked forward to getting underway with some kind of romantic anticipation. I don't know now what I expected, perhaps a magical voice singing whaling songs throughout the ship. We were just so busy. One bos'n's mate came down with a burn and laceration on his hand. On the first time getting underway after several months, forgetting how to handle one of the lines, his hand had been pinned against a capstan during the Sea and Anchor detail, burning and tearing his palm.

THE FIRST DRILL

Through all the paperwork and minor injuries we were seeing in the Medical Department that morning, about 30 minutes after we passed the St. John's Buoy, we heard the call for a man overboard drill. "This is a drill, this is a drill. Man overboard. Man overboard. All hands muster at your battle stations immediately. Up and forward on the starboard side, down and aft on the port side. Man overboard. Man overboard. This is a drill."

Whenever somebody hit the water, a number of things had to happen immediately if there were any hope to save him. At speeds like ours, we could quickly be out of sight of a shipmate who fell overboard. Sometimes, especially in the dark or during rapid operational tempo, somebody might just see a splash, or see something appear to leave the deck. So you might not be certain that a shipmate had gone over. Turning the ship rapidly to come back and get a guy, or launching three or four helos or boats to get somebody is dangerous in itself. Every time you have to dangle a wire down over the water, or put a boat over the side, there is a chance for somebody else to drown or break a leg. Not to mention the literally thousands of dollars it costs to turn a behemoth like an aircraft carrier around. So we don't take it lightly.

The first thing that has to happen when there is a possibility of somebody falling overboard is to verify absolutely that somebody is gone and who it is. That's why one of the main things in a Man Overboard Drill is for everybody to "muster" at a designated spot within 5 minutes. This is harder than it sounds with 5,300 people. An accurate count is critical. Yet, the announcement, "This is a drill," lets some people take it less seriously. The members of the Air Wing are famous for this. Some guys just simply stay in their rack; others never hear the announcement. Some guys don't know what the drill is all about, think it involves somebody else, and never come to the muster. Until we can prove that the ship's man overboard bill works correctly, we can never be comfortable that we are ready to go to sea. So the Man Overboard Drill is something we take very seriously.

While all that body counting is going on, other people are launching boats and helicopters, doing all the things you need to do to find the person. The Medical Department has a couple of crews of corpsmen who go on boats or helos if they have to rescue a the fallen sailor. They get mustered as they pick up their medical rescue bags on their way out.

The drill this day was not going well. At the end of the last deployment, we were able to get everybody mustered in well under 5 minutes. Today, at the end of 12 minutes, there were still a dozen people unaccounted for. Since every work center has a list of all members, those who don't muster in within 5 minutes are easily identified. Of course, that's how you know who is really overboard in a true emergency. It's also how the XO catches the laggards in the Drill.

At about the 7 or 8 minute mark, the XO came on the 1-MC. "Good Morning. This is the XO. The Man Overboard Drill is not going well. Anybody knowing the whereabouts of the following people lend a hand." He then read a list of the people who hadn't been mustered yet. In a real Man Overboard, reading those names would be important. Perhaps a shipmate would need to go into those sailors' racks, or anywhere else they might be to verify who was lost, and how many. Everybody had to be involved. About 4 or 5 minutes later, now 11-13 minutes total, the XO's voice came over the 1-MC again. He had a way of being a little whiney when he was irritated. "This is the XO." No good morning this time. "This drill is not going well at all. We have spoken about it before, most of you guys have been to sea before. This is inexcusable. I want the following individuals to report to XOI." Then he read the list.

Finally, at what was almost 20 minutes out, the XO came on again, "This is the XO again. We are calling this drill off, but at almost 20 minutes there are a bunch of guys who still didn't check in. We're going to keep doing man overboard drills until we get it right." So we had been underway only a couple of hours, and we already got scolded.

In the melee to get 5,300 people checked fast enough, the inevitable hyperenergy of youth finds an opportunity to express itself. Sound a starting gun and the boys want a race. That morning, we had seven guys with lacerations on their scalps from bumping their heads at the top of "knee-knocker" doors, two other guys with bruises, and one with a facial laceration from falling down a ladder. Some are careless, some are inexperienced, but most are just exuberant adolescents with an excuse to run. Maybe they haven't been underway before. Sometimes they forget where metal hangs down from the overhead. The characteristic "man overboard" scalp laceration is a two inch coronal gash right at the vertex of the scalp where the sailor's head hit the top of the door. The "knee-knocker" is an oval opening in a stress-bearing bulkhead, usually up on the O-3 level. The oval opening has a horizontal metal shelf or band around it that sticks out and knocks your knee when you try to go through it. Sometimes they forget while they're looking out for the knee-knocker part on the bottom that there is a similar part sticking down from the overhead. This was our first Man Overboard Drill, and we had seven scalp lacerations from it. By the end of the cruise, we'd only get one or two with each drill.

After we took care of them, I stopped down to the XO's office to fill him in on the day's epidemiology. He was flushed, irritated not only by the Man Overboard Drill, but our general difficulty getting underway.

I noticed the XO had been gaining a little weight since he came to the ship. He was also smoking a lot more. He had bags under his eyes. The pounds he had gained since being on the ship were not surprising, working longer hours, and having an opportunity to munch a doughnut or sandwich while he was working overtime in his office late at night. His khaki shirt was beginning to blouse just a little bit over his belly, so that there was a little rippling around the buttonholes. In fact the same thing was happening to me, I noticed just then. Funny I noticed first on him.

It was getting into late afternoon when I got back to the Medical Department, but I could tell when I saw Father Dux, the Catholic Chaplain pacing back and forth in front of my office with a morose young guy in dungarees slumped on the bench, that there was still more to be done that afternoon.

The padre told me that this young man had been in to see him a couple of times in the prior week. The guy began by telling him that he had discovered the Navy life was not for him. He just couldn't handle the hassle he was getting from his boss, and he realized that the kind of structured life in the Navy was bad enough, but nobody ever told him what shipboard life was like. He told the priest that he had enlisted to try to please his parents, but he just couldn't handle it anymore. Father Dux had been pretty supportive, apparently. Navy Chaplains are trained in counseling techniques and psychotherapy. Of course, they remain ministers above all, but on the ship their role is as much social worker, guidance counsellor, psychologist, and community maintenance as it is religion. Finally, this morning, the young sailor seemed more morose than he had been before, and he told John, "I just can't be responsible for what I might do if I have to stay here." That hits the trip wire. At that point, the chaplain always brings the member down to see the Medical Department. The chaplain and I sat alone with the young sailor for a little while. He was clearly well oriented, not psychotic. His vital signs and physical examination were normal. He wasn't physically sick. After we spoke for a while, he seemed a little bit less sad with each minute, but I asked him, "You know, Chaplain Dux is concerned about your safety. Have you been thinking about hurting yourself?"

"Not really, Doctor, but I'll do anything I have to to get off this ship."

"Now, does that mean injure or maybe even try to kill yourself? Is that what you're telling me?"

"I really don't want to die, Doctor, but you can't keep me here if you think I will."

Neither the Medical Department nor any other place on the ship really has a truly "suicide proof" room. With all the potential hanging places, myriad electrical source, sharp objects, places where you can loop a belt around your neck, and so on, it is hopeless to find a suicide-proof room on the ship. Our safest places are in the brig, but strict rules forbid keeping a patient in there even for safety reasons. The only thing we can do is to keep somebody on guard <u>with</u> the sailor constantly.

Father Dux and I called his DivO and arranged for him to stay in his berthing space with two people with him all the time. I reassured the sailor that we would get him to psychologic counseling the next day when we got back into port.

"What about today?"

"We don't have any planes onboard today. There's no COD, and no way to fly you off."

"Can't we just bring the ship back?"

It may be a kinder and gentler Navy, but we haven't reached the point of being able to turn a dreadnought around for an unhappy sailor.

When his buddies came for him, and his DivO left my office , I saw that HM2 Lopez was waiting restlessly to talk to me. It seems that Rock Tosser was planning to take a guy into the operating room to undo a testicular torsion. Somehow the testicle twists around inside the scrotum in some young men. The vas deferens and the blood vessels attached to the testicle get tied up in a knot, and because of that torsion, the testicle is strangled. A true emergency, it almost always has to be treated by an operation, even when diagnosed promptly. Tosser had already sent a corpsman down to tell the XO, but not me, that he had to operate immediately and he was preparing the patient for the OR. I knew it was going to be another one of those scenes, but nonetheless I had to confront Rock about it. I stuck my head into the ER and asked, "Commander Tosser, can we talk for a few minutes?"

"Not really, I have an operation to do."

"Really, Commander, this won't take very long."

He stormed over across the passageway into my office petulantly. Since he was the surgeon he felt it was a waste of time to discuss the case with me. I asked if he would let me try to manually reduce the torsion. Sometimes with proper angulation, you can untangle the mass. You can tell it is effective if the pain disappears. Usually, the patient will need an operation eventually, because a torsion will occur again if the underlying tendency isn't corrected. My thought, however, has always been that whenever possible really elective operations should be done at a real hospital. If possible, relieve the problem and do the operation under calmer circumstances "on the beach."

Rock told me I could not examine the patient.

"Rock, there is no need of our having a scene. We have a new Skipper now, and if I told him that you refused to permit a 'second opinion' before an operation, he might take a rather dim view of that." (I didn't bother with a "who's in charge" debate.)

The guy had already been shaved and prepared for the operating room. He was twisting in pain on the exam table, sometimes would sit up, then lie down, then stand up and take a couple of paces. The severe pain with testicular torsion is typically grabbing, gnawing, undulant. Victims say it is worse than any ground ball in baseball or knee in football. I asked him to lie down on his back on the exam table with his knees up and apart. Gently pulling the testicles first straight down, and then rotating them both upward and outward, on the right side there was a little give, like clicking a styrofoam bubble, and his facial expression changed. I asked him to stand up, which he did, and he took a few steps around saying that his pain disappeared. Rock stood sulking in the corner and he had nothing to say.

The sailor said, "Gee thanks, Doc. That was a lot easier operation than I thought. Did you already put the stitches in?" HM2 Lopez choked back a giggle, but Petty Officer Casad, who was standing in the background couldn't help himself and he chuckled aloud. I knew that I had to keep Rock happy at this point, too, and it was true that the individual would still need an orchiopexy, the operation to fix the strands inside the scrotum. I told him he would still need the operation, but I would rather he go see the genitourinary specialist as soon as we could send him there. Today's operation was canceled.

I went back to my office to finish up the day's paperwork. In a few minutes I heard the Captain on the 1-MC. I think at CO School, the captains must get a heavy dose of 1-MC immersion. Of course, officers like Thomassy and Pieno were the type who would always try to talk to their sailors without somebody telling them. Still, one had to notice how much Captain Thomassy liked the 1MC. "Good evening, this is the Captain. We're a little over a hundred miles off the coast of Florida, on our first underway period. People are working very hard today, We have a few glitches, but we'll work them out fine. This crew has a fine reputation and I have to tell you I'm proud to be underway with you.

"I need to speak to you, though, about the Man Overboard Drill. The XO is right, that's something we need to improve." The Captain spoke a little about the drill and the need for concentration, but in a more upbeat tone than we had heard earlier. He was obviously letting the crew know that he would be a communicator, so I thought it was fine that he gave a rather long announcement. Most people have to stop or at least slow down their work while the Captain is speaking. So a few skeptics grow restless if the announcement lasts more than a minute or two. He chatted on as though in a casual Sunday afternoon phone call, nothing else going on (all around the ship people were growing restless while they got behind in their work) There were a few customary routine announcements: babies born that day back at home -- of course the first the fathers heard of it, the daily news, major sport scores.

Now the announcement was going a little longer than usual, but the Skipper went on. He was interesting to listen to, and with his congenial accent, he was the kind of person who could be likable as he chatted. He announced a new program, 'Letters to the Captain.' Every day, in the several suggestion boxes around the ship, he invited comments and questions, and promised that he would respond to them every day on the 1MC.

People were starting to chuckle about the length of the announcement. Oh well, first day out. Getting acquainted, maybe there was a lot to pass on.

The Captain finally ended with a pep talk about how good it was to be back at sea again. The 1-MC is really for brief announcements. The bos'n's mates and quartermasters are warned to always "keep it brief." The Captain seemed to warm up the longer he talked, and was obviously enjoying holding that microphone. Amused by the lengthy fireside chat, the crew liked it and they liked the new Skipper. When he closed with ,"and above all, have a Fine Navy Day," the crew knew that he meant it.

It stayed pretty busy the next day and a half, but the first underway period finished uneventfully. The "shakedown" had shown us a lot of things we had to work on, like our Man Over Board response, for example, and a number of issues in each department, but we made it home safe. No big pieces of equipment were damaged and nobody was injured. If we weren't exuberant, we weren't dissatisfied either.

CHAPTER X. MORE WORKUPS

The despondent young sailor was sent over to the Psychiatry Department, and a couple of days later came back with the diagnosis of a Personality Disorder. He knew the difference between right and wrong and had a firm comprehension of Reality. He was not psychotic or sick in diagnostic terms. Although the sailor did not have a treatable psychiatric disease, his personality would remain an obstacle to functioning in the military, so the psychiatrist recommended Separation at the Convenience of the Government, in accordance with BUPERSINST 1910.2.

"Why did they send him back to us if he's medically disqualified?" the XO asked me. It is just as confusing for most doctors as it is for everybody else. There really is a sound logic to the problem, but it is difficult to make it clear.

I tried to give my usual explanation, but I knew from years of experience that it was not very convincing. "The personality is a personal trait, like being tall or being left handed. It's not a disease that we can treat like pneumonia or even schizophrenia. People tend to have certain behavior patterns that they either prefer or just use habitually. If a person is very dependent, or rebels against authority, that's a behavior pattern, not a disease."

"What are we supposed to do with him now? What if he tries to kill himself?"

"XO, he's rational, and the psychiatrist feels he knows right from wrong. You either have to hold him responsible... or with identification of a Personality Disorder you can just Administratively Separate him. In other words, it's a Leadership problem, not a medical condition."

"Doc, that's a cop out, and you know it!"

I had the same discussion later that same day with the Captain.

"Well, then, if it's a Leadership Problem, we'll deal with it that way." Naval officers take Leadership very seriously, and personally. They can accept being unable to cure a disorder, but not failing a Leadership Challenge.

"Captain, maybe I didn't make myself clear in the right kind of way. It's not *just* a leadership problem. Personality once you reach the age of these guys is not that adaptable. This guy is going to continue to be a problem for the Command, and eventually he is going to cause us more trouble by being here than if we let him go."

"People can change, Doc, you know that. If he needs guidance and discipline, that's my job."

"Yes, Sir, but a guy with an Anti-Social personality is not likely to respond."

"Then it's a medical disability," he insisted.

That discussion never got any easier.

The suicide potential added a whole tangled dimension to the problem. Suicide had become one of the leading causes of death among all young Americans. It was about the same in the Navy as the general population, actually a fraction lower, but it was something we were very concerned about. The Medical Department was generally held responsible for the suicide prevention programs, but the chaplains and the chain of command were also critical. Medical needed to be involved in case there were a treatable illness, such as encephalopathy or schizophrenia. Also some people may be injured in an attempt, and the injuries of course had to be treated.

The Captain pointed out that if a guy with a Personality Disorder did kill himself, it would surely be medical at that point. I tried to be respectful but pointed out that once he was dead it was most especially not a medical problem... just like murder wasn't a medical problem. That kind of explanation is not usually taken well by the boss, but Captain Thomassy understood. "Now you're accusing me of murder?" he chided.

We couldn't predict every sailor's behavior, but some of them were more prone to act out until they got what they wanted. Maybe they would not intentionally kill themselves, but in acting out, they could be very disruptive, and might well die in the process.

Two weeks later, the sailor got in a fight with a Chief Petty Officer and hit him with a wrench. When he was hauled off to the brig, he sat and cried in his cell until he was taken to see first a chaplain and then another psychiatrist. The chaplain thought he was depressed. The psychiatrist, a new one this time, concluded again that he had a Personality Disorder. When he came back to the brig after seeing the psychiatrist, he made slash marks on his left wrist with a fingernail clipper. There were a total of eight of the scratch marks made with the clipper, but no bleeding. He was transferred to the Naval Hospital at JAX, where he was admitted for "suicide prevention" and further reevaluation.

After our first ISE, two weeks went by before we went to sea again. Those were two hard weeks for me, because that's when Rick Combs left, and our new Medical Admin Officer, Lieutenant George Lucy, reported onboard. We were back in port just a couple of days when Lucy reported, and he and Rick had a 7-day turnover period. George was about 32 years old, had 6 or 7 years of prior enlisted time in the Air Force, and had been in the Navy about 8 years, although he had never been to sea.

A remarkably good looking guy, he obviously was a weight lifter. Muscles like his didn't come simply by genetics or even just by ordinary athletics. He was only about 5'8", and wasn't so deformed by all of his muscles that he had to wear abnormal sized garments. However, the muscles were such a prominent part of his being, that neither an observer, nor George himself, could ever quite be unaware of them. He had a habit of shrugging his shoulders or slowly flexing an extremity when he spoke with you. Looking at his wrist watch, he would elevate his left arm, maintain a 90-degree angle between the forearm and upper arm, and slowly twist his fist toward one side in order to look at the wrist watch. Kind of reminded me of ancient Egyptian paintings, or of comedians mocking weightlifters. George wasn't joking though. Sometimes, his chin or an extremity would flex slowly, move to one side, not quite writhing, and not quite in a twitch, but like he practiced it, in a way that would make one muscle here or there stand out. It was as though his body, poised ever to unfurl like a great eagle, could not quite be contained completely. George took his body seriously. He probably considered it a temple. Or at least a basilica.

He had another disarming quality, his perpetual countenance of surprise. He looked startled. Easy questions, like what day is it, or where are you from, were ok, but anything harder than that would clearly catch him off guard. The expression, with his eyes particularly wide open in a blank stare would come over him suddenly with any question harder than "what's your name?" I first saw it the day we met when I asked him if his check-in was going all right. His jaw dropped, eyes opened wide -- the way a deer looks when it's caught in your headlights on the highway. A sudden blank immobility with wide open eyes reflecting light, but no comprehension -- deer in the headlights.

If you put that blank deer-in-the-headlights stare together with a twitching movement of one muscle in the thigh or arm, it was sometimes hard to concentrate on what you were trying to say or what he was trying to say to you. George just didn't get it. He either didn't understand, or rather, he understood just slightly off center. It was like you simply wanted to describe a triangle, but George saw the world in nonEuclidian geometry.

I learned that George had worked at a part time job for the last several years, also. He was a professional wrestler on the side. He wrestled under the nom de Tussle of The Blue Pharaoh. This was something I decided not to learn more about any sooner than I was forced to. Meantime, another new officer reported the same month, our new Nurse Anesthetist, Lieutenant Ron Eslinger. Most of the time, the anesthetists, like the surgeons, preferred to be sent to hospital when a ship is in port and only work on board while underway. Understandably, they are concerned about keeping up their skills in the OR, and most of them far prefer the hospital to the ship's environment. Ron had been an anesthetist for over fifteen years. "I've done that long enough that being out of the OR for a few weeks won't make me forget it all. We're going to be steaming soon. I want to be as much part of the crew as I can." He really did talk like that. With Rick leaving, Ron would prove to be our salvation.

Ron and George weren't our only new members. Senior Chief McGowan had left us about the beginning of the year and we had been without a Leading Chief for a few months. HMC Abercrombe joined us when George Lucy did. From his appearance, I figured Chief Abercrombe was a nearly perfect Chief Petty Officer. He was tall, thin, had a straight military appearance and a commanding baritone voice. This would be the Chief who would help us with our enlisted guys, I thought, probably with Petty Officer Womple in the dark recesses of the idea. Rick Combs didn't share my enthusiasm, though. "I don't know, Captain," Rick told me one evening. "Something shifty about that new Chief. Think you better keep an eye on him."

Rick was prone to be skeptical, heck, downright cynical, about strangers, so I chided him about giving the new chief a fair chance. Still, I never took anything Rick told me too lightly.

Bruce Boswell had moved on, too. Although the Air Wing docs and corpsmen were not part of our ship's company, I always considered them members of the department even when they weren't aboard. After all, they would be living and working with us during the deployment -- the real life of the carrier. George McKenna, a new flight surgeon, relieved Bruce. Bill Flynn would be staying on for another year. The night before his first underway period with us, I took George out to dinner in Mayport. He was a **lot** different from Bruce! Curly headed and serious, George wore John Lennon spectacles, the kind we called "social concern eyeglasses in the late sixties." We had something in common almost immediately when I learned George was planning to become a neurologist later. Even though he had never read any of my papers, we had a pleasant evening. I was impressed how intelligent George was. He certainly was serious, though, and there was something else about him, that old Gaelic thing from either Brian Boru or Robert Emmet, Forrestal had it too, something between being intense and very dedicated... no, maybe just: stubborn. Yes, that's it. He was a stubborn cuss.

HASTINGS AND WOMPLE BACK ON THE PROGRAM

One day shortly after our first ISE, we needed an Xray on somebody because of a shoulder injury. Eddie Hastings was off the ship at the time on an errand, so one of the other corpsmen had to take the films. It was taking a long time, so Curt Rosenthal went back into the Xray suite to help. Shortly we had the films. They weren't technically very good, but the shoulder could be seen well enough. We gave the patient a sling and sent him on his way. "HM1, those films aren't very good. I thought we were going to do some cross training on Xray"

"We did for a while, Sir, but lately, it's hard to get Eddie to do the training. He's getting down again."

After our talks a couple of months ago, Hastings had been going to the AA meetings, and his work had really improved. While he had not turned into a glittering personality, he had been congenial, and until the past few weeks had been coming to work on time. Lately, though, he had turned more surly again, and made careless errors at his work. Now HM1 Rosenthal told me he had let the training slide too. In fact, Curt looked like he had more to say. "I think I should get LT Combs and LT Eslinger," he said. Rick hadn't detached yet, and since it was after 1600, George Lucy was definitely already gone for the day. Ron was spending a lot of time with Rick, to my relief, looking like he would be doing a lot of the administrative things besides the nursing and anesthesia duties.

Obviously Curt thought something was bad wrong if he wanted somebody else to have to tell me about it. "We got us a problem, Captain," Rick said. When he used those words, I knew it was an understatement. When the three of them went back to the Xray suite, they discovered that nine months worth of Xrays had never been sent over to the hospital for reading by a radiologist. Back in October, when we returned home, all the Xrays from the deployment, six months' worth, were to have been brought to the clinic immediately. We had very specific discussions about it, and Eddie assured me it was done. Every week, he was supposed to have sent that weeks' films over to the clinic right on the base at Mayport. Workups were starting now, and we were nine months behind. Furthermore, the radiologist ought to be furious to have nine months of films dumped on his lap late and all at once!

We went back into the Xray file room to check it out. There they were. Hundreds of them. Ron inadvertently bumped a locker door open with his shoulder and a brown paper bag fell to the deck. A couple of little white clipped badges with photographic film tumbled out. The radiation badges. As the Xray tech, Eddie was responsible for the handling and recording of the radiation badges worn by selected people in the crew. Himself of course, but also a group of people in the Weapons Dept and the MARDET. Because of the sensitivity of those badges, and the potential health concerns, letting those lag was a much bigger problem than the delinquent Xrays. Eddie was back in trouble, and this time it was serious.

Art was our Radiation Safety Officer. He had to come in from home that night and he called a number of official people all over Jacksonville to tell them about our predicament. I went down to the XO's office to tell him about it. He was on the phone and gestured for me to have a seat, while he continued talking. Ten minutes later, he was still on the phone, so I left. Miraculously, Art had been able to contain the bureaucratic damage. He arranged to have the badges read that evening, and since none of them had any significant exposures, he was able to get us out of an obligatory late report. We spent about two hours carefully wording the accompanying report to some headquarters, and I brought it down to the XO, who was working late as always. In green ink, the color the XO uses, he changed a couple of my verbs, so we had to rewrite the entire report. I would discover that the XO always would change a few words. Why he preferred Navy-speak jargon to real English I could never figure. Nonetheless, the radiation badge fiasco was repaired with much less hassle than we had deserved.

Eddie Hastings and I would have to speak soon.

The next morning I asked Petty Officer Hastings, who had a particularly long face that morning, to come and talk with me. Hovering behind him was the droopy, surly face of Arden Womple. He was nudging his baleful countenance so ponderously into our conversation that he consumed us. "Something seems to be bothering you," I told Womple in what would have been hilarious understatement to anybody else.

"Captain, I just need to talk to somebody right now, I'm so upset." His jowls frumped a little in his pouting.

We went into my office. Hastings, himself growing a little more surly now, waited on the bench out in the passageway.

"Captain, I can't take that man anymore. Dr. Kempf just won't leave me alone. He's always complaining, always running me down."

Indeed, Doug was a demanding guy, and he was often not gentle with the corpsmen. As Womple went on, though, it was evident that he and Doug may have clashed personally, but it was clearly over Womple's insolence and lazy performance. Most recently, Womple had asked Doug for a medical excuse from the Physical Fitness Test and Doug had refused to give it. Apparently besides refusing to write a note excusing Arden from the Fitness Test, Doug had commented on the corpsman's obesity and threatened to take action about it.

"You are obviously upset, Petty Officer Womple. Do you have anybody you can talk with about things that bother you?"

No, he said, he didn't need a nurse maid, he was just tired of being "discriminated against."

"I'll be very careful to look for signs of discrimination, and at least until we work this out, I'll ask Dr. Kempf to go through the Chiefs for a while, but I have to tell you that Dr. Kempf is always one to follow the book on all matters. That includes fairness and respect as well as work regulations."

"Should have known you officers always stick up for each other."

"That will be all Petty Officer Womple."

Hastings was still waiting, but I needed to speak with Doug. He came in and we sat alone in my office.

"I know what this is about. Womple, right?"

I nodded.

"I was pretty hard on him yesterday, but he was rude to a patient and then he was rude to me." Seems that Womple had burst in with his PFT request right in the middle of a suturing job. Doug hates to be interrupted when he is suturing even for a good reason. Anybody who had known Doug for more than twenty minutes would have expected him to be angry with Womple. So all parties concerned recognized that Doug had chewed Womple out. Doug was feeling a little contrite... but only a little.

Suddenly, it was clear to me. This was not a case of the Corpsman being abused. Womple had bullied patients, other corpsmen, even me in a way. We had catered to his personality far beyond what we would do for our other corpsmen. Womple had a long substandard performance record, and he was fatter than ever. I'd had enough, and so had everybody else. It was time for him to become a civilian.

"Don't worry about it, Doug," I told him. "you and I agree that you're a little too grouchy sometimes, but" (His shifting in the chair at that comment meant he did *not* agree) "this time, though, you did the right thing."

Resolving to discuss the Womple situation with Rick later, I then let Petty Officer Hastings in. He shambled into the office without looking at me and slunked into the chair next to my desk. Just like at our last meeting, he sat square in his seat and yet looked slumped somehow. Saying nothing, he stared at the deck.

"Petty Officer Hastings, I don't have time right now just to go over things the way we should. The fact is, things have got bad again. Do you want to talk about it? Have you been having trouble drinking again?"

As though pinched, he started from the second question. He was alert now, and even angry. "No, I haven't had a drop!"

I thought for a minute he was going to be more animated, maybe open up a little. No, his irritation subsided and he lapsed back into deck staring and had wringing.

"Look, this business about the radiation badges could be big trouble. And what about those damned Xrays you promised you would take care of! I backed you up before, but if you don't help me out here, we're going to have to send you to mast this time for sure."

"Everybody keeps looking for me to mess up. I never see any **white** corpsmen in here."

"Wait a minute. You think you've been treated differently because you're black?"

No answer. Just a shrug. Momentarily stymied because I was both astounded and resentful at the allegation, I said nothing and waited for more from Hastings. Finally, he said, "No, not directly, not from the Department, I guess, but it's always there. I got personal problems, too."

"We offered to help you with that once before."

"I can handle it myself."

"Not so far!" I told him. Finally, Eddie, told me how badly he felt about these lapses. He vowed he had not returned to drinking. He knew he was late about the badges and the Xrays, but as he grew more and more delinquent he was more afraid I'd get a notice when he turned the late work in. In fear, he just got further and further behind.

I made him promise to hook up with one of the Chiefs, preferably one from our department, but elsewhere would be all right if he didn't feel he could relate to one of the HMCs. Later, the alcohol counsellor told me that Eddie's attendance at the AA meetings had become irregular the last few weeks, but he still came periodically and did not seem to be drinking.

Sick Call was dragging on slowly that morning. After securing the XO's permission to get rid of those frequent no-shave chits, we also had begun to schedule guys with shaving rashes only on Thursdays and Fridays, our otherwise slowest days. This day was a Tuesday, and one of my patients was a young black guy with a neatly trimmed beard. I tilted my head and stared. Beards had not been legal in the Navy for six or seven years. This one was not baggy; it was short and had a clear margin, right at the angle where the jaw and underside of the chin and mouth meet the neck. "Doctor Sergeant over at the Mayport Clinic said I was not to shave. Said I should give my Chief this chit and tell him I could wear a beard 'cause of my PFB. Then this morning the Chief said I had to come down here to get a new chit."

The place where shave bumps erupt most is right at bends in facial structures or places where the grain shifts... just exactly in the places this sailor was still shaving. The places that Dr. Sergeant over at the base clinic had told him not to shave were places most guys didn't usually get the bumps anyway. That's one of the reasons that just wearing a neatly trimmed beard is ***not*** a solution. The beard is illegal, and if you trim it where beards usually get trimmed, you still get bumps in their usual places, namely the neck line! Lately, though, a bunch of our sailors had been going over to the clinic on the base to get shave chits, because the doctors over there gave them what they wanted -- a chit that said "may wear a neatly trimmed beard." Despite our efforts to spread the word and educate all the chiefs and Division Officers, most supervisors were in the habit of simply accepting anything from a doctor. So the sailors usually got away with it.

I phoned Dr. Sergeant over at the clinic to talk it over.

"Look, Dr. Riley, I understand you see your job as enforcing the Navy's regulations regardless of the effects on the patient. I have to put the patient first, though. I'm not like you. I didn't check my diploma at the door when I came in. The chit stands. He doesn't have to shave."

"Not trying to talk you out of your own approach to things, but you know a doctor's chit is merely a **recommendation** to the command. Over here on the ship, I have to make sure I take care of the sailors and at the same time help them get along with the rules. Just wanted to explain for you what the command is looking for so we can work this together as well as possible..."

"Look, ***Captain***, we know all about you over here. I'm not selling out my standards just to give in to some archaic rules." Notice, he's calling me by my rank; remember that means he doesn't like me.

"Hey, I'm not asking you to sell out anything. I was just trying to explain about..."

Dial tone. Dr. Sergeant hung up.

I tried to explain about the PFB to the patient and gave him our guidelines about shaving every third day with clippers instead of a razor. "The doc over at the clinic said you'd make me shave," he grumped and grabbing the packet of information from me, he stormed out of Sick Call.

When Sick Call finally ended that morning, all the khaki in the department met to talk about what to do with Womple and Hastings. Lucy took up the chair next to my desk, his multi-sectioned notebook/organizer open on his lap. Moving his chin in such a way that his sternocleidomastoid muscle flexed photogenically, he poised his pen over the page as though to show me he was ready to record my every syllable.

The whole team agreed it was time to deal with Womple. Every officer, Chief, and petty officer in the department had trouble with him one time or another. His evaluations were terrible. He was fatter than ever. We all agreed we shouldn't just use the obesity as an easy excuse; his whole performance was so bad, after all. Yet he had more than a year left on this current enlistment. It is hard to get a guy out for performance in the middle of an enlistment. We would push the Ad Sep, but if that didn't work, we would be sure not to recommend him for re-enlistment when this tour was up.

"LT Lucy, when you take over for Rick as the Division Officer, you have to stay in **constant** contact with the Command Master Chief and Admin Officer about this. Besides doing it right, we must be sure we are fair with this guy at all times."

Lucy gave me that deer-in-the-headlights stare, spread the fingers of both hands, looked surprised.

"What do you mean?" he said, "Aren't we **going** to be fair?"

"The Captain means follow all the right procedures," Rick told him.

"That's not all," I said. "We have to make sure that Petty Officer Womple gets all the support and treatment he needs. Doug, since you and he don't get along, you shouldn't be his doctor. As his boss, I shouldn't be either. Art, you should be his primary doc here on the ship, but when the Flight Surgeons are here, be sure you get one of them or the surgeon to go over everything with him. If he ever needs psych, be sure to get him over to the clinic or NHJax."

Next we talked about Petty Officer Hastings.

First, I told the group that Hastings had implied we had racial problems in the department. Chief Carter, the only black man among our khaki said that just wasn't so. Still I planned to talk about it with the corpsmen at Quarters the next day. Later that week, we met with the chaplains and the Equal Opportunity reps in the command to ask them to visit our department. I was convinced our guys were too close for racial problems, but was well aware that as a white guy twenty years older than most of them, my conclusions could be challenged.

As to Hastings himself, Rick said, "Captain, I think he's got you buffaloed. I know Hastings. He's drinking again sure as Hell. We caught him redhanded letting those films and badges go. If you think we got in trouble about those syringes, that was **nothing** compared to what Hell could break out for letting the radiation surveillance program slide. Send him to Mast!"

Lucy's eyes widened. His left biceps flexed along with his right shoulder. He began to realize what the DivO would have to deal with every day as the DivO in the department.

"I think he means it," I said. "See, he's different from Womple. Hastings knows he's done wrong and he admits it. He says he's going to try and I want to stand behind him. Womple just doesn't accept his own role."

Ron Eslinger had been paying attention. "I agree with you in principle, Captain, but I don't know either of these corpsmen yet. One thing, though. Are you sure you're not willing to stand by Hastings because he's black?"

I admitted I had some reservations about Hastings, but except for Rick, everybody else agreed with me that we'd give Eddie another chance. He needed to be supported, though, and we had to keep Master Chief Shulman, the Command Master Chief, involved.

MORE HELP FROM THE MAYPORT CLINIC

New people were still coming to the ship every week. We had to capitalize on every opportunity to use days in Mayport for any training or repairs. An example was fire fighting over at the Fleet Training Center on the base. Everybody on the ship had to have fire fighting training, so we had to make sure all newcomers and those needing refresher training went over to the FTC. Always a demanding program, fire fighting was even tougher in the heat, but at least the instructors paid a lot of attention to heat and smoke hazards. They were careful, even anxious about both of those. To a fault some said. It was springtime, now, the days were getting hot. Wearing the long sleeves and the heavy rubber OBAs made it worse. On an already hot Florida day, wearing all that gear inside a metal box, surrounded by flames and smoke was hard work and it was stifling.

The teacher-to-student ratio in firefighting is high so that each student has somebody looking after him, avoiding burns, watching for unsafe movements, protecting him. A flustered student might be inclined now and then to pull a mask off so he can wipe his brow, so the instructors guard against that most of all. Smoke inhalation is a constant focus of instruction, and great worry to the people who run the school.

Teachers have to learn too. Some sessions train instructors how to instruct. Those sessions have lots of pupils of both kinds. That week, there were a crew of new instructors along with our couple of dozen FID students. It was well over ninety degrees. Everybody in Mayport was uncomfortable. Even down in the Medical Department it was warm despite the air conditioner. I remember wiping sweat off my forehead when I got the phone call from the Quarterdeck.

"Doc, we just got word that a bunch of guys were injured over at FTC, firefighting. They activated the base Mass Casualty Plan." A Mass Casualty Plan means about the same thing for a base that it does for a ship at sea: too many or too badly injured for the resources at hand. Triage was necessary to prioritize treatment, and help would be sought from others.

With the controlled setting at FTC, there must have been an explosion to injure that many. How many must it have been, I wondered? With five or six doctors on duty at the clinic, and four ambulances, to overwhelm them, it must be severe injuries and many of them. With Doug on Leave and Art over at the hospital with a patient, I was the only doctor on the ship that day, and there were a couple of people in the Emergency Room, so I couldn't leave right then. Phoning the clinic, I was told "This is HN something-or-other, the clinic is in Emergency Status, please call back later... [dial tone]." He' hung up without even letting me talk.

We gathered all the corpsmen we could spare that day and sent them over to help at the clinic. I tried to concentrate, taking care of the minor injuries in our ER, while I worried about the burns, and maybe life-threatening injuries on the Forrestal sailors from the firefighting school. After about an hour, Curt Rosenthal brought me in a new HN who was reporting this week.

"Captain, this is HN Clay. You should let him tell you about the Mass Casualty."

Clay's story was interesting. There had been six students in the tower when one of them complained to the instructor that he was feeling faint. The instructor asked two others if they were feeling ok, and they both said they were "hot," too.

.."Wait a minute," I asked Clay. "Just ***HOT***? Nothing else. Not weak, hard to breathe?"

"Oh no, Sir, nobody had any trouble breathing!"

"What about this Smoke Inhalation? Did you guys take off your OBAs? Did some of them malfunction?"

"No. Mine worked all right. I think they all did. Oh, no, Sir, we weren't allowed to take them off. you get in trouble if you do that!"

Did somebody pass out, I asked him?

No, everybody was walking around, and doing all right after they left the tower.

How about burns, or coughing, or shortness of breath? No, none of that.

"Well, where did the idea of Smoke Inhalation come into it, if everybody was wearing their OBA, and nobody had any trouble breathing?"

"Dr. Sergeant, over at the clinic, he's an Emergency Physician, and he said you never can tell with Smoke Inhalation. He said that FTC was very dangerous, and so he was not taking any chances. He sent four guys over to Beaches Hospital for admission."

Still nobody had called our Medical Department. I tried once again to call the clinic. Dr. Sergeant was too busy to talk to me. About that time, Art came back from NHJax, so I could go over to the clinic myself. By this time, none of our sailors were still at the clinic. Except for the four sent to Beaches, they had all been discharged. Every one of their medical records had the diagnoses of heat exhaustion and smoke inhalation. They were all told to return the next day to the clinic for follow-up, not to the medical department on the ship. Every one of them had undergone an arterial puncture to measure blood gases -- all normal -- and they all had complete blood counts done. Most of them had blood electrolytes and urine analysis, all also normal. It was 1430 in the afternoon. Dr. Sergeant was gone home for the day.

Growing skeptical about the clinical acumen from our "Emergency Physician" at the clinic, I went down to Beaches Hospital to check in after our sailors down there. The doctor in their emergency room greeted me warmly. "Dr. Sergeant," he said, "Nice to meet you!"

"No, Terry Riley," I corrected him.

"Well, nice to meet you, Terry. Dr. Sergeant was very helpful. I guess it's a good thing they got all those guys over to the clinic. He says the doctor on the Forrestal is a real bozo. Who knows what would have happened to those poor sailors if he'd been treating them."

"Yeah, who knows?" I went along. "What about the patients you've got over here?"

"Well, we got gases, Xrays, 'lytes, and UAs on all of them. They were all normal. We released all but two of them."

"What's wrong with those two."

"One's a 'rule out cerebral hemorrhage' and the other a 'rule out hypoglycemia.'"

"Cerebral hemorrhage?"

"Yeah, he had a headache, and Dr. Sergeant sent him over for a 'rule out' so we did a CT scan. It was normal."

The term "rule out" had always troubled me as a buzzword for usually sloppy or automatic thinking. This afternoon was giving me no reason to rethink my opinion.

"But," I asked, "was he groggy? Was his neurologic exam abnormal?"

"I don't know, really. But with the history of the fire and the headache..." So far, there was nothing that sounded like a hemorrhage or a need for a scan to me.

The patient with "rule out hypoglycemia" had a blood sugar of 55mg/100ml. Who knows why they checked his blood sugar, but it was around noon on a hot day. He'd worked all morning in the heat and hadn't eaten lunch yet. So what!

I went to visit our sailors. The young man with the headache said he'd had a headache from the night before. He got headaches a couple of times a month. This was just an average one for him. The other guy was feeling fine, but he was in the middle of a five hour glucose tolerance test (on the same day as the admission! "Either one of you guys breathe in any smoke?" I asked them.

Oh, no! They hadn't dared take off their OBAs.

"Can you release these guys tonight?" I asked the doctor on duty.

"Well, in the morning, if they're stable. I'm kind of afraid for them to go back to that ship. From what they tell me over at the clinic, I'm worried about the medical care on the ship. Sounds shoddy. Dr. Sergeant wants to make sure he takes care of the follow-up himself to keep them away from that doctor... What's that guy's name anyhow?"

"Riley," I told him and left. Since my back was turned, maybe I didn't hear him, but I don't think he said good-bye.

All of our sailors were back the next day. They were all fine. About a month later, we got the bills from Beaches hospital. For the CT scan and all the labs, it totalled over $3000. I tried a few times to phone or visit Dr. Sergeant the Emergency Physician, but he was never in when I called or visited. He had not been to the firefighting site. I called Jim Gentry, the XO over at the Naval Hospital, and suggested maybe the doctors at the clinic should visit the place. Seeing an OBA might be interesting for them too, I said.

GETTING UNDERWAY AGAIN

About a week later, we were preparing to get underway again, for our second Independent Steaming Exercise. Except that the new Combat Officer, Rookie Word, had to suddenly fly off because of a potential emergency in his wife's pregnancy, the departure went much more smoothly than our first time. We had a couple of Man Overboard Drills that didn't go very well but a lot better than the last time. During this exercise, we had a number of observers and advisors from AIRLANT. They were there to check out whether we were ready yet to take on airplanes up on the flight deck, and whether we had mastered things like GQ that would be important for upcoming exercises.

In the Medical Department, we had conferences about our Mass Casualty Drills that we were planning to practice this week.

The second day underway, while we were still within H3 distance of the beach, a member of the AIRLANT team came down to the ER because of tight pains in his chest. He was a Chief, in his forties. Stocky guy. A smoker. He was having a general dull, pressure-like ache in the region of his sternum and he was sweating. Of course, since he was an engineer-type, where he was working it was hot, so the sweating didn't necessarily mean much. From his EKG and exam, we decided he had angina pectoris, a sign of coronary artery disease, but not a myocardial infarction, not a "heart attack," at least not now. Although we were able to alleviate his pain rapidly, and he was stable, he needed to go back to the beach where he could have a complete cardiac evaluation and definitive treatment depending on what could be found. We could take care of a patient with an acute myocardial infarction, but in peacetime, a little over an hour from a full service cardiology department, if the patient were stable enough to travel safely, we were really obliged to send him to a hospital.

In the department we discussed whether we needed to give him TPA, Tissue Plasminogen Activator, a new drug that seemed to help dissolve clots in acute heart attacks. If it is ever to be effective, it needs to be given in the first minutes that clots are forming in coronary arteries. After consulting together and going over a few papers we had reviewed as a group within the past few weeks, we decided not to use TPA since this wasn't an infarction. However we all agreed that the Chief needed to fly off to the cardiac department at the Naval Hospital, where we could have him within a couple of hours. I went up to talk it over with the Skipper. This would be my first encounter with the new boss about a Medevac from sea.

I quickly grabbed my ballcap. You are always covered (wear a hat) when you enter the Bridge. There are ten decks between Medical and the Bridge, so I was always breathless by the time I got to the Captain's chair. Flight Ops were going on. Captain Thomassy, I would learn, always was very attentive to the flight deck during every flight cycle. This, however, was in the very earliest phases of workups, so he was especially focused that morning.

"Permission to enter the Bridge," I panted out to the Junior OOD, and saluted. Entering the Bridge requires a protocol not unlike coming aboard the ship. Granted admission, I struggled to slow my breathing, to seem as "in control" as I could. Trying to hold my breath still only made me feel more breathless. With the panting, and the dark sweat stains streaking my khakis I felt pretty rumpled when I came up to the Captain's chair.

"How bad is he, Doc?" the Captain asked me.

"He's stable, now, Captain. In fact I don't think he's actually had a heart attack. It's too early to be certain, though. He definitely has coronary disease, though. With your permission, Sir, I think we need to send him back to the hospital."

"How soon can you get him up on the Flight Deck?"

I should have worked that out before now. Quickly, I calculated the time to unhook all his wires, hook him back up to the portable monitor, get the elevator...

Uh-oh, the captain wanted an answer. You could see he was impatient that I hadn't anticipated his question. "Twenty minutes," I blurted out, having finished my calculations.

"OK, Doc, twenty minutes. Thanks."

Down I went to get the patient ready. I asked George Lucy to arrange for the elevators up to the Flight Deck. Startled expression. Wrist and shoulder pose. Silence. Lucy hadn't a clue. "I'll take care of that, Sir," Petty Officer Del Rosario said. I examined the patient again, then was called back to my office. Somebody called to ask if I could write a refill on an antihistamine prescription, and somebody else had a skin rash. I told those guys to call back. Ron Eslinger was running around getting oxygen sets and monitors set up.

"Hey, why isn't the Chief going!" I shouted to nobody in particular, but everybody who could hear.

"Captain, we've got to get his records together," Curt Rosenthal said. Rosenthal was the only guy who kept us within bounds on all bureaucratic stuff, but sometimes it seemed to slow us down.

"Captain, phone for you. It's the MiniBoss"

"Hey Doc, where's your patient? We're holding flight ops up."

"I told the Captain twenty minutes, Mini. I've got seven minutes left."

"All I know is we're holding things up. Can't you move it along?"

I didn't have time to argue. Had to go check the patient again. No pain. Lungs clear. Finally, they had him on the gurney rolling out into the passageway. Bill Flynn would accompany him on the flight.

The elevator wasn't ready! The twenty minutes were just about up now. I called the Gun Boss, because the weapons elevators that we would need to get to the roof belonged to his department. He said he'd take care of it.

Finally more than six minutes later, Bill and the patient were on their way up to the roof.

The Captain called again. "Hey, Doc, we're holding up these flights."

"He's on the way up right now, Captain."

"Look I counted on what you told me. Next time I'd appreciate it if you wouldn't just pull a number out of your rear end."

Oh, well, the patient was stable and he was on his way. "Yes, Sir." Excuses wouldn't help. Taking care of the patient was the most important thing, but all the same, you'd just as soon not irritate the Captain in the process.

The rest of that week was uneventful. We got home without any more injuries and tied up in Mayport without a hitch.

THE ELUSIVE BILLY DORSEY

Our second night back in town, I was busy in the Emergency Room with a sprained ankle and a sailor who thought he had swallowed his high school ring. HM1 Grant, our lab tech, was the leading petty officer that night. When I sent the bos'n's mate with the swollen ankle over for his Xray, Petty Officer Grant came to tell me about a phone call. "He won't say who it is, Sir, but you're the only one he'll talk to."

We were too busy for me to enjoy a prank, but I was afraid to not take the call. It took a few minutes to reassure the caller that nobody else was listening, but by then I could tell who it was, I thought. "Doctor Riley, this is Airman Dorsey."

"Airman Dorsey. Are you all right? Why are you calling?"

"I've been drinking."

"Sorry to hear that. I thought you'd stopped. Are you drunk?"

"You could say that."

"Where are you?" I asked him, fearing he might be UA, run off somewhere.

"Afraid I can't tell you that," he said, his words a little slurred, but still with that childish charm. You could almost smell the stench through the phone. There was a lot of activity and laughter in the background. Probably a bar or pool hall, I thought.

I asked him to tell me where he was so we could send somebody to bring him back to the ship. "Oh, I don't think that would be in my best interest," he said in remarkably grown-up syntax. We talked for a while, and I was able to determine that he hadn't been fighting and did not threaten to hurt himself. Gradually I recognized some of the noise in the background.

"Now, Airman Dorsey, I can tell you're at a bowling alley. Are you on the one here on the base?" I took the long pause for a yes. "Now listen, Billy, you stay right where you are. I'm going to send somebody to get you and bring you back to the ship, so you can get in bed tonight without any trouble."

"I'll be in trouble with my Division, though. I don't think I should come back right now while I'm drunk."

"But you don't have overnight liberty right now. You'll be in <u>more</u> trouble if you don't come back."

All right, he agreed. I hung up and called base security. It was easy to persuade them that giving this young man a ride back to the ship while he was just a little drunk would be better than what we'd deal with later if he got worse.

Half an hour later, they called back. He wasn't at the bowling alley. He had been there, witnesses said, but nobody could find him now. I started to worry. Billy didn't have any close friends. If he were feeling helpless, and was drunk, I worried what he might do in a desolate mood.

Never should have worried. Ten minutes later, he was back on the phone. "Billy, where **ARE** you?! "

"Right here. Bowling alley." He was perplexed. Why hadn't I sent somebody like I said I would. Well, yes, he had been in the head for a while. He thought he might have fallen asleep in the stall. Maybe that's why the MAs couldn't find him.

"OK, now AN Dorsey, listen very carefully. Do you hear me?"

I made him promise to stand right there at the main counter, fall asleep if he had to, wet himself if necessary, but **DO NOT** go a single foot from that point. The base police refused to go after him again. "Sorry, we're not a cab service, you'll have to send somebody else."

The JOOD got one of the ship's vehicles and sent a couple of watchstanders from Dorsey's division to go after him. They were back in forty minutes. Empty handed. No Billy. "Just refused to come, Doc. He said you ordered him to stand right there and not budge for any reason until you got there. He said he promised you he wouldn't move."

Finally after three or four more phone calls and another couple of hours, Dorsey was back on the ship. He was more sleepy than drunk by then, I thought. Cleaner than usual under these circumstances for Billy, his red hair wasn't even too badly tousled, and he hadn't been in a fight. We had somebody tuck him in for the night, like a little cub scout who fell asleep during the bedtime story.

Besides Level II, I thought Billy Dorsey might need Antabuse.

CHAPTER XI. GETTING READY

It was late spring, but felt like midsummer in Mayport. A surly young Fireman had just slammed angrily into the chair in my office and dared me with his frown to take a history. Doug Kempf opened the door just enough to show his face. "Captain, when you're free, can I talk to you?"

I glanced at the patient, FN Tyrone Hill, I guess to check his permission to even answer, since he seemed so angry. He must have read my mind, because he shrugged just a tiny grudging permission. When Doug closed the door, I asked, "OK, FN Hill, what seems to be the problem today?"

"My feet. I have flat feet. They hurt all the time. My Mama says I'll have to leave the Navy."

"Well, let's see... you've been on the ship for about seven months now, been in the Navy a little over two years. When did your feet start to bother you?"

"Always have. Just worse now on these steel decks all the time."

I looked at his feet. Sure enough, almost no arch. The soles of his boots had a normal wear pattern, though. Mobility and bulk in his feet were normal too. "Your feet look OK to me, FN Hill. Why don't we get you a set of arch supports, try those a week or so and look at it next week?"

"Knew I'd get a run around down here! I want to see a specialist!"

"Well, let's see how it goes for a week with the arches and then we'll decide OK?"

"You can't make me deploy if my feet hurt. I can ax to see the Captain." I realized it wasn't just his feet that made FN Hill angry, but it never worked to argue with the young sailors while they were agitated. So I sent him out with the arch supports we both suspected he wouldn't like and made an appointment for the next week.

Doug had become more friendly during the work-ups. While I could never take John Bigbee's place, Doug knew how much I counted on him and his devotion to the ship spilled over to me a little bit. When he wanted to chat, as he did this morning, I learned to be glad for the opportunity. He came in now, after Hill left and took the same chair. Often, with Doug, you had the feeling your English teacher or your pastor was about to explain something about basic manners or deportment to you. His posture was straight but not rigid. His gestures were not cold, but they were deliberate. He had an air a little bit like being **proper**, or maybe it was **correct.** It was natural in Doug, though, not at all pretentious. He was just a **correct** kind of guy.

"You know Dr. Pompadour, my relief?"

He waited for me to nod. Summer was coming, and Doug would be transferring in July. We had a copy of orders on a young physician named Gary Pompadour, a D.O. presently at the Navy Hospital in Orlando. Of course I was a little anxious to be losing Doug, but he had already stayed a year longer than most GMOs.

"I think you'd better watch out. My friends in Orlando say he's bragging that he'll get out of the assignment. You might want to think about getting somebody else."

I told Doug that Pompadour's visit to the ship a couple of weeks before went well enough. However, I never told anybody that I was troubled about why the young doctor avoided eye contact. Pompadour also spoke about coming to the ship in the subjunctive mood. That seemed curious to me too, but I didn't share it with anybody.

"Also, I might as well tell you I called him last night," Doug continued. "He wouldn't tell me when he was going to report, and that bothered me." Of course it did. Doug does not tolerate uncertainty. "I tried to tell him about uniforms and things he would need, and he acted like he didn't care. So I told him, 'Look, if you think **I'm** tough, you better watch your step, because Captain Riley will kick your ass!' " Doug's face widened in a proud smile when he told the story. He thought he had flattered me. He also figured he had given the new young doctor fresh motivation.

I winced. If Dr. Pompadour had any doubts at all, I suspected Doug had solved them. What irony. Should I celebrate that Doug had become so fond and loyal to me, or should I wonder what I had done to let him think "kicking ass" was a virtue. Regardless, Doug was so proud of their little talk, that I decided not to question it right then.

When Doug left, I remembered I had to call Dan Eardley too. Tosser, our surgeon, would be leaving even before Doug, and Eardley, the new surgeon, never would give me a firm answer about when **he** would report either. Dan was nice enough on the phone, but I just couldn't pin him down. "Hey, we've got underway periods in August, and I have to know when you're going to get here?" He didn't seem to be as shifty as Pompadour, but why wouldn't he ever give me a simple, straight answer?

This afternoon, his wife answered the phone. She was a lot less reticent than Dan had ever been. "I'm not crazy about the idea of a deployment, I can tell you that!" She said. "Why did the Navy send us here to Newport if they expect him to go to a carrier in Florida?" (actually, not a bad question, I admitted to myself).

"Uh, I don't know, Mrs. Eardley, I'm just the doctor on the ship."

"Well, Dan's out now. I don't know when he'll be back."

Happily, Art interrupted me to see a patient. We were about to get underway the next day for a little over a week, so the department was starting to get busy with all the pre-steaming maladies. Art's patient was Tommy Cage the first-class Photographer's Mate I had met during my orientation to the ship the year before. Cage was old for an enlisted sailor, in his late forties. Like me, he had returned to active duty after years as a reservist. He had run his own insurance business for years, put some money aside, and was happy to be back at sea. He was having attacks of "tightness" and "trouble breathing."

"At first I thought it was asthma or cardiac, Skipper, but it just doesn't fit," Art told me.

Cage looked fine, except a little anxious, maybe depressed. "Doctor Riley, these attacks come on me suddenly, like I'm tight all over. It's hard to breathe and my ankles swell up real bad, see?" Cage looked well-groomed even in his dungarees, the work uniform. His wavy pommaded hair reminded me of Tommy Edwards, a singer from the 50s. He insisted his ankles were swollen, but they weren't. His work boots were slit up the sides.

"What happened to your boots?"

"Have to cut 'em like that so there's room for my ankles when they swell up this way." The ankles were not swollen. No edema.

His lungs were clear. Heart sounds, pulse, ECG, Chest X-ray, all were normal. As we spent more time on the history, the sudden panic quality impressed me. For a man in his late forties, we needed to be sure we checked his heart and his metabolism, but I was thinking about Panic Attacks, maybe a Panic Disorder. We arranged for Petty Officer Cage to be examined by an internist at NHJax, and I arranged for some blood tests, including his thyroid before he would see the specialist. On my note to the internist I suggested considering a stress test as part of the evaluation.

Later that week, we were preparing for Advanced Phase Training a ten day cruise with the Air Wing and the whole battle Group. It was late the night before an early morning departure. A Gunner's Mate had pain in a very tender testicle. He could scarcely stand, and his testicle was so tender he was jumpy when I tried to examine him.

It wasn't red or swollen. The pain seemed to begin early that morning, but it wasn't too bad at first, so he stayed at the beach with friends, but it grew so severe a few hours ago that he could not bear it any more. Rock Tosser was off the ship until morning.

I called NHJax to speak to the duty urologist for the night. It was Dr Savorini. Good. Of the two at the hospital, he was the cooperative one. He returned my page in about 30 minutes at a little after 2300. "Dr. Savorini, thanks for calling. We're getting underway in about seven hours and I have a sailor with a very tender testicle. It could be epididymitis, but I'm concerned about a torsion, and regardless we can't take him with us in the morning."

"What did his urine analysis show?"

"He hasn't been able to void, yet, but..."

"You mean to say that you called your ***Urological Consultant*** without even checking the basic laboratory tests on the urological system!" Indignant outrage. I think I was supposed to be embarrassed. I had been about to say that I would have to send him to the hospital regardless of the UA in his condition, but Savorini had interrupted me. He continued then to lecture me about the logic of medicine and about how **real** doctors consider the thoughtful, ethical use of consultants' time.

Silly me. I had thought Savorini was the nice one.

"Well, Doctor Savorini, it's almost midnight. This guy is in a lot of pain and your hospital is almost an hour from here. What would you like me to do?"

"That's the kind of question I expect from a medical student, not a practicing doctor. As I said, you should do a UA and then if you still feel you need a consultation call for one at that time."

Almost 30 minutes later, the UA was done. It was virtually normal. We gave the patient some pain medicine and transported him to the hospital in the morning before casting off. From that day forward, anytime Dr. Savorini and I spoke, he addressed me as though I were an idiot.

This was late in the work-up cycle, and we were becoming a very proficient crew again. Our Man Overboard drills were going much better, for example. That is they were going better in the XO way. Sailors still loved to run down those passageways. We still had scalp lacerations and falls, even if fewer than before. On this first morning at sea, a Messman came to the ER after the drill with a cut on his knee.

"You shoulda seen it, Doc," his buddy said. "That fork was sticking right out there. Just like a dart in a dartboard." Running down the chow line for the Man Overboard drill, he had somehow jammed his fork into his knee. It left a 3 cm cut and it seemed to go deep.

I irrigated the wound profusely and contemplated whether to suture it closed. We are reluctant to suture closed puncture wounds usually, especially if they may go into a joint space. We don't like to "close in" any bacteria. This guy worked in a dirty place, though. Rock and Doug were doing a procedure in the Operating Room, so I couldn't get Rock to look at it before deciding. I went ahead and sutured the wound and the guy felt fine. Just then the Division Officer and Leading Chief from E Division brought Philip Williams in for an exam and I forgot about the guy with the knee.

"He won't talk, Doc. At first I thought he was just being stubborn," the Chief said.

"That's what we both thought," the DivO added, "but this isn't like him. He's usually one of our best guys."

Williams and another electrician had a fight, and when they were disciplined later, Williams just stopped talking. "Could this be a shock or something, Doc?"

I asked them to leave us alone and first I examined the sailor. Except for not speaking, his neurological exam was normal. He could understand very well. He just sat quietly, fingering a notebook that he looked at longingly. Williams was a handsome man. He had fine features like a model. Every strand of his uniform lined up perfectly. Even in a uniform, only somebody who really **cared**, really **thought** about his appearance would be that neat. He also had a shiny silver cap on one of his front teeth with a stylish cutaway heart design in it.

In a few minutes I could tell he wanted his book to be noticed. "What's in the book Fireman Williams?"[11]

He shrugged.

"Can I see it?"

He let me take it easily, although he didn't quite hand it to me. The book was full of rhymes, mostly one or two pages long. The margins were trimmed with drawings of roses, trees and women's faces. A lot of the words were misspelled, but the handwriting was flawless and beautiful. The meter was forcibly iambic in every line. Either all lines or pairs of lines rhymed. There were three subjects: his mother, love poems, or violent fighting against oppressors.

"It looks like you spend a lot of time with your writing."

Another shrug. He liked that.

"Do you think you would be able to speak if you read some of your poems?"

He took the notebook and was able to read a short rhyme about his mother. "You can call me Philip," he said.

Philip and I decided he was mostly just hurt from being lumped in with that other guy in the discipline. His DivO and Chief were relieved he wasn't sick. We agreed Philip would come by to see me for a couple of days and we would see if he could get a little better. He decided he could go back to work.

VIP AVIATORS

The Florida weather was beautiful this time of year. So the beautiful days together with the short trips and nice flying guaranteed that we had a steady stream of VIPS, not as many as at the end of a deployment, like last year, but still quite a few. Congressmen and important people in the Department of Defense always have some important information gathering that they can only do at sea for a few days at a time. We were always proud to show off our ship, and these are invariably charming people (how do you think they **get** those jobs?) so we enjoyed showing them around and answering their questions.

During this at-sea period, a tall dignified man in his fifties, whose name I have forgotten, was on his first carrier trip. He was something along the lines of an Assistant Secretary of the Navy or Deputy Assistant for something or other and he seemed fascinated by everything, especially the flying. After dinner one night, I was shining my shoes and watching CCTV in my stateroom when Kevin Myette, the AIMD officer knocked. "Hey, Doc, do you have a jet helmet?"

Yes, I told him, I did.

"Oh great! Nobody else seems to have a big enough head size for Mr. Bigwig. Can we try yours?"

---

[11]*He was an EMFN, Electrician's Mate Fireman, so he would be addressed directly as "Fireman." When promoted to E4, third class petty officer, he would become Electrician's Mate Third Class or "EM3."*

"What's this about, Kevin?" I asked suspiciously, but I already knew the answer.

"Oh, no problem, Mr. Bigwig wants to go for a ride in an F-14."

"Jesus, it's night, Kevin!" Nobody but essential crew flies over the water at night!

"Well, he's leaving early in the morning, so they can't do it tomorrow."

"What about his NATOPS? Water survival? Does he even have an up-chit?!"

Kevin was obviously a trapped middle man. "Hey, Doc, I don't know! He says he got all his clearances before he came out here. He's in great shape. Runs five miles a day."

I gave Kevin the helmet, but I frowned. I called the XO to complain.

"Don't worry, Doc, Mr. Bigwig says he got clearance before he left DC."

"Has anybody seen his NATOPS sheet or up-chit, XO?"

Who was going to ask an Assistant or Deputy Assistant Secretary of the Navy-for-something-or-other to see his up-chit? Half an hour later Kevin called to thank me for the helmet, the only one on the ship big enough.

I watched on the flight deck monitor as the Tomcat with Mr. Bigwig took off.

On the climbout and ascending left turn, Mr. Bigwig told the pilot he had some pain in his abdomen and they ought to land. Turns out he had an inguinal hernia repaired two weeks ago and didn't tell any of us that. Seems he forgot about it. Being the cynical Missourian that I am, I suspected at the time that he may have forgotten that he never really got an up-chit either.

Naturally, they brought him right to the ER. I was there to examine him. The hernia had not recurred, the operation was well healed. Just the ordinary G-forces of the flight caused local pain in the region of the recent operation. I reassured Mr. Bigwig that he was all right, and he left the Medical Department with no apparent embarrassment.

Thirty minutes later the XO called me. "Hey, Doc, Mr. Bigwig asked if we could have the Surgeon examine him. No offense but he feels a surgeon should make the decision, OK?"

When he came to the exam room, Rock had a pressed, clean uniform newer than any I had seen him wear before. When the Assistant Secretary-for-something-or-other lowered his trousers, Rock knelt down like Lord Essex or Sir Walter Raleigh in front of Queen Elizabeth. He closed his eyes and bowed his head to keep out any distractions, and as he prodded and examined -- about four times longer than I had ever seen him before -- he nodded his head, yes, yes, as though responding to a message only he could hear.

"Who did your operation, Mr. Bigwig?"

"Hal somebody or other."

"Yes, I know him," Rock said with a knowing but slightly forgiving smile. "He's very good." I thought to myself, this politician will be glad to know our thirty year old surgeon approves of his private doctor. "But, I don't think he got the hernia absolutely closed. Only an experienced surgeon would be able to notice that. I'm not surprised Dr. Riley couldn't tell. Nothing wrong with that. He's not a surgeon, that's all. I don't think it came loose in the flight, though. You'll be fine, but I think you should call Dr. somebody or other this week. He probably won't need to do the operation over again. This isn't a major problem. Some surgeons would consider it good enough."

"Well I am certainly glad I asked to have The Surgeon examine me."

"Yes," Rock said, "I am too. So often other doctors are reluctant to ask for help when they need it."

That ended a generally pleasant evening for me. A politician went for a jet ride he shouldn't have, concealed his medical history without being embarrassed by it, and a young surgeon was able to come to his rescue. The good part was that nobody got hurt.

A couple of days later we were steaming up to New York for a port call, and the young man with the puncture wound to his knee came to the ER. The whole knee was swollen and red. I had been afraid of that. I shouldn't have closed that wound. Probably should have left in a drain or a packing. He didn't have a fever, nor much pain, happily.

I removed the sutures, and a small amount of clear thin fluid came out. No pus. As much as I hated it, I called Rock immediately to come and see the patient. I thought then, and I still do, that irrigating the wound, leaving in a drain, and giving antibiotics was what the wound needed at that point. However, since it was my treatment that caused this complication, it was my responsibility to follow the consultant's advice now. We needed the surgeon.

Predictably, Rock said, "He has to go to the Operating Room right now. If we're going to save that knee, we have to open it up immediately." I wasn't surprised at what he said, but I was glad that once in the OR Rock did not carry the theatrics as far as I feared. He did not open the joint space. He irrigated the wound, put in a drain and started antibiotics. The guy was healed fine in a few days. He always asked for somebody other than me whenever he came to the Medical Department, though.

We steamed into New York the next day in a cloudy drizzle. I stood up on Sponson One when we slipped into what seemed like a shoebox berth on the West River. By this time Tommy Lennon, former CO of the VS 28 "Gamblers" had taken over from Bohunk as the Navigator. Bohunk wanted to stay assigned to the Forrestal as long as he could, though, so he had arranged to fly ahead to New York to help with our port call there. He was waiting for us on the pier, holding a brick in his hand.

At that moment I began to despair about Bohunk's steering skills. Recalling his driving in Benidorm I began to panic when I saw him running back and forth on the pier waving to the bridge and to the tugs, and speaking rapidly into the brick while he scurried around. Was this guy who couldn't keep a Mercedes in the traffic lane going to direct us into this slip, I wondered. The 75,000 tons turned, but not enough, and began to push the big flat starboard side of the ship into a big sharp stabbing edge of a granite and concrete pier. It was right below me. Like in slow motion on a tragic movie, and yet too fast for me to cry out, I saw us slide right into certain puncture. Twelve feet, six feet. Here it comes!

I closed my eyes and crunched down.

We didn't collide. I'll never know why. We slipped in just like Cinderella's foot to that glass slipper.

New York City welcomed Forrestal. Liberty call set the Hangar Bay and quarter deck abuzz with departing sailors and visiting New Yorkers.

On the first full day in port, when it was time for Rock Tosser to leave the ship for good, he didn't come to say good-bye to me. HM1 Rosenthal said, "I think he's on his way up to the brow now, Captain." So I ran hurriedly up to shake his hand. We didn't agree much of the time but after all we had been shipmates. I got there just before he stepped out to the quarterdeck. Rock looked right at my hand, but not at my face. He turned to ask the OOD permission to leave the ship, saluted the ensign, and left. I never saw him again.

Several thousand visitors had guided tours of the ship that day. First they passed a greeting board with photos of the Captain, the XO, and the ten department heads. Then they toured the Hangar Bay, Flight Deck, and Mess Decks. The only excitement that day was when the XO stormed into the WardRoom and asked "OK, Who did it?" He had just discovered that the 7000 visitors that day all wondered why there were ten pictures of the XO (with moustaches drawn in ballpoint pen) on that greeting board and no other officers' faces. I don't know if the visitors ever figured it was because the Department Heads thought the XO was a micromanager, but I think he did. I don't know who did it myself. Really I don't.

About a week later, back in Mayport, we were busier than ever trying to balance everybody's final leave before the last time at sea, and treating all the sailors who didn't think they were well enough to deploy. FN Tyrone Hill came back to see me one morning in Sick Call. "These things don't do me any good." He threw the arch supports at my desk.

"Now, you're going a little too far, Fireman! You stand up now and get control of yourself."

"I'd like to know if you'd talk that way to me if we weren't on the ship!" He said.

"What do you mean?"

"Just what I said. I wonder if you'd have the guts to talk to me this way if we weren't here where there are other people to protect you."

"If you mean am I afraid to fight you, of course I am! You think I'm nuts? I'm 43 years old, man! On the other hand it's kind of bad judgment on your part to ask me that." I reminded him how much trouble he could get into for threatening an officer. Once again I explained about flat feet to Hill and arranged for him to be seen by a podiatrist. Hill left satisfied. He knew as well as I did that if he wanted to get out of the deployment, he would eventually find a way.

Just then George Lucy came to the door with Gary Pompadour. Lucy flexed both shoulders, the left a little higher than the right, and looked momentarily speechless. Pompadour, though, was as smooth as ever. He tipped his head back a little, raised his left eyebrow in a friendly gesture, and stuck out his hand. "Lieutenant Pompadour reporting, Sir." Was he smiling or smirking? I'm still not sure.

Only as an automatic platitude, I said "How are you?" Didn't really mean to ask a question. It's just an expression.

"Well, my knee's a problem, you know. They wanted me to have an operation, but I'm putting it off as long as I can."

"I thought it was your shoulder." In fact I had called Joe Ricciardi, the clinical director and an orthopedist at NHOrlando, his last duty station. Joe told me that the guy complained about his shoulder but didn't have a real orthopedic problem.

"Well, they both are problems, but I'll get by." The reason Gary came by that day was to get permission to move some things the following day, which was going to be our Family Day Cruise.

"I'm really going to need some help. Without you I'll be the only doctor with all those civilians, some of them children and old people."

"Hey, I'm really sorry but I just can't make it. I'm not officially on board yet anyway."

A quick couple of phone calls to the detailer revealed that Pompadour had put in a letter requesting exemption from sea duty because of his shoulder and knee, without telling me. The waiver had been turned down because he couldn't get orthopedic verification. Also, I learned he had not closed out his apartment in Orlando. That kind of worried me.

Stewing about Pompadour's future was interrupted by new problems with our X-ray tech, Eddie Hastings. I had been worrying about him for a few weeks. After our last set of problems, Master Chief Shulman, the Command Master Chief, had been couselling Eddie like a Union Stewart would. Eddie had been really through complete Level II now, and although Master Chief Shulman was serving like Eddie's Sea Lawyer to assure we would not hassle him, he also insisted Eddie stay sober. True to his long time pattern, Eddie had perked up and was a sharp, good worker for a couple of months. Lately, although his work was still acceptable, he had been avoiding me, though. I found out he had been avoiding all khaki in the department. When I stepped into the Xray room that afternoon to check on a patient with a sprained ankle, I smelled liquor on Eddie.

"Petty Officer Hastings, do you have something you want to tell me?" No. He knew what I was asking, though.

"I just had a couple of drinks last night, that's all."

I grimaced for him. A doctor for 17 years, I knew that smell was more than a two-drinks-last-night smell. "You're in AA, Petty Officer Hastings. They agree with any drinks?"

"...Sometimes," he lied, even knowing that I knew it.

He went up to see the CAAC who suggested Eddie start Antabuse. There are a lot of limitations to Antabuse, and serious side effects for some people, so I never prescribe it unless the patient really is willing. Eddie wasn't. And even though I didn't need it, Master Chief Shulman phoned down to my office to tell me Eddie could not be forced to take Antabuse.

"Looks like Level III, Petty Officer Hastings." He pouted about that for a week, but we put in the application.

Two days after we sent in the application for Hasting's rehab, Master Chief Shulman was knocking on my office Door.

"Captain Riley, Petty Officer Hastings came down to tell me you've been harassing him."

The Command Master Chief's job includes being more than just an advocate for the men. The CMC in some ways is like a parent, in others like a union stewart.

"He's been drinking again, Master Chief."

"Says he hasn't been."

"I smelled it on him this week. His job performance is slipping again."

"Captain, did you do a Fitness for Duty on him? Get an alcohol level? Notify the Command?" Master Chief Shulman called me "Captain" whenever he was stern or wanted to lecture me.

"Hey, Master Chief, I notified the CAAC! What is this? If you **care** about this guy you'll help us get him treated."

"He still hasn't had a full Level II, Captain. If you just force him like this, it's discrimination, and I think he can make a case for harassment."

That week, Master Chief Shulman, the CAAC, and I met about four times, three of them with Eddie Hastings present. Finally, the ship's lawyer came at the Master Chief's insistence and we had to drop Eddie's Level III application.

Two weeks later, during sick call a beaming FN Tyrone Hill was waiting for me. He had refused to be seen by any of the corpsmen or the WOPA Bob Willmore. "No I got a note here just for Doctor Riley from the specialist."

The note from the podiatrist said that the fireman had constitutionally flat feet due to lax plantar tendons, and that he could be administratively separated from the Navy according to our old friend 1910.2. I called the phone number on the consultation form.

"Captain," the podiatrist explained, "there's nothing we can really do for this, and really FN Hill's feet shouldn't be causing him pain, but if he keeps pushing this, he'll eventually get out. You can't stop it. It's not worth fighting it."

The podiatrist was right, of course. Experience had shown that eventually there would be enough angry letters -- from lawyers, relatives, congressmen, that the sailor would get out eventually. The myth of the flat feet is a powerful one. It hurt the ship, though, because Administrative Separations, whether for physical reasons of unsuitability or for personality disorders, did not entitle the ship to a replacement. The ship's company would remain short until the separated person's tour was supposed to end. It was inevitable, though, so I took a deep breath and sent the fireman back to his departmental office with the initial paperwork.

About 0900, as Sick Call was winding down, HM1 Dunwoody came to tell me Eddie Hastings had failed to report aboard that morning. We had to go bring him back from the Day's Inn where he had passed out the night before.

"I guess you were right, Doc," the Command Master Chief admitted with no contrition at all. He called me "Doc" when he wanted me to feel that he liked me or wanted me to agree with him. Finally we were able to get Hasting's into the residential Level III treatment.

FAMILY DAY CRUISE

I had dreaded the Family Day Cruise for months, even before it turned out I would be the only doctor on board. We had a screening questionnaire to exclude very sick or immobile people or people with unstable conditions. We discovered, though, that people falsified them or the XO overruled me. So we had a menagerie of several thousand innocent and not-so-innocent family members climbing all over the ship while we steamed from eight in the morning to three in the afternoon.

An F-14 was going to fly by and break the sound barrier alongside at 1300. That was the only thing I insisted that I must see. I was resigned to be busy, but I underestimated the load dramatically.

Forget it. It was all such a blur that I can't even recall the day's events coherently. A woman had an hysterical seizure on the flight deck while a middle aged man with angina fell down a ladder on the hangar deck. Lots of people smashed fingers in doors, and a dozen or so felt overcome by heat up on the flight deck. A few got sunburned although we warned everybody about sunburn and provided free sunscreen.

The two things I remember clearly are Chief Abercrombe ("You'll have to watch that guy," Rick Combs had told me) being missing all day, and the lady who broke her knee on the flight deck.

Amid the melee of getting everybody signed up and counted while getting underway, LT Lucy came to me agitated. Striking an anxious pose with an extended left arm and flexed left quads, he began with his characteristic eloquence. "Uh, Umm, I mean..." Momentary shrug. "Captain, we can't find Chief Abercrombe."

That of course is an impossible sentence. No such thing as you can't find the Leading Chief.

"Did you check his rack?" Of course. "Chief's mess?" Yes.

"Well, what about the head down by his rack?"

"Sir, we've checked all the heads in Chiefs' Country! He's not onboard." That can't be. Chiefs just don't go UA. Couldn't find him all day. We had to report it in case he was injured someplace out in town. As the day went on and we looked everywhere, including his rack and the heads over and over, it became clear. He was gone.

About noon there was a 1MC call, "Medical Emergency. Medical Emergency. On the Flight Deck. Medical Emergency. This is not a drill."

A very large woman about seventy years old tripped on the arresting cable and fell on her knee. Her family was huddled over her. "Are you the doctor?" one daughter about 40 years old asked before I could introduce myself. Yes, I told her. "Are there any civilian doctors on the ship?" No, that's why we took histories before signing people up for the trip.

The rest of the family, about seven of them, buzzed in the background, while the boss daughter kept asking me questions. Please, I said, let me examine her first to make sure she doesn't have anything else wrong. "You mean like....? " and she silently pointed to her heart. Well, yes. That and other things. "Oh well, you don't have to worry about that. She doesn't have any heart trouble. But I'm worried about that leg. At her age, you know you have to worry about the hip too and I think she broke the knee anyway don't you?

We took the lady, who was very nice herself, and had little to say, down in a Neil-Robertson stretcher very carefully to the medical department. There now seemed to be about ten members of the family buzzing, and the boss daughter now had a deputy boss helping her with the questions. "Are you going to take an X-ray?" Yes, as quickly as we can. "Will that do any good if you don't have a radiologist on board?"

"Can you give her anything for pain?"

Finally, out of innocent curiosity I stopped what I was doing, looked up to stare at Boss Daughter, and asked, "Are you from New York?"

She was offended by the question and yet not quite surprised that I would ask it. "Yes I am. Why should you ask me that?"

"Just wondering," I said, but I wished I had asked it sooner, because she slowed down the harangue a little after that. We never found any fractures in the mother's limb, but I missed the supersonic fly-by.

We pulled back alongside Charlie pier about 1500. After the ship was all tied up, people were walking on and off, and we sent the large woman and her family off to the civilian hospital of her family's choosing. Shortly after Liberty Call around 1630, who should saunter down the starboard passageway but HMC Abercrombe!

"Chief, where have you been all day!"

"Down in Chiefs' Berthing. I was sick this morning."

"But the guys couldn't find you down there."

"Must have been while I was in the head. Bad diarrhea."

He was smooth. Like Rick Combs said, "better watch him." But even watching him he was going to be hard to catch.

I went out for a walk around the base to relax that night. I needed some fresh air and a walk on grass. When I passed the softball diamonds, I saw Tyrone Hill. He was playing third base, jumping around, moving his feet just fine. When he saw me, he quit jumping, but just looked away and stayed in the game.

The next day Gary Pompadour reported for duty officially. He was different now, though. He wore a bright blue rubber support brace around his right knee -- on the **outside** of his khaki trousers! And he was limping. "You OK, Gary?"

"Oh, yeah, it's just that old knee, you know."

That afternoon, he changed into civilian clothes after regular work hours. He was a little surprised that you had to wear a uniform all the time, even when you weren't at work. When he realized I wasn't joking that you're **always** at work while you're on the ship, he was even more surprised.

Gary wasn't a bad doctor. He had a very pleasing personality, and the guys liked his manner. Several people asked me during our last underway period whether the poor guy with those braces should have to be on sea duty. Besides the limp and the bright blue knee brace on his right knee, he now was wearing a big rubber sling brace on his left arm. He often carried a cane around the deck too and seemed to use it whenever he climbed a ladder. He didn't complain aloud at all even though his limp seemed to worsen daily, and he was a good worker in sick call. I was still curious why he had not closed out his rented apartment in Orlando, or moved his boat to Mayport, but I had to admit the crew and the corpsmen liked him. He made a lot of friends on our ten day trip to St. Thomas.

On the way back to Mayport one day, the 1MC alarm called "Medical Emergency, Medical emergency, Hangar Bay One Starboard Side. Medical emergency." I ran up to the hangar as quickly as I could. I passed Pompadour in the Dental passageway, dragging his left leg with the blue brace on it like Lon Chaney in the "Mummy" movies; I don't think he was even going toward the emergency. Up on the deck, there was a gaggle of people kneeling over the patient. It was Tommy Cage. "Says he can't breathe, Doc."

"Feet. My feet are swollen again. I think I'm having a heart attack," he almost panted out.

He wasn't sweating. Pulse was normal at about 80 beats per minute. Although his chukka boots were slit up the sides, his feet were not swollen at all. "Now, Petty Officer Cage, the specialist over at the hospital said he couldn't find anything wrong." The internist had done a stress test, checked a bunch of labs. "Your exam is normal now, too. I think you're just anxious. Try to calm down," I told him. There are litters everywhere in the hangar, so we put him on a litter and took him down to Medical. His EKG was normal again.

This was one of the most fascinating cases of panic attacks I had seen. The attacks are uncommon among people this age, but I thought it showed how frightening, how extreme, the feelings can be. It also emphasized that they can happen to people who seem "normal." The clinician has to remain vigilant. When Tommy calmed down, I reviewed this with him, and he agreed.

"If it's not physical, I sure feel terrible when that happens to me. If you say I need to see the psychiatrist, that's what I'll do."

He agreed too fast. That should have tipped me off. He rested for a while and then was able to go back to work.

My last order of business that day was being summoned down to the XO's office where Master Chief Shulman and FN Tyrone Hill were waiting for me.

"Doc, Fireman Hill says you're keeping him from getting his disability."

Disability?

"Yeah, I got to leave because of a medical problem, that's supposed to be a Medical Discharge. In Personnel, they told me you were trying to make this just an Administrative Matter."

He had a letter from his congressman asking why he should be denied his rightful medical disability.

"Mrs. Hill called me this morning, Doc, and she was pretty upset," the XO said.

Once again, I explained about the feet. I brought them the podiatrist's note, explained that the sailor didn't have a disease, and that he had brought his flat feet with him when he came to the Navy, so this would be an Administrative Separation, not due to a disease.

"Oh, no!" Hill raised his voice in the anger that was by now becoming familiar to me. "My feet never hurt me until I came to this ship, and nobody here wants to help. They just treat you rough or try to kick you out."

I showed him and the XO his entrance physical. He had flat feet then. Still had them.

"OK," the XO said. "There's nothing we can do about this, FN Hill. You can go back to see the specialist when we get back to Mayport, but I don't think this is going to qualify for a disability pension. Doc, I want you to call his mother when we get back and put her mind at ease." Hill was still not happy.

Later that night, lying awake, I reviewed something that stuck in my mind -- wasn't Gary Pompadour's brace on his **left** knee tonight?

THE DEPLOYMENT NEARS

Dan Eardley finally arrived in August. Somehow I had expected not to like him, I guess because he was uncertain about when he would arrive. When I first met Dan, though, I knew he was a keeper. Unassuming, affable, and pleasant, Dan was a former nurse who had partly paid his way through medical school as an RN. I had not been home for many months, so Dan and Gary agreed to watch the Department to let me spend a few days with Ann and our daughters.

The second day up in Boston, I got a call from the ship. Gary fell down a ladder, couldn't move his left shoulder, and would have to permanently be off sea duty. He was alone when he fell, so he was the only witness. The orthopedist at NHJax couldn't find anything torn or broken, but he said that without shoulder motion, a man was unfit for sea duty, and he transferred Gary to the care of an orthopedist in Orlando. "After all, he still has an apartment there," the Jacksonville orthopod said, "and since he can't be assigned to your ship, he might just as well recuperate in Orlando as in Jacksonville."

I called Frank Trumble, the hobbit-like, but useless AirLant medical officer. "Gee, Terry, I wish you had told me sooner you had problems with your staff. It's too late in the year for us to get a relief now. Sorry. You should have let me know before this."

"Come on, Frank, don't you remember you told me that I wasn't being fair about this! We've talked about Pompadour four times." In fact, Frank had even scolded me for doubtng the young doctor's motives at one point.

"Funny," the hobbit-doctor said, "I just don't remember talking about it. Oh well, you'll have to do the best you can."

So we would have to get along without a GMO. Once I thought that just losing Doug Kempf was bad. Little had I suspected we might actually have to get underway without a GMO altogether!

Finally, it somehow became late September, the last in-port period was almost over. My phone call with Tyrone Hill's mother was generally unsuccessful. I was calm and tried to be helpful, but she remained convinced that her son was cheated out of a Navy disability pension. At one point, I suggested that if he couldn't get a pension, perhaps he would like to stay in the Navy. She pondered that briefly, but eventually ruled against it. Shortly Tyrone became a civilian and we suggested he inquire about his disability from the Veteran's Administration. I never heard from him or the VA.

We would be getting underway on the deployment the next week. So Ann came down to visit for a few days and we had a picnic on the beach for the corpsmen and their families. While we were at the picnic that afternoon, I thought about Hugh Beaumont. Apparently he and his wife were going to divorce. The psychologist decided Hugh's anxiety and his reactions were troublesome, all right, but not unexpected around the break-up of a marriage. There hadn't been any more trouble from his hanging around. Still, the scene of this picnic with all the children touched me. Perhaps it touched me selfishly; my kids were older teenagers now, and they were up in Massachusetts. It touched me for Hugh, too, though. He had seemed so close to them when we met on the beaches down in Daytona last October.

Eerie that I should have thought about Hugh that day, because when we came back to the department, one of the corpsmen said, "Captain, HM1 Beaumont and his brother are waiting for you."

The two of them were sitting in my office. Hugh had lost weight over the months. His eyes were red, and he sat expressionless but vaguely morose, just staring at a wrinkle in the bulkhead. His brother was a handsome man who looked like Hugh. His outgoing charm reminded me of what had been so appealing in his brother the corpsman when we first met. "Captain, I don't think Hugh is in any shape to go on this deployment." Such a simple declarative sentence, and yet I found myself preparing to debate.

I thought better of it, though, and looked at immobile, staring Hugh. "Petty Officer Beaumont, what do you think?"

"Tell you the truth, I'd rather go. Their transmitters can only reach a few miles. If I can just get away from here, she and her so-called friends will finally have to leave me alone."

"Your wife?"

"She calls herself my wife, but she's not, and she knows that I know it, too."

His brother said, "Ask him her name."

"You can talk right to me, Bill, I'm right here," Hugh said. "Linda, Grindl, Lindl, Grinda. She uses them all. Sometimes they call her Elesandra, sometimes they don't use a name. They have their reasons."

Hugh's brother was obviously right. Hugh had to go to the hospital. We were able to arrange it that afternoon.

Ann was able to stay another couple of days. The weather was good, we spent some time on the beach, had breakfast at the SunDog restaurant, just relaxed. I took Ann back to the airport the day before our departure. Since it would be six months before I'd sleep ashore again, I kept the BOQ room we had rented for one last night on land.

Besides the bedroom, another thing we wouldn't have for six months was a bathtub. Feeling a little lonesome, I climbed into the tub about 2200 that night for a long hot soak. After about twenty minutes, though, just as my ligaments and muscles were sagging into warm laxity, the phone rang. In the distance I thought I could hear sirens too.

"Uh... Captain Riley. This is HM3 Davis. There's been a fire on the ship, and we're vacating the Medical Department."

I looked out the back window of the BOQ and saw smoke rising from Charlie pier.

Back at the ship, the smoke only seemed to be coming out of the island up on the Flight Deck, and the starboard Hangar Bay doors. Hundreds of sailors were smoke stained, smaller numbers coughing, but mobs and mobs of people milling around. Water ran off the starboard side of the Flight Deck and the Hangar Deck, but there were no flames. The Captain was there and the XO. Everybody was doing his job, there was no shouting, but facial features were expressionless granite. Everyone remembered "Trial by Fire." Every FID sailor always remembers July 29, 1967. We remembered it that night too. This time, nobody was seriously hurt and even the smoke inhalation was not severe for anyone.

It was a situation where somebody had to take charge, and nobody liked being in charge as much as HM3 Arden Womple. There he was up on the Hangar Deck barking orders, "Keep to your right please! Don't go down there, you guys, what do you think you're doing? Let me see your I.D."

Over the next several days the investigation showed that the fire had started in what was supposed to be an empty machine room on the starboard side right under the island. We weren't told many details about the investigation, but most of us figured it must have been sabotage. One young sailor was escorted off the ship a few days later without explanation. Nobody died or was even badly hurt, but thousands of wires and cables leading from one important part of the ship to another were destroyed.

We couldn't get underway in the morning. In fact, it took a month with our own and extra contractor crews working around the clock to fix the FID so we could start our deployment. It felt like a new SRA on the second deck with hoses, welders, ropes, and barricades everywhere again.

In the first week of November, when it seemed as though we'd finally be able to start the deployment, we learned that one of the officers in the Engineering Department had nominated Womple for a Navy Achievement Medal for his role in fighting the fire. I called the new CHENG, Greg Sanford. "Hey, Greg, Womple is a problem in our department. Don't your guys get a departmental endorsement for awards?"

He told me he would look into the matter.

Two days later there was a formation in service dress uniform up on the Flight Deck for all the people getting awards. On my way up the ladder, LT Lucy stopped me. He was agitated. First his right shoulder, then his left, shrugged up and forward, and his left biceps lifted his left wrist. His neck and chin dipped to the right as the muscles on his neck stood out in photogenic relief. "Captain, Captain!" he almost shouted, then paused for a brief vacuous stare. "Captain, Petty Officer Womple has locked himself in the pharmacy and he won't come out. He says you have bullied him so badly he's going to kill himself."

We ran back to the pharmacy where the door was indeed locked. "Petty Officer Womple, are you in there?" I asked.

First there was no answer. Lucy shrugged his back and thigh muscles anxiously. I would not have suspected Womple would kill himself. Then from behind us, two doors aft, in one of the storerooms, came a muffled bass voice. "I'm not coming out!"

"Lieutenant, he's not here, he's back there in a storeroom." Deer-in-the-headlights. "Oh. I thought that **was** the pharmacy."

It took us two painful hours of negotiations to get Womple to come out. Only after being promised he wouldn't have to see me, Womple agreed to leave the storeroom so he could be transported to the psychiatrist at NHJax. The psychiatrist said he was depressed. Although probably not suicidal, Womple would need to stay in the hospital and could not deploy. We asked the Ship's Secretary to inform the hospital that when Womple recovered, he still should be separated from the Navy.

Dr. Pompadour was off the crew a lot faster than he had joined it, our Xray tech was off to Level III alcohol rehab, Arden Womple was admitted because of his frustration or depression, and Hugh Beaumont was being treated for a major thought disorder. This was not the right time for those four to go to sea, I decided, but it sure was for the rest of us. The team was short four players, but we needed to go.

Finally it looked like we might be able to get underway.

Chapter XII. GETTING UNDERWAY AT LAST

If God had not already created Navies, the human race would have invented one for a day like November 5, 1989. You could see all the way to Nebraska, the sky was so open, and it had just a few slashes of high cirrus clouds, like the marks Zorro used to zap into a silk curtain. It was definitely an aircraft carrier day. Charlie Pier was crowded with a festive mass of TV news people, local politicians, and family members by the thousands. A Navy band was playing, people were waving banners. From the flight deck or the bridge, there were two views. Down on the pier, all the cheering people, dressed with lots of red, blue and silver, looked like the stadium at a football game. There were even vendors selling Cokes, popcorn, and ***Forrestal*** souvenirs,just like at a stadium or a circus. From the nine stories up on the flight deck, or twelve up to the bridge, if you looked over to the port side or aft, to the east, the sky and the spear clouds pulled your vision to the horizon, the ocean.

Down on the pier, an hour ago, all the sailors and officers had said their good-byes, had the long hugs, and for the very young ones (likely who just met the girl this week) long movie-like kisses. The brows had been pulled up then and every one had to be on board in time to get everything ready. The Admiral came on board in the last few minutes, and for him and any last minute details, the last of about four brows waited until just before departure. Six months is a long time. Those who had never been through a prior deployment would fret about how a separation hurts, but those who had survived many before knew better all the pains and challenges ahead. The crying and working it out had been done over the past weeks for those who were able. A lot of other veterans and their families just didn't indulge in the departure festivities. Too hard. They had said good-bye at the house, did the crying there if they had to, and just drove to work. For those families, it wasn't a matter of ignoring the situation. They knew the pain too, usually from six or eight prior deployments. For the kids, better to start today knowing we are going to take on the routine, face every day ourselves and do it right, even if Dad's not here. Dad had probably cried on the way to the ship and they all cried when they closed the door behind him. Even if they cried behind the door they also started the coping right then. They didn't want to let the sailor or the strangers on the pier see them crying in public. Not that they had some phoney facade; they wouldn't *deny* the crying, they just didn't need to *share* it with strangers.... and they didn't want to make the departure harder for him. (While at the same time, not always even knowing it, they were resentful at him for going. Again.)

Plenty did show up for the occasion, though. Departments and Divisions had family groups with banners and signs painted on sheets. Lots of cameras. Many of the women were dressed up, although a lot less provocatively and wearing a lot less red than we all knew they would when we would arrive in six months. Hundreds of crew members had ordered roses from a few florists who were there to deliver them to wives and sweethearts that day. Some of the small children were awestruck, as all small children had to be, by the size of the ship, but most especially by the gala, the motion, all the noise. All of the excitement thrilled most children, especially those under four and over fifteen. But a lot of school age youngsters had wet faces, clung anxiously to their mothers, and wanted either the day to go away or the whole idea to be a mistake. An hour before, a lot of "No, Daddy, don't go!" or "Daddy, we want you to stay, PLEASE," were heard before everyone had to get on board. Now, scattered crying and shaking shoulders could be seen, but these were partly obscured or hidden among lots of crying babies -- who were just tired of being held so long -- and overshadowed by all the other youngsters caught up in the great patriotic spectacle.

Getting underway is a critical, busy, and dangerous time. Many people on the ship have a lot to do, especially the Deck Department. The Boatswain's Mates scurry from one sponson or station to the next. Line handlers and working parties on the pier and hangar wells throw and pull the 8 inch lines, always laying it in careful order so it can be moved and not be tripped over or caught in a knot by casual movement. Machinery and gear are everywhere, some of it whirring or moving, all of it skulking or sprawling someplace waiting to knock someone down, tear a trouser leg, or break an ankle. In the mass movement and activity, chances for people to fall off the ship or trip on the pier are always a concern. We had teams of corpsmen stationed with their Unit One first aid kits at critical places on the hangar deck, and among the crowd until the brows came up. The Mayport Clinic positioned an ambulance at the pier for the event. Sure enough, one fat fortyish woman fainted and had to be carted off to the clinic, and forty minutes later, a bald man in his sixties who had been warned twice not to smoke on the pier, had sudden chest pain and was taken off presumably toward Beaches Hospital.

Running everywhere through all this were the two busiest men in the crowd, the XO and Ed DeMartini, who was now the First Lieutenant, since Warren Lobs moved on. Both of them were carrying on continuous discussions with their bricks, while their heads swiveled everywhere. The XO, with his Dress Blue jacket bulging at the buttons and streaked tight across his waist and hips, searched for trouble from the crowds, looking to be sure everything was stowed, and preparations were going well. His gaze was at eye level and often upward. Ed, as First Lieutenant, was responsible for the Bos'n's Mates and line handlers, and all the sailor stuff. By contrast, he mostly had to look down, down and sideways, as he moved here and there, back and forth, pointing at things, yelling at some guy, speaking in the vernacular peculiar to Bos'n's Mates, longshoremen, and Marines.

Then somehow, it was obvious, like the day your term paper came due, that it was time to go, and everything seemed to know it and somehow everything was ready. All the activity didn't have any obvious connection to the being ready. The activity seemed kind of disembodied, like it was a ballet or something, and the ship just got ready by itself, like when a bud on a branch is ready to open. The time just arrives. First Ed, then the XO, came over the last brow, the crane took the brow away. The crowd grew a little quieter, and a few of the rentacops moved among them, along with some Shore Patrol uniforms, and the margins of the crowd drew back a few feet. Some lines were tossed from the ship to the pier, and a few others slurped up into the ship like long strands of spaghetti. The rails were all manned, with sailors dressed for recruiting posters, at parade rest, all along the flight deck and up the walkways on the island. They looked just as you would expect only better. All straight, kerchiefs flying, hats whiter than if they were a thousand ivory teeth in the line. At the bow, in the straight line at the end of the flight deck, in front of the number "59," the place that only shipmates can call "the pointy end," it was Marines at parade rest in their dress blues with white gloves. The crowd on the pier got very quiet for some reason. Then, gradually, in a breath, you could tell why. The ship moved just a little, with a sideways sigh, not jerky at all.

Suddenly, next came the Captain's music, first Willy Nelson singing, "On the Road Again...I Can't Wait to be On the Road Again... Makin' Music with My Friends. I Can't

Wait to get ON THE ROAD AGAIN..." Loud on the 1MC and the speakers on the pier. Now the crowd is rowdy and every shipmate smirks a little, but at the same time he wonders, "How did the Captain know..." The ship moved in earnest then, finally with a... a little shudder. The crowd whoops, a few wives and children jump up and down or do little dances while they wave.

The tugs pulled the ship out into the turning basin and started to turn her around, to face the ocean. I scrambled up to get as high on the island as I could to take this all in.

About the time I got up near the Signal Bridge, as high as you can go without going up a tower, the music stopped for a moment. From where I was you could see the swirls of sand bottom contours under the blue ocean in the St Johns Inlet. It kind of set off the paler cirrus slashes up in the clearer but paler sky. The crowd quieted now, because we were about to leave. Music again. First a real short prelude from an organ. Then in a voice as clear as this day, and as rich as her memory, Kate Smith sang ***"G-O-D Bless A - MER-i-ca..."*** The cliche says, "you really had to be there..." Well, for those of us who were there that day, most would confide that it was probably a little like Fatima or Lourdes (of course, being there meant we were zealots, anyway, so our objectivity as observers was tainted). By the time she reached "From the Mountains... To The Prairies, " the Forrestal was turned and if there had been a single Communist in Florida, he would have converted and joined the rest of us in the orgy of patriotic tears. We were underway.

I stayed up on the Signal Bridge for about a half hour, watching Mayport shrink and fade. The view was hypnotic. Knowing there was going to be a steady diet of 18 hour days for the next six months, and that it was going to be worse without a GMO, I let myself linger for a while, enjoying the fine mist sea mist and the view up here about a hundred feet above the white caps. Finally, I decided I should go ahead and take my departure photos and get down to the Medical Department. No film in the camera. I had forgotten to load it when I left the stateroom a couple of hours ago. Was that an omen? Oh, well, time to get to work.

On my way below, I got off on the O-3 level to cross over to the port side so that I would pass my stateroom on the way to the department. There I could change from blues to khakis and drop off the camera. I could cross over on O-3, the hangar deck, or the second deck, and it was more or less random which one I would take any time. The O-3 level was pretty busy on departure day, with a lot of traffic coming and going from Strike Ops, where daily plans were organized, and a lot of business in the Ship's Office. Most especially, though, the O-3 deck was where the Staff lived and worked. On departure day, the Staff had reasons to be out bothering and bossing everybody. I was greeting and glad handing Tom Fitzgerald and Ed Dicey, a couple of the Staff guys I liked, when suddenly there he was in all his 6'2" gaunt sobriety: Oliver Leen. My circuits erased, I was speechless. Tom and Ed must have wondered how I went from effusive camaraderie to abject catatonia in midsentence. They had not seen Leen, who came down the passageway behind them. Even if they had seen him, they probably didn't know why I would go into brain arrest. I tried to speak, to be confused, to be angry, to have an opinion or reaction of any kind at all. I think I said something along the lines of "b'duh...b'duh...b'duh." How did he get here? Almost a year ago, John Seibel, the head of Internal Medicine at the Navy Hospital Jacksonville had signed his Medical Board to keep him off sea duty.

CDR Leen seemed a little bit startled, but a lot less befuddled than I was at the moment. He had been expecting an encounter probably. He quietly turned and left, so Ed and Tom never knew he was there. They looked at each other and telepathically agreed that this conversation was not a rewarding one. We halfheartedly mumbled some platitudes about how nice it was to see each other again, they quickly ducked back into the Flag offices and I scrambled down to my office on the second deck. I had to see Leen's medical record. If he was a stowaway or had altered his medical record, I was going to go straight to the Admiral. His own health and the concern of a lot of other people were involved.

When I got to the department, there was a crowd in the amidships passageway between my office and the Emergency Ward. A couple of MAAs with their big white belts and their bricks squawking were milling around with two Chiefs and a jg. A seaman was sitting on the bench with a Jimmy Cagney half grin, ***Forrestal*** ballcap tilted back on his head, and a semi-dirty t-shirt wrapped around his forearm. "Don't tell me," I said. "You cut your wrist, right?" He nodded and the half grin became a victorious but small smile. The seaman knew that we were within helo distance of the beach, he would be going back to Jacksonville before long. We would examine him and do a detailed medical history and psychiatric evaluation, all right. Yet, when we had finished, either he was earnestly suicidal and would need to go for treatment, or even if not a likely risk, he knew that we would never gamble or play tough with these stakes. We would have to send him back.

"It's his buddy I'm more worried about, Doc," his Chief said. There was another seaman in the Emergency Ward. Bob Willmore was with him. The second seaman had a characteristic stack of very, very superficial scratches on his left wrist, too. Since most people are right handed, they hold the pocket knife or razor blade in the right hand and make the tentative slicing attempts on the left wrist. A little bit more blood on this guy than on Jimmy Cagney out in the passageway, but the marks were still way too superficial to need sutures. This guy was weepy, morose, incommunicative. He spoke only with reticent semiaudible grunts. His name was Warner. He had only been on the ship a couple of months and didn't have any real friends. Always a loner, people took little notice of him. He did his work acceptably, but was not a standout. In fact, his Chief had begun to notice a few weeks ago that he kept to himself a lot and didn't mix with others. When we started getting ready to go the day before, he was seen sobbing a little but refused to talk. Thinking he was alone outside a workspace after we got underway, he tried to cut himself, but a couple of friends, including the smart aleck on my bench outside saw him.

They called the Chief, who came right away and called Medical and Security. Just when the MAAs arrived, Seaman Number One took out his knife and said, "I know what he's going through. I can't take it either." Whereupon he made as many tiny little cuts on his left wrist as he could before the MAAs wrestled his knife away from him.

I asked Bill Flynn to help Willmore with the two cases for the present. Besides looking after the patients, there would be reports to the XO and the Captain, notification of the sailors' department head, and arrangements for flying them off if the Skipper would agree, after the heloes arrived.

I ducked into my office and buzzed for Curt Rosenthal. He got me Oliver Leen's medical record. Both to my alarm and yet also a little to my relief Leen was back on the ship legally! His record showed the Medical Board, recommending Permanent Limited Duty, which would have allowed him to stay in the Navy to complete his twenty years but prohibited duty at sea or in duty stations where a hospital was easily accessible. He had gone through the proper appeals route, rebutting the Medical Board to the Central Physical Evaluation Board. The rebuttal included a letter from his (civilian) endocrinologist saying that shipboard duty would be no problem for CDR Leen, who was very capable of managing his own insulin. In all these years, he said, the Commander had not suffered any complications of his diabetes or insulin therapy. The Physical Evaluation Board was persuaded by the rebuttal, and determined he was fit for sea duty. I was chagrined of course that the near-coma ketoacidosis that almost killed him last year showed something that us old fashioned GP-types would have been tempted to call a complication. His hiding severe illness from us was still worrisome (worrisome, hell, it was infuriating) to me. Would that happen again?

Finally, I resolved my feelings this way: The Central PEB knew that he had insulin-dependent diabetes, and they knew that a reliable Board-Certified internist, John Seibel, recommended he not go to sea, that he had a serious case of pyelonephritis. If after weighing all the evidence, the PEB would let him go to see, the consequences were his and the PEBs. We on the ship now knew we would have to be very attentive and frankly, now that we were on alert, I felt comfortable that we would be able to handle his diabetes. While the medical risks were manageable -- especially since we knew about his propensity to cover up -- he didn't really need to go to sea. There were other officers in his special field; there were plenty of jobs he could do on shore duty. With the questionable premise that medical precaution could "hurt" his career or promotion opportunities, he was permitted to go into an environment with more risk than was necessary. But this time, it wouldn't ruin my day. He had followed the rules. I couldn't fault him for that. Ironic; I spent so much of my time the past many weeks with people looking for physical excuses to *avoid* going to sea. Here was the opposite, and I had resisted emotionally. I phoned Leen to tell him I was glad to see him back on the ship, and invited him to come down for a cup of coffee when he had the time. (Four years later, assigned to the Bureau of Medicine and Surgery, I was jogging across the Memorial Bridge toward the Pentagon one sunny February day, and I passed Ollie going the opposite direction. He was going a helluva lot faster than I was. The diabetes had pretty obviously not done him in yet.)

Bill Flynn came in to talk about our two suicidal sailors. One of them was almost speechless, couldn't express what he was anxious about, but Bill was worried about him. He might be depressed, Bill thought, but he might also be psychotic. As long as somebody would stay with him, Bill thought he would be safe, but we had to get him to a proper suicide-proof environment and competent, probably in-patient, psychiatric care. The second character, the smart aleck, seemed to just want off the ship. We had no choice. Since HS-15, the H3 helo squadron, flew on board the first day (while we were still within their range) we could send these two fellows back to the Navy Hospital Jacksonville. I talked it over with the XO. We now had a cellular telephone on the ship, so I was able to arrange with the psychiatrists at the hospital without using the Red Phone.

FLU SHOTS AGAIN

The first day was still only in midafternoon. It was far from over. George Lucy brought the officers and Chiefs of the department in for the 1600 meeting we had scheduled to talk about flu shots. Everybody remembered that I had sworn "no more mass immunizations!" but flu shots could not really be spread over the entire year. Influenza is predominantly a seasonal winter illness, so effective immunizations should be given in the fall. Because the influenza virus undergoes antigenic evolution from one year to the next, the vaccine changes every year, and to be effective must be given annually. Flu is a bad disease, and can be savagely infectious in the confines of a ship. So we had to plan to give flu shots. Everybody on the ship would need them. The best time to do it would be while transiting the Atlantic before operations became very busy. Therefore, we would have to make an exception to my "no mass programs" dictum.

"But I thought you didn't want to give shots anymore," Lt Lucy said. He twitched his jaw to the right and his head to the left, flexed his pecs.

"No, Lieutenant. I said I didn't want to give '**mass**' shot programs again. Giving flu shots is not optional. We still have to do it. I just want to do it smarter. No lines, OK?"

He gave me the deer-in-the-headlights expression again. We talked about how to schedule people in manageable small groups of about 40 in every 15 minute interval, so that nobody would have to stand around too long, the lines would never have more than 40 people in them and we could keep the whole exercise down on the second deck, maybe entirely in the Medical Department. Bob Willmore suggested we could keep the project going almost 24 hours a day so that people who worked night shifts wouldn't have to interrupt their sleep to meet our schedule. "But if you do that won't some people who work in the daytime have to get up at night just for their shots?" asked Lucy, flexing his left biceps. Somebody explained to him that separate schedules could be made for people on various shifts. We decided to schedule shots by alphabet rather than workspaces, so that the shops could spread out time away from work. It was my job to go to the Department Heads and the XO at eight o'clocks to clear it with the ship and all the departments.

That night at eight o'clocks I brought up the subject of the flu shots. Groans all around. "Hey, Doc, my grandmother has never had a flu shot in her life. She's 97 years old and never had the flu. You tryin' to tell me healthy people our age need those shots?" A very popular complaint was this one: "Doc, I don't take flu shots anymore. They always make me sicker than hell. Ever since I quit takin' the shots, I've never had the flu. No thanks." I heard that one more than a dozen times every flu shot season. Another popular stanza was, "Why make us get these shots for the flu? I can see typhoid or yellow fever, but not a minor illness. Nobody ever dies from flu!" Of course, the general public does not understand influenza, so every year we had an educational program about it on the ship, with pamphlets, lectures on the closed circuit TV, and sessions like this one.

The common, mostly trivial, respiratory or gastrointestinal short illnesses people catch from time to time are often colloquially but erroneously called "flu." Connecting those trivial illnesses to the word "flu" gives a serious misimpression about influenza. The real illness is caused by a very infectious virus, spread by close contact and moisture droplets in cough or breath particles. Of course the elderly or people in crowded environments are the most vulnerable. In the world's worst epidemic in 1918, millions died, more than a hundred thousand in the U.S in that single year. There is no cure; as in other viral infections, antibiotics have no direct effect. Although the vaccine is not 100% effective, it prevents an outbreak from becoming an epidemic and significantly limits the severity in those few vaccinated people who do catch the flu. If we would have an influenza outbreak on the FID without immunizations, a conservative estimate might be that more than a thousand members of the crew would become sick, and at least 2/3 of those would be unable to work for a day or more. Case fatality rates varied among outbreaks, but was usually far more than one in a thousand. Influenza is not a trivial disease. If we had more than a thousand sick, probably at least one would die.

Once the Department Heads and XO heard this pitch, the moans subdued, even if they didn't go away. The Department Heads would cooperate and the XO would make the shots mandatory. The Black Shoes always would have gone along. Once I announced that there was a SECNAV (for "SECretary of the NAVy") instruction requiring flu shots for everybody, the "Shoes" would comply immediately. No questions asked. Aviators were another matter. Anything that hurt, other than PT or an airplane crash, aviators were against it. They agreed now, after I spelled out the facts, and while their friends were watching. But when the time came to roll up the left sleeve, there would be sniveling, guys would suddenly remember allergies that weren't in their health records, and some guys would just remember something they had to do immediately. Aviators hated shots. For now, though, I had everybody's consent for the flu shot program that would start tomorrow, the fourth day underway. Admiral Sweetpea Allen, our new Battle Group Commander, had relieved Snuffy Smith, and he volunteered to go first. The Skipper, the XO, and I would be next. By setting the example, we would get more cheerful cooperation from the crew. (Being a Flight Surgeon, I didn't forget that Captain Thomassy and the Admiral were aviators. The more senior they get, the more crafty aviators can be about dodging a needle.)

The fixed wing aircraft from the Air Wing came aboard that morning. In its more private and military manner, this was as impressive for us as our getting underway had been a couple of days before. We had our planes now. The hangar bay filled, the Flight Deck started teeming. The Sleeping Giant Admiral Yamamoto spoke of 47 years ago stirred again.

Later that day we sent representatives around to all divisions to begin the education and information campaign, and to work out the scheduling. Chief Priggemeier down in the Print Shop printed hundreds of schedules so we could post them all over the ship for people to recognize their scheduled times. Even the Captain consented to plug the flu shot program on his daily 1MC address to the crew. He was getting to like the 1MC, perhaps too much. It was getting to be a running joke how long he would carry on. "Good morning. This is the Captain." Who else would it be with that country accent? "We are 800 miles east of Norfolk, and 1280 miles away from Mayport. The weather is clear and mild with a temperature of 52 degrees. We're makin' about sixteen knots and we should be near Rota in about five days. Today we're going to..." Then he would talk about the day's various activities. Next, the Captain would read the notices he had received in the day's message traffic, that included the two to four babies born to FID wives every day. Then he plugged the flu shots for us, "Now I know you guys are like me in not liking to get shots, but Doc Riley and his gang down there in Medical tell me that flu is a lot more serious than you might realize." Captain Thomassy, I thought, should consider a career in politics or radio if he ever retired from the Navy. He had a perfect touch for the crew.

Captain Thomassy then got on to the part of his daily fireside chat that made me cringe, the "Letters to the Captain Show." Ninety percent of the letters were complaints about either the Medical or Supply Departments, with another ten percent about Personnel. The XO now and then gave me and the SuppO leadership pointers. Because of the disproportionate number of complaints to only two departments, the XO saw these as his two "problem" departments. Medical was even one of what the XO called the "minor" departments, because we had so many fewer people than Engineering, Air, Supply, AIMD, and Weapons. The SuppO and I didn't take it personally, though. We realized that most complaints in all ships were about the service departments. Ours were the departments that touched everybody on the ship regardless of their jobs. Since everybody was one of our consumers, everybody had an opinion about how well we did our jobs. They were less likely to have such an opinion about other departments. After all, what could the sailors complain about how the Weapons or Air Department did their business? Medical and Supply were the two departments most directly responsible for the sailor's quality of life. The crew loved it that the Captain welcomed their input, and at the core, the SuppO and I liked it too. We just didn't like what we considered a kind of capricious quality to the process.

On this particular day, Medical escaped. The letter complained about the choice of breakfast cereals. Sure, the complainant said, you could always get eggs and a choice of cream of wheat or oatmeal. But nobody likes oatmeal and cream of wheat anymore, the complainer said; those are old fashioned. The selection of cold cereals was poor. How come we never ran out of cornflakes (almost as stodgy as oatmeal) and the Fruity Pebbles ran out every day before 0700. That wasn't fair. Remarkably, on this ship of war, this supercarrier with more bomb power than all of WWII, the two most popular breakfast cereals were Trix and Fruity Pebbles. The Captain promised the writer that he would look into the matter. The SuppO knew that he would be increasing the inventory of Fruity Pebbles.

While the Captain finished up his 1MC announcement, I was completing the day's reports in my office. When he signed off with his trademark, "...and ABOVE ALL---Have a ***FINE*** Navy Day!" I left the office to go check on something elsewhere in the department. I could scarcely get into the passageway. It was crammed too tight with sailors to permit any movement at all! There was a line stretched all the way down the starboard main passageway, back up our amidships passageway past my office door, doubled back on itself, then stretching all the way back down the starboard passageway up a dozen frames or more. What in the hell was this? I hated lines!

"Get me LT Lucy!," I shouted, hoping some corpsman somewhere might be able to hear me.

When Lucy was able to squeeze through the crowd to find me, he must have known I was angry. Maybe he could tell by the red face or the steam streaking out of my collar or my ears. Perhaps my breathing rate or the foam at the edges of my mouth gave me away. I'm not sure. He knew, though, somehow. I knew that he could tell, because he was flexing and twitching a little more and a little faster than usual.

"Lieutenant, why are all these people standing in line outside my door? I hate lines, Lieutenant."

"We arranged to have forty men every fifteen minutes, Sir, just like you said." He flexed his right thigh and left shoulder, taking on a pose a little like you see in body builder posters.

"But I think there are a couple of hundred people out here!"

"Well, yes sir. We told all the people from 1600 to 1730 to show up a little before 1600, so everything could be in line and ready to go, then we could have a break at 1730 for dinner."

The plan had been for people to arrive in increments of 40, at fifteen minute intervals. Everybody else but Lucy seemed to understand that. I didn't yell at LT Lucy out there in the passageway where anybody else could hear me, but I thought... this proves it. The man has a unique logic board. I got Curt Rosenthal and Ron Eslinger and we went up and down the line together to work it out for people to come back in 15 minutes, 30 minutes, 45 minutes, and so on. Eventually we got rid of the line. I figured I would deal with the cause of the snafu later. I needed some exercise and a good hard run to cool myself off.

A HATCH

Flight Quals were going on up on the Flight Deck, so I had to run on the Hangar Bay. In some ways, I preferred it there anyway. You had to keep your gaze alert and looking everywhere, just like an aviator's scan on the control panel, to avoid banging into a wing or a drop tank hanging below a wing. People pop out from behind yellow gear, bulkheads, and airplanes. If you don't watch carefully you can collide with a shipmate. Periodically we had to treat a fractured arm from two-man jogging collisions on the Hangar Deck. The tie-down chains that held aircraft and yellow gear in place on the deck, were sneaky, dark, and only ankle-height above the deck. All these distractions slowed me down a little but added something to think about while you did lap after lap. The hangar is loud, though. I used to go through and ask all the crew to wear ear plugs when they worked there, so I wore mine when I was running.

Even with the earplugs, though, I heard the 1MC, "Medical Emergency, Medical Emergency. Seven Tack eighty six tack sixteen. Medical Emergency." They had not added "This is a drill." Still in my PT gear, and sweating, I ran forward to the AIMD ladder well as fast as I could down one ladder, back the port passageway and to the ladderwell over the spot. I was the first medical rep there. Looking down the shaft from the second deck, there were four open water-tight hatches and one closed. I figured the sick guy was on the deck down there. I climbed through the hatch to the vertical ladder and started climbing down as fast as I could. I realized suddenly I was going down the same hole where we had found Jimmy Fulford less than a year ago. When I got to the last open hatch, I stopped and looked down. The last hatch wasn't really closed. I could see some guy's dark hair and top of his head sticking out. Was he helping out his buddy who might be stuck on the ladder there? No, that couldn't be it, the hatch was mostly closed. They weigh close to five hundred pounds. When I climbed down closer, it was clearer. The head belonged to the injured guy. It wasn't moving and he was not making any sound.

"This is Doc Riley up here. Anybody down there?" I hollered through what little opening there was.

Airman somebody was down there. he was the one who had called for help. Just then HM3 Ammerman and Ron Eslinger came down the ladder and could help. The hatch was just too heavy for a single guy to lift by himself, and the job was made more difficult because of the trapped sailor. It looked as though he might be dangling by the top of his head. While we lifted the hatch we had to make sure he didn't fall. Most of the vertical shafts like this one had canvas nets draped under the openings, so that if a guy fell, he would only go one level and not plummet straight down the 60 or 70 feet some holes reached. With the hatch closed, though, we didn't know about this one. "Airman," I shouted through the crack, "we're going to lift the hatch, please make sure he doesn't move. Most of all, for God's sake, don't stand where you can get hurt too if this thing slips. One injury is enough. Try not to let him move at all, but especially don't let him fall. Is there anybody else down there with you?"

"Yessir, there are two of us."

I pushed my hands around both sides of the head below us and Ron and Petty Officer Ammerman lifted the hatch. It was almost too heavy for two guys. We didn't know how it happened, so I warned them to be slow. An MAA arrived then and he was able to help. When the hatch came up, we saw that we had an unconscious boy about 19 years old. Both sides of his head seemed pushed in. Blood was coming out his ears and nose. Obvious skull fracture. He wasn't breathing, but he wasn't cyanotic yet. There was indeed a canvas net slung under the hatch, and his right knee was braced against it. From somewhere on that lower deck HM3 Brooks appeared and he helped the other two guys down there slowly lower the patient to the deck while I tried to hold his head and neck. As soon as we had him on the deck, Ron Eslinger came alongside. The Medical Response bags had been lowered down to us by rope. While I checked the guy over for other signs of injury, Ron started ventilating him with an ambu bag.

We learned that his name was Airman Connor Bergen, an Aviation Ordnanceman, AOAN, he worked for the Weapons Department. He and a coworker had been doing preventive maintenance on a hatch just like this one and they needed a spare spring for the latch mechanism. This particular hatch apparently was out of order so Bergen had come to take the spring out. You're never supposed to work on one of these alone and there is a complicated procedure for getting permission. Also, the door was supposed to be "tagged out," identified as out of order.

"Should we intubate him, Captain?" Ron asked. It was clear he was going to need ventilation for a while. A direct tube to his trachea could handle that far better than a facial mask. In the meantime, Ron kept his color up well with the ambu and mask.

"I don't know, Ron, can you get a tube in?" We both agreed that with an apparent basilar skull fracture a nasotracheal tube may be hazardous. His jaw seemed intact. Ron was able to slip in a normal endotracheal tube through his mouth. Breath sounds into both lungs were good. We were able to stabilize his neck and fasten him to a rigid litter. By going just a few frames forward, we were able to get to one of the Weapons elevators, and take him up to the second deck to the medical department. As we rose, I kept studying his face. For the first time, I noticed some pink grey gelatinous material coming out his nose and ears. Brain. Swelling of the brain, or cerebral edema, progresses a few hours after an injury to the brain. This was just minutes after. The crush had fractured the base of his skull and lacerated his brain.

We went straight to the ICU. Ron and Dan Eardley looked after the necessary attachments to the ventilator, and started Ivs. I called the XO. In seconds, I told him the patient's name and told him to tell the Captain it was very bad, a brain injury. I'd get back to him as soon as I could. "Somebody find out what his religion is right now." Without interfering in necessary action, we tried to get the priest, Father Linehan, if Catholics were dying.

We gave him dexamethasone immediately, a drug used to combat brain swelling, and then a load of mannitol, a faster acting solution. I looked into his fundi, the retinae, and saw massive swelling and hemorrhage confirming severely increased intracranial pressure. Being a neurologist, I checked all the signs of brainstem responsiveness that we use to determine brain death. He qualified, but it was an unnecessary academic exercise with his skull deformed and brain tissue in the nose and ears. No operations even at Bethesda would have helped him at this point.

Ron and Dan were busy with the necessary sustainment actions, but they had things under control. The Airman was a Baptist, reportedly a religious young man. I went up to the bridge to tell the Captain.

I described everything we saw and had done, described the nature of the injury. "Captain, I'm afraid he's already brain dead. Sir, there's no way he can survive." the Captain asked how we could know that this soon. I described the significance of the brainstem functions. Did not remind the Captain that I'm a neurologist.

"Well, Doc, do all you can and let's hope for a miracle."

You never close out the hope for a miracle. Not with a family member or a shipmate. Yet, while leaving the role of prayer and hope, it is irresponsible to contribute to false hopes. "Yes, Sir, but that is truly what it would take, I have to be clear with you about that." We were at this point about midway across the Atlantic, a little bit closer to Rota than to the States. It would be two days before we could get into range for fixed wing flights to shore. He couldn't handle the G-forces for a cat shot, though. So realistically, it would be three days before we could be in range of an H-53 helo to Spain.

With this injury, and clinical brain death, if we were in most U.S. hospitals, we would talk to the family about the meaning of brain death, and gently help them reach the most likely conclusion to terminate life support. None of us felt we should do that at sea. The family has a right to participate in the decision, for one thing. For another, we did not want the family to have any worry at all that their son had the fullest chance at survival. Hard as it might be to be told by doctors at a fully credentialed hospital that a loved one was brain dead, we all agreed that most families wouldn't want a ship's medical department to assume that prerogative, at least in a peacetime setting. We resolved to keep him alive and in the best possible condition until he could be taken safely to the nearest hospital, which in this case would be the U.S. Naval Hospital Rota Spain.

Word spreads quickly on the ship. The Captain knew this better than anybody, so he talked to the crew on the 1MC. "Good evening. This is the Captain. Probably most of you know by now that we have had a shipmate injured. It's AOAN Connor Bergen from down in G4. They're doin' all they can for him down in Medical, but Doc Riley tells me he's in very serious condition." The Captain said that everybody should pray for him, and then ended. That was the only short 1MC announcement I recall from the Captain, and one of only two that didn't end with "and ABOVE ALL, have a FINE Navy Day."

Ron and Dan and I took turns staying with him round the clock. Ron looked after the ventilator. His arterial blood gases stayed good until the second day, when he became a little acidotic. Chest films showed some diffuse infiltrates. We had a hard time deciding whether he had pulmonary edema secondary to the cerebral injury, or was developing pneumonia. Dan suggested we start high doses of a couple of antibiotics. In just a few days, a resistant organism would not be a concern, but if he had a fulminant pneumonia at this point, he may not be alive in a few days to worry about it.

When we were a day out I went up to Combat to get on the Red Phone to talk to a doctor at the Navy Hospital in Rota. No radio at the hospital. We had to call a destroyer that was in the port there. They called the hospital, and a doctor came down to the destroyer to talk with me. It took a couple of hours to get it all hooked up and then we waited for the nets to let us in. The doctor was a Surgeon named Harris. I recognized the name. He had just left NH Jax a few months before, in fact he had at one time been considered as Rock Tosser's relief, before Dan Eardley was picked. I explained the patient's condition and that we expected to helo him over the next day. Harris was receptive and pleasant. We promised to send over our detailed notes about Airman Bergen. Harris had no questions and we signed off.

Making the connection between the ICU and the helo would be critical, so we started making arrangements right away. I recalled the time during work-ups when Captain Thomassy was irritated about our coordination for a medevac. This time we needed everything to go perfectly. Bergen was stable, all right, but very fragile. His lungs were clearing up, but he still needed to be ventilated and now we were giving him oxygen too besides the mechanical part. Everything had to be coordinated with the Weapons department for Elevator Seven on the starboard side beside one of the mess decks. The helo would call en route from about twenty minutes out and we would get everything set up. Bergen should be on the helo within five or ten minutes from when he left the ICU. I did not want to use the deck-edge elevators to take him up to the flight deck. They were a little faster, could be used with less hoopla, and we did use them for mass casualty drills. They were jerky and windy, though. Weapons Elevator Seven opened up by the after edge of the island, by what is referred to as the "Bomb Farm" on the starboard edge of the flight deck.

I insisted that we rehearse the transfer a few times that afternoon with HM3 Brooks in the litter. Petty Officer Brooks was about the right size, and seemed to always be cheerful. The first time we tried it, it took us fourteen minutes just to get the simulated monitors in the ICU moved and disconnected and the litter brought back to the mess deck. The second time, we got him back to the elevator in seven minutes, but there was a twelve minute delay getting the elevator crew to crank up the elevator. Finally, on the third try, we got the litter up to the flight deck in eight minutes. "OK, guys, let's not tamper with a smooth system. It has to go at least this well in the morning. Everybody please remember your part."

Back in the department, Dan was his usual well-composed amiable self. I frequently was thankful to have him and now was one of those time. It crossed my mind for one painful instant what it would have been like to have to deal with Rock Tosser at a time like this. Ron was quietly getting a little anxious about the trip. "Captain, I think I should go with him."

"Ron, I know you'd like to make sure his ventilation is maintained. He never would have survived until now without you, but you know we can't spare you." It would be over a two hour helo ride. For the round trip, including the transfer over to the hospital, he would have been gone for five hours. We really couldn't be without anesthesia coverage that long. That's one of the things flight surgeons are for. Even Air Force flight surgeons are trained for medevac missions.

The next morning about 0800, the ATO called to say that the H53 had departed Rota and was en route. Our own H3s would not have had long enough legs to reach Spain until much later, and we wanted to get AN Bergen to the hospital as soon as we could. Even six or seven hours mattered to us. At 0900, the aircraft called to say they were twenty minutes out. The "Handler," LCDR Tony McFarlane had cleared a spot on the waist for the big helo and made sure there was a clear passage between the elevator and the helo. We started getting everything ready down in Medical.

George Lucy had gathered up AN Bergen's personnel and pay records from LT Max Small, the Admin Officer. All the litter bearers were standing by. George McKenna was the flight surgeon who would go. He already had his gear on and was standing by to help us move Bergen to the helo.

"Let's make sure he has enough oxygen," Ron pointed out.

It was all worked out. Ron had computed the amount of O_2 that would be needed last night, a little over one standard bottle, and the helo crew had twice that amount on board. Medical oxygen differs from aviation oxygen by the technique of preparation. They both have to be free of oil and other contaminants, but for flight ops more moisture is added. In medical applications, the amount and type of moisture may be adjusted. "What if they forgot it?" Ron said. "I think we should send a spare tank just in case." About then, the Airboss called down to say the helo was overhead and would be on the deck momentarily. They had to unload the mail on board while they refueled and they'd be ready to go. We should plan to be up on the flight deck in about twelve minutes.

OK, we had a few minutes. Before unhooking the monitors, one of the corpsmen ran back to the EW to pick up a spare oxygen tank. We carefully unhooked the monitors, and attached the portable monitor. AN Bergen remained the same as he had been for four days, completely unresponsive. His color was still good, his face was cleaned and his hair combed. The Gunboss and a few of his shipmates asked to come in just to say goodbye to him. He couldn't hear them, they all knew, but they needed to say it whether he could or not. The Captain came in too. Always considerate, the Captain asked if time would permit him to say goodbye. It would. The unloading up on the flight deck was taking a little longer than we expected. He reached down to take AN Bergen's hand. "Be careful, Shipmate. I wrote a letter to your mother and I'll call her as soon as I can." That's all he said, unpretentious and genuine. We took Bergen on down the passageway to the elevator.

The Weapons elevators were run by G-4, Bergen's own division. They made sure the elevators were running and waiting for us. When we got him loaded on, Ron and I were going to ride up with him, one of us working the ambu bag all the time, since he was detached from the big ventilator now. Before they could close the grate on the elevator platform, Ron ran off back to the Medical Department and asked HM1 Amstutz to help me on the elevator. "Where are you going, Ron?"

"I want to make sure he has enough oxygen. I'll meet you up on the flight deck."

"But they have plenty on the airplane, and we're bringing..." It didn't matter; Ron was already out of earshot and the elevator was taking us up.

When we arrived on the flight deck, they were just finishing unloading the mail and were still refueling. The H53 is a huge helicopter, about the size of a very large mobile home or a boxcar. A huge tail door, about the size of a volleyball court, opens down like a ramp to permit entrance. It's big enough to let in a couple of jeeps. We stood there waiting in the wind for clearance to bring our patient on the helo. The crew was arranging the inside of the helo. I sent somebody into the Flight Deck BDS on the island to bring out an extra blanket for Bergen. Ron came panting up with another oxygen bottle. "Ron, for Pete's sake, you've brought enough!"

"Nothing wrong with being safe," was all he said.

George had gone up to talk to the pilots and check the situation in the back where he and AOAN Bergen would be going. "They're almost ready. They have two oxygen bottles in there."

"That's not enough!" Ron said.

"Jesus, Ron, you said two bottles would be enough last night, and besides, we have three more we're sending thanks to you."

"How do you know theirs are all right?"

We were interrupted then by the Loadmaster beckoning us on. We brought Bergen up through the back and secured his litter. Ron ran out to take the spare O_2 bottle from the Flight deck BDS.

"Just in case," he said. This was getting interesting. We now had 6 O_2 bottles on the aircraft.

Finally, we had AOAN Bergen tied into the aircraft, we all exited and stood along the island waiting for the big H53 to be untied and depart. Ron grew nervous. "It took longer than we expected. He's been on that tank for almost 20 minutes. John: go get another tank!"

"Ron, cut it out. there are six tanks already on that helo. They're just going to Spain, not to Mars."

"If he runs out of oxygen he's going to die. It's that simple."

"Yeah, but that's not going to happen until April with that many tanks, Ron. Let it go."

"Be safe. Hurry, John." So, before we could let the helo lift off, HM3 Delrosario ran up and handed an aircrewman the seventh O_2 bottle.

Finally, they were gone.

We learned the next day that an EEG had been obtained, a flat line confirmed. The day of the injury, the Red Cross had notified Bergen's family in Texas, and the Navy flew them to Rota. His father was a retired Master Chief Petty Officer, his mother a veteran of a lot of deployments. They were there when Connor arrived, and after the EEG, they asked that the ventilator be removed.

First the fire and now this. Not a great start to the deployment.

CHAPTER XIII. THE MED

The next day we arrived at Rota, the Nato base just south of Cadiz, right at gate to the Mediterranean. Here we were going to "chop" with the ***Eisenhower***, the carrier we were relieving in the Med. The ***IKE*** had to extend her cruise by about three weeks because we were late. After our turnover, we would have war games for about a week between our battle group and ***IKE'***s. The ***IKE*** was a "nuke," one of the ***Nimitz***-class big nuclear carriers, only about eight years old, without the maturity, dignity, and character of a ship like the FID. Kind of arrogant with her higher tech propulsion plant and bigger flight deck, but we on the FID knew that newer is not by itself better, in fact not often better.

Ordinarily, the turnover would take place inside the Med. The departing ship would not pass through Gibraltar until we arrived. A combination of Glasnost, with reduced international tensions, and the pressures to get ***IKE*** home for the holidays led to our having a turnover here in the Atlantic. This was the first time since World War II there wouldn't be an American aircraft carrier in the Mediterranean.

Helos brought parties from each ship to the other. On the 1MC, we heard Admiral Allen and Captain Thomassy bonged off to meet with their counterparts on the ***IKE***, "Carrier Group Six, departing. ***Forrestal***, departing." Shortly, a couple of H3s from ***IKE*** arrived on our flight deck with some of her department heads coming to give us turnover information. To our surprise the SMO and MAO from the **IKE** were among them. The XO had told me earlier that there were not going to be any medical reps. That had been unusual and irritating news, but not unexpected. Medical guys are accustomed to being thought of as expendable hangers-on by some "operators." That was never true on the FID -- Mitchell didn't listen to my advice as often as I wanted, but at least he respected and cared about the role of medical services.

So, I was pleased for a couple of reasons to discover that the ***IKE***'s SMO had arrived. For business, of course, I wanted to get the information from the last SMO in the Med. The main reason was personal, though. Fred Spencer, the ***IKE***'s SMO, was a friend. He had not been in the Navy very long, and he was only a Lieutenant Commander. Most SMOs were "full" Commanders, or occasionally Captains like myself, and usually had to have a lot of Navy experience to get a SMO's job. Fred, however, had come into the Navy as an experienced physician only a couple of years before. When he was given the opportunity to be a SMO he had resisted at first, even though confidant of his medical and managerial skills. I had been one of the people who had encouraged him to take the opportunity.

Our greetings were enthusiastic. Not only because we were good friends, but because we both needed some ventilating, too. I reviewed our experiences and the loss of the young airman in the past couple of weeks, but overall, I was glad we were underway. The ship is better when we're steaming, I told him. We talked about a few common clinical problems. One was the suicide question and what to do about suicide threats. The manipulative suicide threat was occurring frequently on the ***IKE***, too, even more often than on the FID. In fact on the **IKE** they had a psychologist embarked for a couple of months, but the number of threatening gestures had not changed.

It seemed that Fred needed to ventilate more than I did, though. Both of my Skippers had always listened to my input and trusted my judgments, and even if the XO gave me more direction than I wanted, I really knew, somewhere just below consciousness, that he was really on my side. This wasn't the case with Fred on the ***Eisenhower***. He was tired, quiet, less eager than usual.

"Maybe you're just overreacting because you're tired, Fred. This is new for you. Maybe you and your Captain are just getting to know each other. Obviously he knows about your medical credentials. I'm sure he has more confidence in you than you think."

"No, Terry, this is different. It isn't working out." Fred had always been successful at everything he ever did. He had once run a state's emergency medical systems and had been a professor in a couple of medical schools. Apparently a couple of times his department had not done some administrative functions the way the Captain had wanted, and on a couple of other occasions, the Captain questioned some diagnoses or some medical evacuation decisions. Fred felt that the skipper did not listen to him. It was frustrating for him to meet this kind of stone wall. Even worse, though, was not knowing how to fix it, how he could win his Captain's confidence.

A few hours after Fred's helo left we heard the ship's bell and the 1MC, "Forrestal, arriving." and then four bongs and "Battle Force Sixth Fleet, arriving," that was Admiral Allen's new title since taking over from the admiral in Eisenhower's battle group. For the next three days, we had war games against the IKE battle group.

The maneuvers ran night and day. Except for an extraordinary attention to safety we used all tactical tools just like in a real war. The Eisenhower was bigger and more modern in design, and she had more ships in her Battle Group. Her Air Wing had more airplanes, too.

News about the war games came two ways, the Captain's reports on the 1-MC, and of course the grapevine. While the grapevine messages may have been factually a little less accurate, they were surely more succinct. Captain Thomassy's reputation on the 1MC continued to grow. Whenever he got that microphone in his hand, the disc jockey lurking inside just had to speak. Once or twice during the war games when Tommy Lennon the 'Gator made the 1-MC announcement, it would be just a brief comment about how many of IKE's planes we shot down. I couldn't tell whether the cheering was for the news -- because it was invariably good; we were clobbering the IKE -- or the brevity of the 1-MC announcement.

THE HOSTAGE

Despite the operational tempo from the wargames, the business of the ships still had to go on. All those things like mail, paychecks, cargo, all had to come and go from the ships like always, squeezed in between the attacks and maneuvers. Among that business was the arrival and transfer of personnel. One day, a nervous young newcomer brought his orders down to the personnel office to check in after arriving on the COD. The Personnelman who checked him in snickered and showed the orders silently to a coworker. The two salty veterans exchanged derisive glances, and went immediately to a back office, snickering and joking in whispers as they went off. The other new guys behind our perplexed victim now joined in making him an outcast, because he was the cause of **their** being delayed, too. One more reason to stand in a line, one more delay from the predicted delays of the day, and one more space between them and dinner.

From the door in the back office, a few other faces peeked out, squinted or stared at the new guy, sometimes pointed at him when they laughed, and then ducked back into the office. About ten minutes later, the Masters at Arms came for the new guy. Although they tried to look stern, the MAAs chuckled and spewed half-suppressed laughs while they handcuffed him. "Seaman Snyder," one of them stammered, because every second or third word broke up, "come with me. Captain Thomassy wants you on the Bridge."

Arriving on the Bridge, he was greeted with a plate of cookies, a photographer and a party atmosphere. "Sit right here in my chair, Seaman Snyder," Captain Thomassy told him, and then the Captain keyed his 1-MC microphone. "Good afternoon,

Shipmates, this is the Captain. I guess you know we've been waxing the ***IKE*** for the past couple of days, and up until now it's been a fair fight, even though we've been winning. Well, this afternoon, they reached the lowest depths and we still beat them. The dastardly villains from the IKE tried to sneak a spy aboard, but don't worry. Thanks to quick thinking and an impenetrable intelligence system we have caught him."

Poor Snyder caught the wrong COD in Sigonella. He was supposed to report to the *Eisenhower*, and came to us be mistake. Later Snyder rode over to the ***IKE*** with a basket of FID cookies as a condolence prize. The FID had humbled the big nuke, and even caught her in her feeble resort to crime.

After our war with the Eisenhower, we steamed east and began to think about our first port call.

The weather was cloudy, cold, and drizzly almost every day. Several flying days had to be canceled. Our moods matched the weather. The crew was ready for liberty. The fire, the delayed deployment, then the death of a young sailor. So far a hard cruise. Now the bad weather. The ship rolled more than we spoiled carrier sailors were accustomed to. I recalled Warren Lobs, the old First Lieutenant, making jokes about the poor job my medical department did in tying down gear. Destroyer sailors, he reminded me, had to be much better at preparing for heavy seas; we spoiled airedales had no idea, he said... Two days before pulling into Toulon, my TV tumbled off its shelf and shattered like a Christmas ornament -- because I hadn't tied it down. We even had a few people who came to Medical for sea-sickness, very rare on a carrier. Most of us had never visited Toulon, and a few days of liberty can be good for attitudes. Shift gears, get out of this bad weather, step into our Forrestal role.

There was also interesting news in the daily message traffic. One day, I misjudged my timing for lunch and found myself trapped at the table when the XO came in. When he started to take over the conversation as usual, I thought, "Oh, no, another Australian sea story," but the subject was world events, and this time they affected us. Recently the Baltic states had been asserting their independence, and with surprisingly little rebuttal from the Soviets. Premier Gorbachev's glasnost was moving along much faster than almost any Americans had predicted. President Bush and the Soviet premier were hinting about a major summit meeting, even very soon -- like this month -- and the President might come to the ***USS Forrestal***! From that day on, the subject grew and took up more and more of every conversation.

One day, the whole Summit had been called off. Another day, they were going to meet in some neutral country rather than at sea. Well, the two of them wanted to capture some drama, some history. The last time a Soviet leader and an American leader had met as friends were back with Truman and Stalin. Yalta, where they met the last time, wasn't neutral though. It was a coastal scene on the Black Sea. To meet at sea, in the Mediterranean, would be symbolic, dramatic. It was **better** than neutral -- it was once considered a potential battle prize! The conference was back on and it would be in November.

We began to plan. Painting got a little more vigorous. There were more meetings. The tempo picked up on the ship with all the preparations, and even competed with liberty for the crew's attention.

Liberty did finally come, though.

The first night on liberty, boating was rough. The sea state was right on the margin of what would allow boating. It was drizzling or raining most of the night, and riding the boats into Fleet Landing slapped the bows up so high, a few guys got knocked down, and a few others got pretty sea sick. I came back to the ship right after my first meal in a French restaurant around 8 o'clock that night. It was good I did, because the camel off the fantail burst loose in the high seas, and boating had to be canceled because of the sea state. Everybody who was still ashore at that point had to stay ashore all night.

THE BOXING SMOKERS

On the second day, the seas were too high for boating still, so liberty had to be called off -- except for the guys who were stranded ashore. However, it was supposed to be a liberty port and we had scheduled some recreation time, so we salvaged the situation with the first boxing "smokers." The name apparently came from back in the days when everybody could sit around and puff on a cigar in the boxing match. There was of course no smoking any longer up in the hangar deck, but the name "smoker" still seemed to fit.

Boxing is a worry to all ships's doctors. On the one hand, fleet boxing programs have been around for generations, and traditions die hard in the Navy. The sailors love boxing matches and the competition between divisions, between ships and even between battle groups or fleets. So it is tough for us doctors to prevent it, even though we all want to. As a neurologist, when I first heard about the idea of boxing on the Forrestal I was distraught. The American Academy of Neurology, and most other medical groups have publically all forms of the sport for years. A couple of years before I arrived, Captain Pieno had agreed to having a boxing program, but John Bigbee was able to talk him out of it.

When I learned that LT "T" Gines, the new Ship's Secretary, a former boxing champion himself, had already secured Captain Thomassy's permission for the boxing team, I resolved to put an end to it. LT. Gines had circumvented me, knowing the doctor would try to talk the Captain out of a boxing program if he could. "You know how doctors are..."

I had learned about "T"'s boxing team plans before the deployment, and went straight away to the XO. "Yeah, yeah, Doc, I know. Doctors are always against boxing tourneys. Let me tell you something. I've been on a lot of ships. Some allowed boxing and on some the doc was able to frighten the Old Man enough to prevent 'em. Never seen anybody hurt. These are healthy guys. It's a Navy tradition. You'll never talk this Captain out of it."

"XO, that's just flat out wrong. The facts are straight forward. Never mind the fact that guys die from boxing injuries, there are hundreds of vegetables in American hospitals from this so-called innocent sport. If you and the Captain will just listen, the data will speak for themselves."

"OK, I'll tell the Captain we need to talk to him. But you're not going to change his mind."

Well, I'm a neurologist. This happened to be something I knew a lot about... I thought. I gathered up all the pertinent medical literature to show the Captain.

After gathering about thirty medical and epidemiologic articles, I found I had to recheck my earlier conclusions. It is true that there are a number of deaths and brain injuries from boxing. However, I discovered that most of my prior information overlooked some critical control factors. The most numerous and severe injuries occurred when there were major disparities in size or experience level of the boxers. The next major factors were poor conditioning and inadequate head gear. Professionals, for example, often use ten or even eight ounce gloves and almost never wear head protectors. Finally, looking at the data, even with all these glaring flaws, boxing has fewer injuries than football, horseback riding, and pole vaulting. The simple precautions of using 16 ounce gloves, alone, brings boxing down to a similar level of risk of injury to baseball and basketball. In series where proper matching of contestants, with 16 ounce gloves, headgear, and a conditioning program are used, to my surprise boxing produces fewer and less severe injuries than most other American sports. With proper screening of participants, and exclusion of people with concussions, the risks fall to much less than unsupervised recreation. The keys, of course, reside in the training and conditioning, the adequacy of the safety gear, and the assurance of proper matching of the contestants.

Reviewing all this with "T" Gines, I learned that he was much more knowledgeable about the entire subject than I was. He was a trained coach. He had purchased super head gear that wrapped all the way around the jaw and had cheek pads and even protected the boxer's nose.

I found myself being the ringside doctor for FID boxing. The second night in Toulon, cheated out of liberty, we had the FID's first boxing smoker in years.

Only a few hundred guys had been able to get out on liberty the first night, so there were over four thousand still left on the ship. Only about a thousand came to the matches, but probably just as many watched on channel 8.

Although "T" had been training them, amateurs is amateurs. Each bout only lasted two rounds for this first smoker. The crowd and cheered just as enthusiastically as if the boxers had known what they were doing. These guys flailed around, elbows almost out at their sides, throwing roundhouse cannonballs at one another, even when they thought they were jabbing.

Although our guys were in very good shape, when you are carrying around a 16 ounce glove at the end of your arm, you tire after a couple of minutes, especially if everything you throw is a haymaker.

After the matches broke up, the enlisted guys went back to their mess decks and lounges, the officers to the Ward Room, everybody sat around eating pop corn for half an hour discussing the aftermath with the same enthusiasm they would have after a Leonard/Hearns bout. They were all looking forward to the next series of smokers. Eventually, "T" was planning to invite boxers from some other ships in the Battle Group over for competition.

The next day, the rain and drizzle continued, but the seas weren't as bad, and boating did permit people to go ashore. We had hired a couple of ferries in Toulon, as we often did, to augment the ship's boats. It turns out that was a good idea. Every battery on the ship's boats seemed to be dead. Ed De Martini was demoralized. He had taken over as First Lieutenant several months ago from Warren Lobs. The Deck Department had been a show case under Warren, but when Ed took over there was a significant changeover in personnel. He still had Senior Chief Jones, the epitome of Chief Bos'n's Mates, but most of the staff was new. Now, Bos'n's Mates are not generally Phi Beta Kappa type guys. The reason that chief bos'n's mates or first lieutenants are so rough and tumble, is kind of, well, because they need to be when they deal with bos'n's mates sometimes. When Admiral Allen came down to get in his Barge to go ashore, it wouldn't start. The Flag Lieutenant and the Admiral's Aide, conspicuously looked at one another and then stared off to the horizon. Admiral Allen wasn't upset by it. He just wanted to go ashore. Ed and the OOD were embarrassed though. Ed called for one of the other personnel boats, making an apology to the Admiral, and said he would send the Barge over to pick up the Admiral as soon as possible.

The other boat wouldn't start either.

Ed sent down to the storeroom to have another battery brought up for the Admiral's Barge, but there weren't any down there that would fit his boat. Finally, they took the battery out of the Captain's Gig, put it in the Admiral's Barge, and after only a 15 or 20 minute delay, the Admiral and his party went ashore. Twenty minutes later, the Captain came down to go ashore in his Gig. No battery of course.

Captain Thomassy in his typical manner chided Ed about it a little bit, but enjoyed the laugh. At this point, Ed did not. By that time the Utility Boat was working, and the Skipper just went ashore in the U-Boat. You could see Ed was going to have a talk with Senior Chief Jones about the boats.

Since boating was open now, I needed to make my visit to the local hospital, so I went ashore the first day. When I got up to the quarter deck, the Boating Officer said, "We're having some trouble with the boats, Doc. You may want to go back to the fan tail and take the ferry. They are running every 30 minutes, there should be one by in 15 or 20 minutes. We're going to be without boats for a little over an hour." As I trudged back through the hanger bay to the fan tail, I saw a lot of guys sniffling and blowing noses. I made a note to myself that we would be seeing a lot of guys in sick call the next couple of days, what with this foul weather, and guys maybe staying out in the drizzle too late at night.

Toulon was a major port for the French Navy. At the pier we could see their air craft carriers ***Clemenceau*** and ***Foch***, tied up. The ***DeGaulle*** was apparently going to be commissioned soon, but was not around when we came to town. Some years ago, the French unified the medical departments of all of their military services so they just have one military medical department, like Canada and a few other countries. St. Anne's is no longer a naval hospital, but is called "l'hôpital des armées", a hospital of the army. Military medical people in France may wear the uniform of whatever service they have spent most of their career with, I guess. Most of the people at St. Anne's were in Navy uniforms, although when I went to meet the commanding officer, he wore the uniform of an Air Force General.

After I met the commanding officer, the Chief of the Medical Staff, Dr. Picard, took me around the hospital. He was a Naval Flight Surgeon, too, and enjoyed talking about his experiences as a SMO. They were much like mine. He told me, in confidence, how much trouble he had with the XO on his last carrier. It seems the XO never listened to his advice, and always told him how he thought a flight surgeon should practice medicine. I smiled and told him I was glad I never had that kind of problem. "Yes, you are lucky you don't," he told me.

By this time the FID had been at sea for a little over three weeks, and we had accumulated a lot of plastic and medical trash. I discussed this with the folks at St. Anne's, and even before I could finish explaining the background, they nodded knowingly. Medical waste and plastic trash was a new problem for the French Navy, too. They agreed to take over all of our medical waste and our plastic trash, and to dispose of it in their system, which had national rules about the same as the United States.

"You don't have any sharps, though, do you?"

"Yes, we have quite a few sharps." In fact, we had done flu shots on the crossing. (A numbing recollection of the results of flu shot needles from 18 months before crept over me.) Could they not take our sharps?

After some deliberation, it turns out they were able to take them as long as we had them in properly marked hard containers. We did.

The next day I came back to St. Anne's with a couple of my petty officers, and we unloaded about 12 large, plastic bags of trash from the Medical Department and five hard containers full of needles and other sharps. The clerk we handed them to was a little puzzled as to why we want a **receipt** for the **trash**. If he had been in Mayport for the investigations aa little over a year ago, maybe he would have understood a little better. At any rate, we made damn sure we had somebody sign a receipt for all of the bags and the sharps. When we got back to the ship, we put that receipt right in our disposal logs.

The final night in Toulon all of the department heads went out to dinner with the Skipper. Toulon is a beautiful, picturesque city. Winding round cobblestone streets lined with shops, houses, and restaurants right on the street. For some reason, all my life I had heard the French were unfriendly. It certainly wasn't visible anywhere I went that year in France, most especially not in Toulon. The French people were happy to see us, would cross over a street to shake the hand of an American, always had a smile or a greeting. They seemed to enjoy it when an American tried to speak French. Whenever I stumbled, those who spoke English happily inserted the missing part or would speak a sentence or two of English to get me back on the track; but then they **did** expect to continue the conversation in French.

After dinner, knowing it was the last night in town, the Captain wanted to walk around town and visit with the FID sailors in liberty. We walked over to the part of town where the clubs and bistros were located. A ship with 5,000 sailors can increase the nighttime population of any town, even one the size of Toulon. Business was good that night, and the French customers mingling eagerly with the FID sailors. All of our guys were behaving well, nobody was making too much noise or creating any problems.

When our party of 12 or 13 older guys walked down the street, the sailors would see the Skipper, and ask him to join them for a drink. It reminded me of the way kids will clamor around a favorite teacher on the playground in grade school. The sailors loved Captain Thomassy.

Just physically, he made the sailors happy. A tall guy with silver hair, straight posture with his shoulders back, almost always smiling, and with a ready joke for any sailor, he just made them like him. The Captain's affection for his sailors was obvious, and theirs for him.

"Hey, look. There's the Skipper!" Five or ten of them would run out of the bar to shake the Skipper's hand, and out of courtesy the hand of whoever was standing near him.

They wanted to introduce the Captain to their new French friends, or to show him some curious thing in the shop or restaurant where they were. Ten or eleven different sailors offered to buy the Skipper a drink that night, but he had to refuse them all since we were going to get under way the next morning. He always called people "shipmate."

"No, shipmate, thanks. You might have had enough tonight, too!" Laughs all around. I don't think we ran into a drunk guy that night, but the Captain made little jokes with everybody about how much they had to drink. Everybody laughed at the jokes, but they knew they were being reminded not to overdo it.

It was well past midnight, and the rest of us department heads wanted to get back to the ship. We wanted to make sure everything was okay in the departments, and for God's sake, get to sleep. The Skipper was reveling in the company of his sailors, though. He had allowed liberty to continue until 0200 for second class petty officers and overnight for first class and chiefs, so there were still a lot of sailors out in town at this point for him to mingle with. The rest of us were tired as Hell, and we were hoping he would finally run out of gas. Finally, a little after 0100, the Captain decided to go back to the ship. I noticed he was sniffling, and a lot of the sailors we saw had been blowing their noses. It was still a little drizzly, but it wasn't raining.

Finally when we got back to the Gig, it was pretty cold, and we noticed that the boat crew had the lid off the engine in the back of the boat. Ed De Martini was there with them, looking a little bit flustered.

The Gig wouldn't start. It was 0130, we were all tired, the ship was getting under way the next day, and the Gig wouldn't start. They had radioed back to the ship half an hour ago on the brick for a new battery, and it was reportedly on the way back now with one of the ferries. Ed mumbled some kind of an apology to the Captain, who just chuckled, made a half-hearted joke about it, but then we all just sat down on benches and waited for the new battery.

By the time we got back to the ship, it was well past 0200, and we were due to get under way early the next morning. It had been a great port call. We were going to see more of France during the cruise, with port calls in Marseilles and Cannes, and just like the rest of the crew, I was looking forward to it.

On the way back to my stateroom, I passed by the Emergency Room and was sorry to see there were four or five guys standing around to be seen. They were all wiping their noses, and a couple of them coughing. George McKenna was on duty, so I stopped in to help him.

"Seeing a lot of respiratory symptoms, Captain."

"Mostly just congestion?"

"No, a fair amount of bronchitis and a lot of systemic symptoms. It looks a lot like the flu to me."

Looking at the Medical Department logs, more than 12 guys had come in with symptoms of sore throat, nasal congestion, or bronchitis that day. The "Toulon Crud" was arriving. In Sick Call a couple of mornings later, we had over 100 guys with a symptom complex that was going to be with us for the next 3 to 4 weeks. The symptoms were a raspy and slightly painful cough, but not a lot of phlegm, usually some congestion of the ears and nose, but most especially a general sensation of fatigue. About a third of the cases had sore muscles and a low fever, seldom over 100 degrees.

On the first week out of Toulon, we had 200 or 300 cases of this illness who came to Sick Call. We knew by taking surveys on the ship that over 600 people had symptoms of at least a mild degree, but not bad enough to seek treatment. Only 65 guys had fevers, a little over 120 had sore muscles, and over the course of the next 2 or 3 weeks, fewer than a hundred had to miss any work with their illness.

During that entire month, we didn't have a single case of pneumonia as a complication, but 15 or 16 guys had to be admitted to the ward so that we could keep their hydration up and look after them.

It was the right time of year for influenza, and the influenza was going around Europe at around that time. After all the complaining we had about flu shots, I was surprised that I wasn't hassled more by people in the crew about whether the flu shots worked.

We weren't able to get immunologic studies to prove what was the agent of the "Toulon crud." However, the flu that year was particularly severe. If this **was** the influenza, having no pneumonia and only 15 guys who required admission was the best proof you could ask for the value of the vaccine. Left unchecked influenza could devastate a closed population of 5,000 people locked together on a ship. Closed breathing compartments, close contact with one another. Influenza would spread like fire. Even counting the people who had mild symptoms and did not come for treatment, fewer than 20 percent of the ship caught the "Toulon crud." That's a lot lower than the influenza would do without the shots.

SWEETPEA ALLEN, THE RED ROTATOR

Admiral Allen had been one of the first guys to get his flu shot, which I had greatly appreciated at the time. When he got the crud, I made it a point to go up and see him everyday in his cabin, almost feeling guilty that he even caught it, since he took the shot.

Sweet Pea Allen was called the "Red Rotator" by people who had worked for him before, and by some of the senior officers in the ship's company. A man with an immense capacity for facts and details, he got the nickname "Red Rotator" because of his hair color, and a reputation for spinning up action from the people who worked for him. As the ship's doctor I never saw that. Sweet Pea always came to church services on Sundays, and made it a point to meet everybody on the fo'c'sle. He had an outgoing personality and a ready smile. Admiral Allen's staff didn't invite the Medical Department to their morning meetings like Admiral Smith's staff had, so I didn't get to know Sweet Pea as much as I did Snuffy. I liked him as much for what I knew of his background as I did for his friendly personality, though.

Admiral Allen had started out as a Nav Cad. Years ago, when the Navy really needed pilots, some young hot shots who qualified could go down to the Navy recruiter and apply for flight training. If they passed all the IQ and physical tests, they could get into flight training, but as Cadets, not commissioned officers. Those who washed out of aviation training simply became sailors. Without a college degree, most NavCads were not likely to have very successful military careers. When their flying days ended, they didn't go very far, usually. A few of them, like Sweet Pea, went ahead and finished college, but for the most part they were a little bit behind their running mates who had college degrees before they started.

I always enjoyed speaking with aviators about their flying experiences and their training. Sweet Pea kind of looked out towards the distance, although we were sitting in some small room, and said, "Yeah, that was quite an adventure for a young man, I liked it a lot." He flew A-4 Sky Hawks for a while and during the late sixties, he switched over to the A6 Intruder, which was being more and more important for Naval air warfare. He must have been recognized as a promising young officer, because the Navy sent him for a degree in engineering in 1969. When he came back to fly again, some flight surgeon noticed that Sweet Pea needed glasses, so he switched over from being a pilot to being an NFO, a bombardier-navigator. That was kind of an unusual transition.

As we have discussed before, pilots and NFO's are pretty definite about the difference in their two vocations. Most pilots, if they can't fly anymore, just take up some other kind of specialty like air craft maintenance, Intelligence, or Operations. We have spoken about the different viewpoint between being a single seat attack pilot, and being a member of a two-person cockpit. I was always fascinated by Sweet Pea's ability to make that transition. He obviously did it well, too, because he became not only a Squadron CO, but a Wing Commander, and a very successful Flag Officer.

When Admiral Allen healed up after a few days, I was much relieved.

About the second day out of Toulon, Bob Willmore asked me to see a quartermaster who had been in twice that day. He came in for Sick Call because of pain in his abdomen after he fell down on a ladder. Bob couldn't find anything wrong on examination and thought he reassured the sailor. He came back around noontime saying that he had been a little bit nauseated and didn't feel like he could work. Once again, Bob found his examination normal. He was a pretty squared away guy, but he had kind of a long and sad face. Bob still couldn't find anything wrong on examination, but he was troubled about the story, so he asked me to examine him, also.

"Good afternoon, Petty Officer Wolff, I'm Dr. Riley. What's the problem?"

"I still have this pain right here in the middle of my stomach, Doctor." He pointed just to a place well above the belly button, a little bit off to the left, not where the spleen is, usually. He wasn't tender there. I began poking gently, and pushed harder, watching his face to see what his reaction was. Usually with real tenderness, the patient will wince, hiccough, or something, to give you some sign of the real pain they're having. He showed no signs of discomfort.

"Does that hurt?"

"Yeah, that's pretty uncomfortable, Doc." When the patient's report and his facial expressions don't match, the doctor is usually concerned.

I was bothered a little bit, too, but I really didn't think he had anything wrong. Even so, we had to take abdominal complaints pretty seriously. It took us an hour to get Xrays and lab tests done. By then Petty Officer Wolff said that his abdomen was more tender but his examination remained normal. This just didn't fit, and I found myself getting a little bit suspicious about whether this was a guy who just wanted some time off from work. I think I was a little bit snappy with him.

"Petty Officer Wolff, everything looks normal. If there were any damage inside your abdomen, it ought to show up on either the examination, the lab tests, or the X-ray. Why don't you go lie down for a couple of hours and check back with us after dinner? Don't take any solid foods, and let me have a look at you around 1830, all right?"

That sounded okay to Wolff. That was another reason to worry me a little bit. Usually a sailor who was looking for a way out of work would not be satisfied if you told him you thought he was going to be all right and ask him to check back later. He would usually want you to write a note to his Chief, or to admit him to the ward. Wolff was cooperative at all points, and just looked a little bit sad. So we sent him off to his rack to rest a little bit and asked him to come back that evening.

Dan Eardley was out in the passageway, so I nabbed him then to talk over the case about Petty Officer Wolff.

"I sent him back to his rack to check with us in a few hours, Dan, but I wonder whether we should tap his abdomen?"

Dan was so much easier to talk to than Rock had been. "No, I think you did the right thing. If he has normal bowel sounds, and his abdomen isn't rigid, you can watch him for a while."

"Well, I really don't think this is anything serious, but I'm a little worried about him. Do you have time to see this guy now?"

I don't think Dan ever said no the whole time he was on the ship. He didn't find anything different on examination, either. However, Dan said he could have a perforated viscous.

"Without any rebound? Without a rigid abdomen?"

"I've seen that sometimes," Dan said. He agreed, though, that we didn't need to tap the guy right away, but should watch him for another couple of hours.

Wolff was still tender after dinner, though. "Are you having any nausea?" I asked. No, he wasn't.

It was getting to be nighttime, and the guy was still tender. We repeated his X-ray, it was still normal. Even so, Dan thought we should tap his abdomen.

With blood in the abdomen we had to operate. I trudged up to talk it over with the Captain. Like Captain Pieno, Captain Thomassy was always behind us. He never hassled me when I told him we needed to operate.

To my surprise, Dan found a perforation in the proximal ileum! It was a contusion that opened a tiny window into the small intestine. When Petty Officer Wolff fell against the brace on the ladder well, it hit that part of the abdomen just enough to bruise and tear at that point. The reason his symptoms were so mild was that there had been no significant blood loss and only microscopic leaks of intestinal juices. A tear in the bowel usually would make a person much sicker than Wolff had been. The peculiar combination of circumstances could have continued to hide this injury from us until it gradually reached a dangerous stage. It scared me to realize that in doubting the severity of his symptoms, I could have let him get much worse. Dan was able to repair the perforation without an ileostomy.

He healed up fine in a week or so, but for the rest of the cruise, I was a little sheepish every time I saw him because of doubting his symptoms earlier.

While the Toulon visit had been good for the crew, as I had hoped, the Crud played itself out pretty slowly over the next four weeks. We didn't let it dampen our spirits, though. We didn't have time. Thanksgiving was coming, and then a short visit to Naples, and in the first week of December, the President would come aboard.

One morning after sick call, Bob Willmore asked me to see a patient. "I think you've seen him before, Dr. Riley. He's got some kind of attacks. He went to see the psychiatrist for them back in Jax and just flew out to the ship this week."

"Oh, Tommy Cage," I guessed. I had grown fond of him, so it would be good to see him and check his progress. When Bob brought him into the office, though, I almost gasped. How could we have missed it! The man was gaunt. He had a tiny little tremor, bulging eyeballs, and his now-thin skin was a little moist. His pulse was around 105.

Tommy Cage was the most florid example of thyrotoxicosis I had ever seen, certainly the most florid case I had ever missed! To think I had called his problem panic attacks!

I tried to stay calm as I greeted him, but I don't think it worked. "Petty Officer Cage, have you lost some weight since I saw you a couple of months ago?"

"Oh, yes, Sir. My wife noticed it too."

While we talked I leafed through his Health Record. It didn't comfort me too much to note that several of us didn't make the diagnosis of his thyroid disorder. We had at least checked screening levels for two thyroid hormones twice. He was florid now, though, and this condition could be fatal. We should have been seeing him more often I thought. Then he told me he just came back to the ship this week. He had been back in Jacksonville for the last month. Several doctors had seen him for months; how he reached this stage before we recognized his condition still puzzles me.

We went to Naples for a couple of days at the end of November so we sent PH1 Cage to the Navy Hospital where they started his treatment and sent him home to recover.

While we were in Naples, I paid a preemptive visit to Bullis Butts, the CO of the hospital. Remembering last year's visit, I decided it would be a lot easier on me to visit him this time. To my surprise, the visit went so well, I invited him and his wife, along with Captain Gil Vasquez, the Sixth Fleet Surgeon to come to dinner on the ship when we would return in January.

That morning on the ship there was a message from CDR Jesse Harrahill at AIRLANT that I should call him as soon as I could get to a telephone, so they let me use one at the hospital.

"Captain, I'm sorry to tell you this," Jesse said after the requisite opening pleasantries, "but it looks HM3 Womple has a malignant tumor on his arm, and he's going to need an amputation."

My heart sunk. Poor Arden. Why couldn't we have been more gentle with him, I thought. But I hadn't heard the worst yet...

"He says he went to see you about it and you told him it was nothing."

WHAT!!

"He says he was working out a lot because you were harassing him about his weight. When he showed you the mass on the back of his right arm, he says you told him it was just new muscle tissue."

I immediately hung up and called the Navy Hospital at Jacksonville. The surgeon there said, "Yup, we biopsied the mass and it was a sarcoma, but we sent him up to Portsmouth for oncology. Do you remember how big the mass was when you examined him?"

"I never examined him. I try not to treat the guys who work for me. You probably noticed there was no note from me in his chart."

"Well, that's part of the problem. He says somebody from the ship tore out parts of his Health Record to protect themselves."

I was beginning to lose part of my sympathy for Arden. How could we tamper with his record? It stayed with him when he left the ship before we deployed.

We had to get underway the next day, so I couldn't track it down any further for a couple of weeks. It worried me every day, though.

Once we got underway the President's visit was dominating every moment outside of Flight Ops, but it affected everybody on the ship a little differently. All the young guys wanted to see the President, and maybe to get their faces on the news back home. All the aviators were basking in the arrival of the first President who was a carrier pilot. The Captain was probably going to escort him around. It was fun for all of them. For us Department Heads, and the XO, though, it was another story. We had hoops to jump through, and official inquiries to write.

If we ever thought that conventional VIP visitors required our attention, they paled by comparison to an Presidential Advanced Party. As demanding as some of the younger staffers could be -- and the younger they were, the bossier they were -- they were simply cherubic compared to the press. One well-known network anchorwoman stepped off the H3 with an open umbrella, that she had been told was very dangerous and forbidden on the flight deck. She was wearing high heeled shoes, that the press had also been warned would be dangerous on the ship. Kevin Myette was assigned to escort her. When she tripped leaving the helo, Kevin asked, "Do you have a pair of flats?"

She retorted, "No. Do you have a pair of heels?"

It may be that The Staff caused more excitement about this than the White House, though. Here we were in the Mediterranean with just a couple of weeks to plan for the President's visit, flying jets off the deck every day, and our Commanding Officer had to answer daily questions about the red carpet. Captain Thomassy, the SuppO, and the XO had to answer a new question about the choice and exact tint of the red carpet every day. Thirty six inches wasn't wide enough. No, not Crimson. Red. No, thirty feet isn't long enough, has to be forty or more.

Then there had to be rehearsal after rehearsal for the President's arrival. Was it a visit, or a coronation, I started to wonder?

Finally, after the long wait, the day arrived. In the back of my mind I stayed troubled about Petty Officer Womple, but like everybody else I was excited about having the President on board.

President Bush was the pilot of the huge TBM Avenger torpedo bomber when he was a very young man. When he came to talk to us in the Hangar Bay, he called us "fellow Navy men," and he said words like "grape" and "midrats." He said the ship looked good, but added tartly that he still could recognize "the smell of new paint." Oh, we loved him. I've told you already that I'm an old-fashioned New Deal Democrat, but that day, I loved George Bush as much as the rest of them. When he walked through the hangar after his talk, I stretched out to shake his hand as far as I could. Every day I still wear the Presidential tie bar his medical staff gave me when we worked together.

After his speech, the President went down to the mess decks to have an uninterrupted lunch with the enlisted guys. They locked the place up. No officers, no Secret Service agents. Just George Bush and the sailors. They tell me he enjoyed it even more than the sailors. He took off his jacket, rolled up his sleeves and relaxed. He stayed forty five minutes longer than scheduled, so somebody from his staff had to go down to get him.

A few days later, after the President and the Press left, the glow lingered for most of us. What the President and the Premier had worked out transformed our world, and we on Forrestal felt that our ship had played a big role in it for thirty five years and most especially that week.

The glow wasn't as bright for me. One of my corpsmen was about to lose an arm to a cancer I may have failed to find, and he was accusing me of neglecting it.

We were steaming to the island of Mallorca for a port call in a couple of days, while I read the request for a Quality Assurance Investigation about Womple's leg. Ron Eslinger and Dan Eardley were trying to cheer me up.

"Captain, everybody knows you have a policy that the other doctors are supposed to treat members of the department," Ron told me. "Our medical records will stand up to anybody. Nobody took anything out of that record."

LT Lucy came in just then with a stack of bills the Ship's Secretary sent us. It seems that the Navy Hospital in Naples was putting people in local hotels at a cost of around $150 per day and food costs over $30 daily rather than admitting them. "They say these guys can be treated outpatient," George explained. Tommy Cage was one of the patients. The bills totalled over $3000, and the ship had to pay them.

"Lieutenant, can you compare this to what happens to our guys if they go to Rota?"

"I already have, Sir," he said with a coordinated flex of his right thigh and right forearm that reminded me of a classic Charles Atlas photo. "No charge. In Rota they usually admit them or put them up in the barracks."

"We also get nice discharge summaries from Rota, and either nothing or sloppy handwritten notes from the docs in Naples," Dan added.

"Arrogant too," Ron reminded us about Naples.

PALMA

As soon as we got to Palma de Mallorca, I went straight to a phone to call Jesse Harrahill. "Anything new on Womple's arm, Commander?"

"May be some good news, Captain," Jesse answered. "This may be a benign tumor. They say Womple wants an operation, but the docs say it may not be so bad."

Womple first showed a lump on his arm to his psychiatrist in NHJax. The psychiatrist called one of the general surgeons, a friend of Tosser's, to do a needle biopsy. The pathologist at Jax called it a malignant fibrous sarcoma, the doctors told Womple it was a very malignant cancer, he would lose his whole arm and still maybe not survive, and they sent him immediately to the oncologist at Portsmouth, Virginia. Since the radiation unit at Portsmouth was having some repairs, Womple was sent to Bethesda, where the pathologists and oncologists thought the mass was a benign tumor called a neurofibroma, and had probably been present for fifteen or twenty years.

Womple was so angry, he called his congressman and forced the doctors at Bethesda to send him to Walter Reed, where the pathologists and oncologists reached the same conclusions. Inquiries from Arden's congressman and lawyer finally forced a repeat of the biopsy that showed the same thing. They told him to ignore the mass because it would never bother him, but cutting it out could hurt his radial nerve and paralyze. Arden said he wanted it cut out anyway. The doctors refused and tried to discharge him from the hospital, but he refused to leave for two weeks.

Finally, one day I was able to reach Dr. W. Hudson Berrey, the orthopedic oncologist at Walter Reed who was treating Womple. "Oh -- Crazy Arden!" he said when I mentioned the patient's name.[12]

While a part of the guilt and worry were off my shoulders, I was still concerned. What if Arden could eventually find somebody to cut his radial nerve? What could we have done sometime before this to give Arden more than the hope of a malignant cancer to feel important about?

The next day, Father Steve Linehan and I went on a tour of the island, including the Abby where Chopin and the writer George Sand lived. That night the crew bought a lot of tickets for dinner at a big tourist nightclub. I was sitting with the Captain and some other old guys over in one corner, laughing and relaxing as we recalled the work of the last month. A patch of red hair off the left caught my attention. It was Billy Dorsey... and there was a bottle of wine in front of him.

"Airman Dorsey," I said with as much supportive enthusiasm as I could muster, "Good to see you!"

Billy kind of looked down. At any rate, no eye contact. He just mumbled a quiet inarticulate hello.

"How did Level II go?" I asked him.

"OK."

"You better not be drinking, do you think?"

"I can do what I want here. I'm not on restriction. You're not in charge of me."

His table mates didn't seem like long time acquaintances, but they also seemed a little defiant. "If you guys are real shipmates, you won't let him drink tonight." They all just shrugged.

I didn't want to make a scene for Billy in front of the Captain, so I left him alone then, but determined we'd have to talk to his Chief or DivO in the morning.

As the evening wore one, Billy grew more effusive. Every time he saw me looking at him from across the room he toasted me with his wine glass and took a big gulp.

When we left, Billy was passed out on his table. Only one of his new buddies was still there. He and I carried Billy back to the bus.

The next week we sent him to rehab again.

---

[12] *A couple of years later, Hud Berrey and I crossed paths in Saudi Arabia during Operation Desert Storm. I told him we had spoken before, and mentioned Womple. In exactly the same inflection, he repeated, "Oh -- Crazy Arden!"*

CHAPTER XIV. END OF THE TOUR

Shortly after we left Palma, we had another boxing smoker. We hosted a team from one of the cruisers in the Battle Group. Their skipper came over, so Admiral Allen, Captain Thomassy, and our Chief of Staff, Captain Lane attended. "T" Gines' training was starting to bring about a little improvement in our guys, and they had a little better showing than the other team. One of our guys, Bos'n's Mate Woods, was turning into a pretty poised heavyweight.

For some bizarre and utterly inexplicable reason, George Lucy talked "T" into allowing a comic wrestling demonstration with the Blue Pharaoh and some hapless volunteer dressed up in cowboy gear. George wore his professional Blue Pharaoh outfit: blue leopard leotard tights, a skin-tight blue spandex tank top shirt, and a hokey blue silk head and face mask. That get-up really **could** have been comical, except that everybody knew George usually was serious about it.

The whole act was so embarrassing the crew, and especially the Medical Department, tried to hide our faces. I prayed nobody would recognize who the Pharaoh was. When he started prancing and flexing his well-formed muscles, though, everybody knew instantly who it was. Suddenly, the context for his familiar muscle flexing was evident. Prancing up in the ring with his high steps, he flexed one arm, then both, turned this way and that to ripple his muscles for the audience. We have all seen it in professional wrestling on TV, but it didn't seem as funny or as entertaining here. What cheated away some of the slapstick, paradoxically, is that everybody could tell, somehow, that even though this was being called a joke, poor George underneath was really, pathetically, serious about it.

So, the Admiral and the Skipper sitting on the front row tried politely to appear amused at first, but then they like everybody else started looking at their watches, over their shoulders, wondering when was this going to end? The Blue Pharaoh and the cowboy stumbled through their choreographed pseudomayhem. Their timing did not call to mind Larry, Moe, and Curley, but we suspected their intellects did for a while.

Then it got gruesome. The Blue Pharaoh reached around one corner of the ring and brought out one whipped cream, and (ooooh) one blueberry pie. A thousand spectators suddenly realized the tragedy that was inevitable at this point. Oh, why didn't the Blue Pharaoh just stop? Or maybe couldn't time just skip ahead about twenty minutes and leave this out? I guess he wouldn't have been who he was if he had any insight, though, would he? As the Pharaoh awkwardly stalked the hapless cowboy around and around the ring too darned many times, his hands with the pies rose above his head. The cowboy... The ***cowboy*** was supposed to be the stooge! They knew that, they allegedly even practiced it. We all cried out internally, "please don't." But sure enough the whipped cream pie hit the visiting Commanding Officer right in his shiny black shoes, and the tragic blueberry pie splattered across the faces and chests of the Admiral and Captain Thomassy.

It was so quiet.

Should have been funny, you know. Blueberry pie right in the kisser of the Admiral...

The Admiral just got up quietly and went away. Captain Thomassy pointed to LT Gines who ushered the Blue Pharaoh away. The rest of us just looked down at our shoes until the boxing started back up.

We arrived in Marseilles two days before Christmas, ready for a long port call and the holiday seasons. We were still basking in the fun and warmth of the President's visit, and although we had been busy for the last three weeks, they were not overwhelming. Everyone was looking forward to plenty of rest, some site-seeing tours, and for many, trips to Paris. Many had arranged, as I had, for their families to fly over to meet us at Christmas.

Marseilles lived up to all of our expectations. It was winter, after all, not the time you expect to come to the Riviera for a holiday. Yet the Christmas and New Year's weeks in Marseilles are at least as balmy as they are in Jacksonville. In fact there was snow that week in Jacksonville, but in Marseille the temperature ranged from 45° to 65°. The commercial harbor in Marseilles is deep and huge. We were able to tie up right on the pier, so sailors could come and go without boating, just like they could in Mayport... but here there were buses that could take them straight into town or to the picturesque "old harbor" full of sailboats, brasseries, bakeries, and shops.

The day after Christmas, the MWR department had arranged a bus tour of some of the picturesque landscape and countryside around Aix, including a tour of some of the vintners, and some historic caves. We bought tickets, and I arranged to have the day off so that I could take my family on the tour. Two hours before the trip, though, the XO called me to his office. A FID sailor had been murdered the night before, and the XO wanted me to coordinate the investigation with the local coroner. "Doc, they're going to do an autopsy this morning and the Captain wants you to be there."

My initial reaction was that the Skipper and the XO didn't realize how excellent French medical standards are. To think I would have anything to add to a skilled forensic pathologist was naive. (I also wanted to go on that trip). This was one of the few times I was circumspect enough to keep my mouth shut and listen to the XO, though. "You speak French, don't you, Doc?"

"Yes, but I'm not good enough to follow complicated medical studies like a post mortem."

"We know that, Doc, but there are no other American medical reps in town. If this should later have any important ramifications, FBI, NIS, National Security investigations, we need to be sure there's a member of the service there. Didn't you tell me that you studied pathology and even did autopsies for a while?"

"Well, yes, XO, but that was almost twenty years ago..." Reluctantly, I was beginning to understand that the XO was right. I needed to be there.

So, I sent Ann and my daughters off to the tour, where they had a great day. I learned all I could about the murder before I went over to the University and city morgue for the autopsy. The victim, although an American sailor, had been raised in Sierra Leone, and he had friends who had come to the growing Sierra Leone community in Marseilles when he went to the States. Sitting in a bar with his countrymen that night, he was mistaken for a well-known local drug dealer and shot dead in the back with two shotgun blasts.

My French, it turned out, was entirely adequate for the autopsy. The forensic pathologist's techniques were almost identical to the ones I had learned back at the University of Missouri years ago. In fact, during the procedure, when it was difficult to find the precise mechanism of death, I found the pellets and aortic tears that had killed him. One can't say that we "enjoyed" working together, I guess. Notwithstanding the ugly circumstances, however, my French colleagues and I recognized that we had shared a meaningful day's work. The police caught the murderer a couple of weeks later.

When I gave my report to the XO about the autopsy, it was evident as usual that he couldn't wait for the talking to stop so that he could get on with some other work, but naturally he wanted a written report first thing the next morning.

"By the way, Doc, how come it costs so much for our guys to be treated at the Navy Hospital in Naples?"

"It's a little convoluted and complicated, XO. Some of it has to do with lack of barrack space in Naples, and some of it has to do with command policies there. We have a plan..."

I was going to explain that we were going to try to send most of our consultations and transfers to Rota, but the XO broke in first, "Wouldn't it be better for us to send our guys over to Rota? With the log flights, I can get them there from any place in the Med usually."

"Good idea, XO," I said. "Rota's a beautiful new hospital, too." Well that was good. Not only did I have the XO's backing for our new plan, but he thought it was his idea, too.

Even with the autopsy and the paper work, I was able to take a week's leave with my family. We drove over to Monte Carlo, spent a couple of nights in Nice, and took the train up to spend New Year's Eve in Paris. It may have been winter, but it was still Paris. When I put them on the plane in Paris, the deployment was almost half over.

A few nights after we left Marseilles, Philip Williams came to see me. He had been letting me look at his rhymes and ventilating a little. Without pushing him too much I encouraged him to read some poetry we found in the ship's library, but he didn't like it if it didn't rhyme or "have a beat," so I let him go at his own pace.

"Doc, why do you suppose they make people who have other talents stay on the ship? You know I got friends back home who can't get a job, you know. They'd be glad to work. This isn't right for me, you know."

We talked about obligations, whatever Philip's earlier expectations had been, what his expectations were now.

"See, Doc, I got this agent back in Jacksonville. I think I got what it takes, you know, for like show business."

"Philip, we'll be back in Jax in just about four months, man. If you start polishing up your material, you might be ready for a couple of bookings on the weekends when we get back."

That wasn't what Philip had in mind, exactly. He pouted a little. "No, Doc, that ain't it." He didn't want to talk any more, so he left, shoulders hunched down a little.

A couple of weeks later, we came to our next port call, the big industrial city of Valencia. No American carrier had been to Valencia for more than ten years. We heard the city was looking forward to our visit, but there were reports that the Greenpeace organization might picket us alleging that we could have nuclear weapons aboard. Even most of us didn't know whether we did or not, of course. Longstanding American policy at that time was to neither confirm nor deny the presence of nuclear weapons.

The port in Valencia seemed to me to be even larger than Marseilles. They were both large enough for us to tie right up at the pier. That alone is unusual anywhere in the world for such a big ship. When we pulled into the harbor a few Greenpeace inflatable boats tried to block us, but the Spanish Navy and police gently guided them away.

People lined up by the thousands to try to see the ship. We sold more Forrestal ballcaps than we did in New York City. Thousands of friendly Spaniards crowded up to see the ship and try to meet Americans. Because of the reports of the Greenpeace demonstrations, though, we had to be careful. Extra Shore Patrol, Marine, and Master-at-Arms patrols wandered up and down on the pier, trying vainly to look inconspicuous and unconcerned.

Finally, on the third day, the protests started. A truck drove up on the parking lot with about six young people in the back. Two of them came to stand in the bed of the truck with bullhorns and started to give speeches, one in English and the other in Spanish, about nuclear weapons. Before they could finish two sentences, a squad of Spanish policemen appeared from nowhere, ripped their bullhorns away, and carted them off in a paddywagon that materialized as mysteriously as the police had. Twenty other protestors suddenly appeared down by the fantail, and threw big balloons at the ship, bursting open with fluorescent chartreuse and yellow stains. A bos'n's mate up on the catwalk drove the balloon painters away with a fire hose, knocking only one of them down.

My worst fear was that an angry American sailor or Marine would punch one of the young protestors, or strike them with a club, and aggravate a mob. Our guys had been well coached, though, and maintained an almost amused aloofness and calm. The Spaniards who had come to admire the ship and meet the Americans were more angered by the protestors than we were.

On the third night in Valencia, I was awakened well past midnight by the OOD. A FID sailor was injured and had been brought to the University Hospital downtown. There were no details at first, might have been an auto accident. I had one of the corpsmen wake up Jose Blanco, the Nurse Commander who relieved Ron Eslinger to come down to the hospital with me and find out about the sailor. As usual, the ship had rented a handful of cars for official business during the port call, so we were able to drive down to the University Hospital. Jose and I had been down to visit the hospital the day we arrived, something I did in every port call. I was glad we knew the place already. My impressions of Spanish medicine were already favorable just from my visits to the small hospital in Benidorm over a year ago and the community hospital we had visited in Palma a few months ago. The University Hospital in Valencia was very impressive. First, the magnificent architecture had wide hallways with pretty columns, and sweeping stairwells, a proud grandeur just in the building. The main buildings of the medical school had been built in the thirties. There was a seven foot bust of General Franco in the main entrance foyer of the medical school. We wandered down past the anatomy wing and some of the lecture halls, impressed all the way how much cleaner and neater were the surroundings in this "academic" part of the institution than in most American universities.

To get to the Emergency Room, we had to go back out the other side of the wing we were in, cross a court yard, and then step into a busy ward indistinguishable in every respect from an American ER. A clerk greeted us none too friendly and said something unenthusiastic. When Jose smiled his characteristic smile and started to answer, an apparent supervisor clerk intervened. Even though I don't speak spanish, I know the supervisor said, basically, "For God's sake, look at their uniforms! They're obviously here to see the American. Let them in!"

Our sailor was in a cubicle with his leg elevated in a traction splint. With the fracture immobilized he had very little pain. He had obviously been medicated too. A friend was with him. They were a couple of guys from the Air Department. "Hey, Doctor Riley! We're glad to see you."

"Broke his leg, Doc," the friend said, in a classic recapitulation of the obvious.

When the doctor came to talk to us, it was clear that he was finishing a long shift from the preceding night. He had bags under his eyes and was sipping a cup of coffee. Very friendly, though. I probably didn't need Jose as a translator at least right then because the doctor wanted to practice his English, which seemed to be at a level very near my own ability in French, which I considered pretty good.

"He has a mid shaft femoral fracture, as you can see," he said as he showed us the X-rays. Did not break the skin and the bone is not..."

"Not comminuted, not shattered," I inserted.

"Yes, comminuted, thank you. It is not comminuted. Our orthopedists have seen him, and they say he can go back to the ship."

Back to the ship!

"Oh, I'm afraid you may not understand, we cannot really treat him on the ship."

"But don't you have a surgeon? An operating room?"

This was kind of hard to explain. In absolute terms, or in wartime, all of the doctors on the ship could put a pin into or through the bone and place the femur in traction. The young man would probably heal with the treatment we could give, especially with Dan's direction, at about a 90% cure rate. We could meet the standards of, say, 1955. However, if there would then ever be an emergency on the ship, we maybe wouldn't be able to get such a guy in traction off in a hurry, or into a survival raft. Besides, in 1990, in peace time, 90% was just not acceptable, especially since we and the patient were right here in a thoroughly competent University Hospital with a full orthopedic department, who could give him definitive treatment and prepare him for proper transport over to the Naval Hospital in Rota.

We discussed this with the ER doc, who seemed perplexed. When he learned that we had all those doctors on the ship, why wouldn't we just put the pin in and keep him in traction on the ship? I did feel a little guilty, momentarily, when he asked me that, but I had to explain our concerns about safety and the importance of always thinking whether a sailor could escape in an emergency. OK, then we summoned the Orthopedic doctor.

This doctor spoke even better English. He had studied in Cleveland, and once had toured an aircraft carrier. "But I've seen your departments on those ships. You have a good ward, no? I'll show your surgeon how to handle it." I explained again that we couldn't keep a guy on board who would not be able to escape in an emergency. Like a footnote in my frustrated thinking, I reflected how difficult it sometimes was to explain these same points to our own U.S. Navy doctors. The escape issue is not so farfetched, and something we never forgot on the Forrestal. July, 1967, had been vividly reinforced in all our minds with the fire just a couple of months ago.

The spanish orthopedist wanted to go home. It had been a long night for him too. "O.K.," he said, "we can set the thigh properly in a traction cast that will give him excellent, perfect stability. Then he will be safe to return to the ship and moderate movement will not be a problem. After a month or two, if he is not healing well, you can re-evaluate whether he will need an operation."

"Thank you, that is the most important, of course, to get him the treatment he needs. However, even if stabilized, if he has a cast, especially on a lower extremity, he wouldn't be able to escape in the event of an emergency!"

"Ahh, escape! Now I understand." Finally.

We agreed that the orthopedic department at the University Hospital would treat him and we would arrange for him to be flown to the Navy Hospital in Rota. The orthopedist went off to get some of the orthopedic residents and start arranging for the case. I had to go and speak with one of the hospital administrators.

"How are you feeling, Airman?" I asked, as much to hear how sober he was at this point as to know the answer.

"Hey, great, Doctor Riley, considering how lucky we were!" He was absolutely sober, even with the pain medicine on board. I figured the alcohol must have worn off. We by now had learned that he and his buddy were walking in town after dark and had been struck by a railroad locomotive on the tracks downtown. He apparently had been thrown to one side a distance of about twelve feet. To only break one thigh rather than be cut in half or lose a leg was remarkable. The buddy, too, had been thrown aside, but remarkably had only mild injuries.

I stood by while the patient called his parents, so that I could tell them what to expect, while Jose went to an adjacent room to interview the friend. We were surprised to learn that these two young sailors had consumed no alcohol that day or that night at all. At first I was skeptical. How can a healthy young man be run over by a train in the middle of a clean city without being drunk ... or deaf. Yet it was clear. Gradually there were witnesses who had seen them around town. The two were beginning to be offended by our questions about alcohol. They had just not been drinking! In fact, there were few alcohol incidents in this port or any other among the FID sailors.

Eventually the sailor went to the O.R., where they put a pin through the end of the femur, which was held in place in traction by a big cast that extended from his hips down to his ankle.

We came back the next day to arrange to transport the patient to the airport so he could fly to Rota. It seems that in Spain, ambulances are still independent, private businesses. They aren't owned by the hospital. The hospital calls them though. So the driver met us on the ward, and he knew immediately how to get to the medical evacuation plane at the nearby airport. No problem. He wanted cash first, though. But our ship was going to pay the hospital, and the hospital would pay the driver.

No, not in Valencia. Cash first, in pesetas, please.

"But we don't have a way to do that." And the plane would be ready to leave shortly. "Wait here," I asked, and I ran off to make arrangements with the administrator. To avoid a confrontation, we were able to agree on a way for the hospital to pay the driver, but when we got back, he had gone. He put out the word that this trip was not a cash deal, and none of the ambulance drivers in Valencia were willing to come. Finally the Spanish Navy arranged transportation for us, and we got our sailor to the plane two hours late.

When it was all over, the cost of excellent medical care, even if we had calculated a price for the airfare to Rota, was less than comparable treatment would have been in an American hospital, and much less than the various related and peripheral costs of treatment, lodging, and logistics at Naples.

After another week, we were back in Naples. We had a rash of guys who needed outpatient evaluations by specialists, but by prior arrangement, anybody who would need an operation or admission to hospital was going to fly to Rota.

On the Sea and Anchor detail pulling into the molo, our star boxer, BM3 Woods fractured his right ring finger just across a joint surface. Curt Rosenthal escorted him over to the clinic at the hospital and one of the orthopedists pulled them out of the line and scheduled Woods for an operation to pin the finger the next week, and then a month of therapy in Naples.

When they got back to the ship Rosenthal and Woods came to see me. If the big Bos'n's Mate was going to be off the ship for a month or two anyway, he might as well be back in the States in his own home. It would cost us thousands to put him up in Naples, and he wouldn't be on the ship anyway. The only worry was that there was a narrow window of about four days in which the operation had to happen. If delayed beyond that, the likelihood of contractures and nonunion went way up. We discussed it with the patient, the XO, and the ATO. We knew we could carry it off.

So I called over to the hospital and asked them to cancel the operation scheduled for four days hence. Less than five minutes later, the orthopedic surgeon Dr. Wilson was yelling at me on the phone. "If this guy doesn't get his operation in the time window, I'll see you get kicked out of the Medical Corps. Do you have any **idea** what you're doing!" My goodness he was angry. I have to admit that it sometimes amuses me when other people -- especially surgeons -- get mad.

That evening the Vasquezes and Butts came for dinner and a tour of the ship as we had arranged a month ago. Hard as I tried to be the knowledgeable host, though, it became apparent to even me that Gil Vasquez knew a lot more about aircraft carriers, this one included, than I did. Whenever I would stammer or be uncertain about any question on the tour, he would gently, even unobtrusively, ask a kind of reminding sort of question that would hint to the answer that I could slip in. I began to appreciate some of the differences between him and Captain Butts... who never seemed to defer on any subject.

We ended our tour up on the flight deck. It was a classical Naples early spring evening. With the purple and yellow dusk shades streaming over the harbor, Naples took on all the grand beauty that history intended. Looking across from our elevation to the evening traffic and building lights, and then to the dusky silhouette of Vesuvius, it felt as though the cool spring breeze had been ordered for the occasion. The careful angles and sweeps of the airplanes posed against this setting seemed surprisingly fitting. It was a very harmonious evening and I was enjoying the company of our guests. They thanked me for the evening and Mrs. Vasquez surprised me with an invitation to bring a bunch of my guys to dinner a couple of days later.

A QUIET EVENING IN NAPOLI

Ron had departed back in Marseilles. Although I would miss him much, LCDR Jose Blanco had relieved him and promised to leave his own colorful stamp on the department. So for the dinner trip, we had Jose, George Lucy, Bill, Dan, George McKenna, and Will Everett, our recently acquired temporary GMO. Dress was discussed a good deal that day. I requested ties and jackets, although one of the guys suggested that Navy people in Naples seemed to favor a more leisure style. No, I said, a sport coat would never be overdressed, and coming to the home of a senior officer called for this level of decorum. So, the evening of the dinner, we all assembled at the quarter deck turned out for a drive to the other side of town, where we would watch the sunset from off the Vasquez' balcony.

After the brief ferry ride over to fleet landing, we turned to George Lucy, who was to have arranged for the van we could drive over to the Vasquez' house. "Sir, we just go over to the Beach Guard office and sign up for it." My heart sunk. Sign up? We were expected for dinner in less than an hour, and we were just going now to sign up? "No problem, sir, there are plenty of vans."

We walked the two blocks over to the transport desk that the beach crew set up. Nobody there. LT Lucy walked the two blocks back to the main beach det office while we waited. When he returned ten minutes later, he showed us the keys with an attached license number and said, "It's a white Fiat, supposed to be back here on the back lot." Good, ready to go. We looked for about twelve minutes, beginning now to be concerned about being late for dinner, and with seven of us looking couldn't find it anywhere. Finally, I took the keys back to the main desk, to tell them we just couldn't find the van.

"Doc, they're back over at the transport desk now. They were just out for dinner before. You'll have to check with them." Dinner break, eh? I was wondering if we were going to make it to dinner.

"I don't know why he gave you those keys. That van's not even around here. What you have are the spare keys. The XO and some other guys have that van going out to dinner. We just don't have any transportation for you, Doc."

I looked at George. "Lieutenant, I asked you to arrange for a vehicle for this two days ago." Deer in the headlights. Flex left shoulder, twitch chin to left.

George was going to remain stunned and paralyzed for the present, so I tried to negotiate. "Isn't there anything we can drive? We are late for an invitation to the head doctor on the Sixth Fleet staff. How about a supply vehicle?"

"Well, if you want, we have a cargo van, but there aren't any seats except the two in front." We had no choice.

Jose volunteered to drive. He said "Captain, you don't want to drive, and these people are like my people. I can get us there faster."

Will and George McKenna were a little hesitant to get in. No seats, no seat belts. Two wooden pallets on the deck, bits of cabbage and little metal parts, like wing nuts and angle irons rattling around too in the dusty rear of the van.

Driving in Naples is like a bumper car concession in double speed. It would be a painful cacophony of horns and shouting if those noises were not drowned out by worn-out mufflers and the sound of collisions. Add to that, Jose Blanco, for all his personal charm, goes into a cinematic trance whenever there is a steering wheel in his hands. I guess Jose can't help it, it seems automatic whenever he drives, even in normal settings. His eyes take on a flaming glint, his left eyebrow raises, and his head jaunts forward just so. That day the opportunity to enter the great Neapolitan traffic adventure overtook his very being, and Jose became one with the passion. Darting a Lamborghini or Alfa Romeo in and out may be artistic, but a big commercial Toyota van is a waste of such wizardry.

In the back of the van, the young officers were being thrown around like dice in a cup. George McKenna was getting irritated. Bill, when he could catch his breath, called, "Jose, can you make those turns a little more grad...(banged his head) ouch...more gradually!" I looked back now and then to ask if the guys were o.k. When their bodies were stationary enough for me to focus on a facial expression, I could see grim resolve on Dan and Will's faces. Those two always made the best of any situation. George McKenna and Bill were starting to get angry. Lucy was using this adventure as a way to do some novel isometric contortions. He wedged a shoulder against one bulkhead and a knee against another then tightened his muscles to anchor himself in.

"Jose, maybe we ought to take it a little easier."

He made a characteristic, and I must say very winsome, shrug of his shoulders, turning both palms up (Turning both palms up in this traffic melee, of course, left his hands off the wheel for a moment. That added a certain flare to the gesture, but a bit of anxiety to me. I was glad the guys in the back couldn't see it) "Captain, there is nothing I can do about it. This is just Naples." Just then felt the vehicle lurch to the left with a bang, and looking back I saw Will actually inverted bouncing off the left sidewall. Will and George McKenna were wearing Navy blue blazers that were beginning to get some dusty marks.

About this time, we departed the busy urban traffic and got out to the outskirts hillside nearing the Vasquez' house. Now, however, the roads took on a romantic, almost sinusoidal curve pattern going up and down the hills, back and forth from one valley to another. Evening was coming, casting beautiful shadows on the gnarled Italian trees and shrubs on these lovely hills. Jose hopelessly succumbed to the devil inside him that made him attack the curving narrow roads like in a grand prix or a James Bond movie. Now it wasn't as rough, exactly, as it had been in the heavy traffic. However, in this big commercial van, I saw the tires bite over the edge tauntingly over the cliff now and then. The undulating turns now more rhythmically rolled the guys around in the back than before, but they were now getting sick, I thought. Also, we were climbing at a pretty steep angle. Suddenly the back door popped open from their weight against it. Dan slid out, hanging on to the wooden pallet as his feet dangled out. George McKenna or Will vomited, somehow missing Dan with the load.

"Stop, Jose, they're falling out," I told him.

"They're just teasing you, Captain."

"Jose, I'm not kidding."

About that time a big dog, looked like a cross between a police dog and a retriever, started chasing us. At first he was barking at Dan's dangling legs, then he caught up and jumped into the open back door. George Lucy reached back to try to pull Dan in, but when he did that the other wooden pallet slid out to the road, knocking Dan's left hand loose. The dog leapt up to the front, barking loudly, as though he enjoyed this immensely. He took a sudden interest in Jose, and jumped up to his lap wedged against the steering wheel just as we entered another sharp bend in the climbing road.

With the door flapping in the back and the dog barking into my left ear, I couldn't hear the conversation very well, but it sounded like George Lucy was calling some instructions to Dan. Suddenly the van lurched forward a little faster and then Jose finally threw on the brakes.

Looking back, I saw what had happened. Following Lucy's advice, Dan fell out, followed by LT. Lucy. Seeing that in the rear view mirror, Jose slammed on the brakes, breaking the windshield when he slammed forward. On the hill behind us was the record of our accomplishments. A quarter mile back was the splintered remains of the wooden pallet. Stalled behind it was a small collection of traffic. The pallet had fallen into the grill of a truck full of dogs. I still don't know if it was a dog catcher or what, but about twenty dogs of various sizes were running all over the neighborhood. Two tiny little terriers and a lumbering big sheep dog were now coming up to meet their scout friend from our vehicle who in turn was now running down to give them a report. They were all yelping and barking excitedly. Assorted motorists were yelling and making Neapolitan gestures behind the blocked truck.

Dan was back there fifty yards or so, somehow being his unflappable gentlemanly self, now with holes in the knees of his trousers and not-quite-tattered sport coat. He was dusting off his sleeves as though there had merely been a spilled salt shaker. Somebody else vomited again out the back.

Oblivious to the entire scene, Jose looked at the map in his hand and said, "We're almost there, just two more blocks." Everybody filed back in without a comment and we drove up to the Vasquez' villa.

Gil Vasquez greeted us warmly at the front door, in an open collar shirt and short sleeves. "Oh, you guys didn't have to dress up to come over here. I told you 'casual.' " The five guys from the back of the van glanced down at their variously dusty, rumpled, or torn sport coats. They all made prim little smiles and then menacingly made eye contact with me one at a time.

"I hope you had no trouble finding the place or getting here," Mrs. Vasquez said.

"No, none at all," Jose told her. "It was a lovely drive."

The evening at the Vasquez home was wonderful. Mrs. Vasquez is an accomplished linguist and like her husband is conversant in a wide range of literary and artistic subjects. Everybody truly enjoyed the conversation and an elegant meal. Of course, knowing that a trip back to the pier in that van would come next, they could have even enjoyed a night in Newark.

Thanking our host and hostess, on my way out the door, I was handed an envelope by the Captain. "This is from Bullis Butts. Don't read it until you get back to the ship."

Dan offered to drive back.

Before Jose could even answer, George McKenna and Bill Flynn hooked his elbows and threw him in the back.

Back at the ship, I opened the lettered from Butts. It was handwritten, and on the surface simply a collegial letter of advice. He said "In these troubling times, we always have to be concerned about the costs of medical care," and he talked of the line dividing quality care for our patients from fiscal constraints. In the case of BM3 Wood, Butts said, "I think you crossed that line." He understood the need to "satisfy your XO," but it would be wrong to let "a few bucks" to get in the way of treatment for a patient. Finally, he closed by saying he was worried for my career if I kept making patient judgments based on cost.

At first I was infuriated by the letter. He had clearly not understood anything of what I had told him and seemed not to understand the way his doctors acted toward the patients and the rest of us. Was the Naval Hospital there to serve the Fleet, or was it the other way around?

Gradually, I grew more philosophical. It was at the least considerate of him to take the time to give me what he considered good advice and warning. Finally, I just let it go. Doctor Butts and his orthopedists had no idea what the needs of the Fleet were, and no real grasp of the situation for BM3 Wood, either. They were just in a different Navy. I threw his letter away and forgot about it.

********* ********** *********

A couple of weeks later, just after Flight Ops ended, Dan and I were inspecting some of the gear in the Operating Room, when the 1-MC called "Medical Emergency, Medical Emergency. Engine Room Two." Dan ran to his post in the ER and I ran out to the port side passageway and aft to the special doors down the engineering spaces about half way to the Ward Room.

Down in the loud engine room, back on one of the grated false decks in behind the top of a stack of pipes and machinery, a gaggle of snipes in blue coveralls were standing around a guy on his back. None of them were kneeling, though, like people usually do around a fallen person. As I ran up closer, I could see why. He was having a seizure. Seizures frighten and confuse onlookers. They often stand by more as sentinels, rather than touching the patient the way they might for other conditions. (This is just as well. There's not much a lay person can or should do until the seizure stops, anyway.)

Well, maybe.

At first I couldn't see his face, but I saw the arms and legs shaking. This would be a pretty long grand mal seizure, I thought. Allowing for the alarm, the announcement, and my response, this was probably five minutes or more into the alarm.

When the witnesses saw me they stepped back and uncovered the patient. It was Philip Williams, the unhappy would-be rap star. Above him there was an open high power junction box. But there was no tool box near by.

Philip's seizure was not a typical tonic-clonic convulsion. He looked more like a fluttering catfish on the bank. His
hands and wrists were slapping up and down, a little bit like he was slapping out a rhythm on the grate. His knees and heels were kicking up and down, but reciprocally, not synchronously: right, left, right, left. His eyes weren't just closed, they were clenched, and yet his face was expressionless.

Speaking loudly, so that Philip would know I was there, I asked, "Who saw it happen?"

"I did!" one of the frightened sailors said. "He just walked right up to that junction box and stuck his hand right on those wires. I'm telling you he did it on purpose sure as hell. There's something like 400 volts in that thing, Doc. He's an EM. Knew what he was doing. Did it on purpose!"

Philip's right eye opened for an instant, and I thought the shaking pause briefly while I caught him glancing at me.

"All right, everybody, he's going to be OK. You guys leave us here for now." Just then a couple of corpsmen arrived.

I kneeled down to be close to him. "You can stop now, Philip. This is not a convulsion," I said as quietly as one could say anything in the 90 decibel Engine Room.

FN Williams stopped shaking but his eyes stayed clenched.

"You're fine, Philip. It's over now. I'm a neurologist, shipmate, and I can tell this is a fake." Philip stuck to his performance, but his eyes opened.

"Where am I?" he asked, as naively and moronically as in a grade B movie script. "Who are you?" he asked slowly and sluggishly, although he had seen me daily for the past several weeks.

While I examined him for any trauma, checked his vital signs and his neck, I asked HM3 Brooks to have somebody from E-division come to check the junction box.

Philip was fine. He was acting groggy still, but not shaking.

"There aren't any lines connected to that box at all, Captain," the EMC who came to check it said. "No telling how long it's been unhooked but it doesn't even show on the current diagrams." Only an electrician's mate could have known that.

"Did you put your hand in that box to kill yourself, Williams?" his Div-O asked just then.

Williams' stupor appeared to worsen momentarily and he nodded yes slowly.

"Well, since there's no juice in the box, we know you didn't get shocked, and I can tell the seizure is a fake, so let's go on back to Medical, OK, Philip?" I suggested.

"Not... fake... really tried..., " Philip haltingly groaned out, still sticking to his script. When we tried to help him to his feet, he swooned and flailed out his arms. Philip was not a very skillful thespian. However, I was afraid in his acting out he might injure himself or somebody else so we brought him up to Medical in a litter.

The electricians verified that there was no power to the box. Philip had no burns on his hand nor his shoes. As the night went on, his speech was inconsistently telegraphic, but he continued trying to convey a slowly recovering encephalopathy.

As hokey as it was, we had to be as careful with this fake suicide attempt as we would with the most sincere attempt. I went down to see the XO to plan to fly Philip off as soon as we could.

"But that's just what he wants, Doc!" the CHENG said. He was right, of course, Philip wanted to hurry back to Jacksonville to the rap career he thought was waiting for him.

"This is as clear a case of malingering as you can get," the lawyer said. We could do a Summary Court Martial.

"What if he raises the ante next time?" I asked. "Whether he's faking or not, the next time he might really hurt himself, or even really get way with it if he thinks he needs to convince us."

The XO agreed. Philips' performance was a little sillier, a little more flagrant than most, but the majority of our suicide gestures were just acting out. They were usually pitiful scratches on the left wrist that didn't even bring much blood. And they were usually done by some of the immature trouble makers. I was becoming convinced that this was a different phenomenon from the rising numbers of suicides among young males in American society. These futile threats differed in degree and in the entire setting. And yet the whole spectrum, the feeble gestures and the real suicides, had something in common. The pernicious and growing respectability or acceptability of the suicidal idea was somehow at the base of both. At any rate, they all had to be dealt with surely and safely. If Williams, or any sailor, felt his first attempt didn't win our attention, if this was how he wanted to win it, the next try might be worse.

That week, Philip flew off the ship with a friend, and went to the psychiatry department at an Army hospital in Germany. Eventually, he returned to Florida... five weeks after we did. He never was charged, but he also never staged a suicide act again. The psychiatrist said he had a personality disorder and an adjustment reaction. I don't know if his music career ever took off. I wish we could have persuaded him to stay out the cruise.

ACROSS THE ATLANTIC

The translant return trip seemed a little less hectic than the one eighteen months ago. No flu shots or catch-up immunizations this time, and the 3M Inspection was done a few months ago. I had been on the job for a while now, too, so I knew what to look out for every day. We still had a gaggle of politicians, VIPs, and reporters coming to the ship for **Fact-Finding** trips across the Atlantic, and they required attention and escorting. In general, though, the tempo was slowing just a little.

I took advantage of the respite to get up to the Flight Deck a little more. The Fly-Off was even more impressive to me than last year, perhaps because I knew more of the people now. When the Red Rippers zoomed past at deck level we all squared up a little. At this point, though, the main benefit about the Fly-Off was to liberate the Flight Deck for joggers. The running was now unrestricted, no tie-down chains, taxiing aircraft, rolling tractors. A fellow could have a good run finally, so there were dozens of us up there most of the time whenever we could fit it into our schedules.

The Hangar Bay was busy, though. Since the Fly-Off there were no airplanes left in the hangars, so the Supply, AIMD, and Air Department guys were turning the hangars into huge industrial warehouses. With their fork lifts and tractors pushing tons and tri-walls of industrial volume into staging corridors for the coming off-load, the cavernous bays became more crowded than they were when full of airplanes. Like a maze in a Kafka story, a person could be lost among the stacks if he wasn't very careful.

One day when we were about three days away, I ambled off the Flight Deck happily fatigued from a windy run. After peeking in to chat with the corpsman in the Flight Deck BDS, I stopped for a moment to watch the frenetic shuffle of fork lifts and stuff in Hangar Bay II, and then down the starboard ladder to the second deck. It was about 1700 and I had to get ready for dinner.

About the time I stepped on the ladder, the 1MC said, "Man Overboard, Man OverBoard. Starboard Side... " I didn't have to hear the rest of the announcement. The Captain and XO came running past me up the ladder, elbows in front of them to get to the Bridge as fast as they could. I hurried to Ward II to check in and get the Medical Department ready in case we would have work to do.

All our drilling on Man Overboard was finally effective. Within six minutes all but one member of the crew was accounted for. The lookout stationed on the fantail who called in the alarm had a strange report. He saw a black guy in the wake waving to him, as though just waving farewell. The guy had a purple shirt, a "grape," one of the guys who worked in fuels. That he was in the wake at least meant he hadn't been sucked into the screws, one of the main worries about falling overboard.

His name was Johnnie Travis, an airman who had been on the ship about two years. He was due to leave the Navy in a few months and planning to go to college.

One of his buddies was a fork-lift operator who had seen him up on the starboard deck-edge elevator in Hangar Bay III a little while ago. At first he thought it was a little curious, but then he thought Johnnie was "kidding around" somehow. Johnnie was standing on the edge of the elevator, like he was staring at the ocean go past. Not looking upset, just transfixed. He waved to his buddy and stepped behind a stack of gear. The buddy didn't think any more about it and went on about his work.

You're not allowed on the elevators underway without a flotation vest. Had Johnnie been wearing his? His buddy and the lookout weren't sure. A grape's vest is purple like his shirt. The vest would have bright reflective patches on the shoulder, but the witnesses just couldn't recall.

We launched the rescue helo within about fifteen minutes. The marker buoy thrown by the lookout was found quickly, but no sailor. We checked the water temperature. He should be able to survive almost forty minutes here without special protective garments. A second helo went up within another ten minutes, and a third one shortly thereafter. The ship came almost to a stop. The maneuvering has to be done in such a way that turns don't throw the stern and the screws over the victim immediately -- not a likely problem this time -- or put the ship either out of sight or on top of the victim in a circle.

Besides the helos flying carefully designed search grids, every pair of binoculars on the ship were being used on the Signal Bridge or the Captain's Bridge, and hundreds of us were searching from the Flight deck.

An hour went by and the first helo, not topped off when it launched, had to refuel. Checking about the water temperature, I called the Bridge. "Captain, if he hasn't drowned, we are passing survivable hypothermia." The skipper knew that, of course, but survival data was part of my job.

There should not have been much of a shark threat in this area. Some garbage had been thrown out just before he went over, and the helo crews reported it was still floating and there were no sharks seen. No purple shirts either.

Travis' bunkmates were rounded up and interviewed. No, most of them said, this guy would never kill himself. He had a weird sense of humor, one buddy said... he **might** do something like this for a lark. Could that be why he waved to the fork-lift operator and to the lookout?

The XO pointed out how pilots sometimes become so fixated on another airplane while flying in formation, that they just fly into it. Could Travis have become hypnotized by the rushing water as he stood on the elevator edge?

Two hours went by, then four. Then it was dark. It was three hours beyond his survival time just by temperature alone. We recovered the helos. The Captain sent a message to the Fleet and prepared a letter for Travis' mother. Our quiet ship headed back to Florida.

When we got back to Mayport, we found that BM3 Woods' finger healed up fine. Petty Officer Womple didn't have cancer; he finally left the Navy a year later. I still get inquiries periodically from a surgeon or oncologist about a new workup for Arden's mass. He nearly had one surgeon persuaded to amputate the arm, but the doctor was sent to jail for doing too many operations on old people in a nursing home, so the operation was cancelled that time. Arden is still looking for a surgeon as far as I know. George Lucy broke his neck in a Blue Pharaoh performance over in Orlando one weekend the next summer and had to leave the Navy.

A month after we got back to Mayport, Tommy Lennon fleeted up from Navigator to XO, and Mitchell Vaughan left the ship. About a month after that, it was my turn. Somebody told me later that when I left, they bonged me off, but I didn't hear it. When I saluted the Ensign, I didn't turn around to look back at the ship. After I drove off Charlie Pier, though, about a mile away I had to stop and look back for a few minutes. My desk was cleared and I had completed a good turnover with Bruce Bohnker, my relief, but somewhere under the stack of the day's thoughts it felt like I'd left some unfinished business somehow. No, I guess I felt as though I'd left something back on the ship.

In October of 1993, Ann and I went to the decommissioning ceremony for ***USS Forrestal*** up in Philadelphia. We didn't find Captain Pieno, but Captain Thomassy, now an executive for McDonnell Douglas, was there and five or six other former skippers. Six months later, I learned that Captain Pieno was there too. He wouldn't have been hiding of course, but I suspect the Cajun was as distracted that morning as the rest of us, an unfamiliar thing for him. There were several hundred FID sailors there from all across the country. Their memories and sea stories about the First of the Supercarriers covered thirty eight years.

Not many of us had been in the ship's company at the same time; even a stranger could tell we were all Shipmates though. That day I realized what it was I had left on the ship back in Mayport, and I knew I wasn't supposed to have it back.

After the ceremony, I walked back to the fantail where I finished a lot of days the way Myron told me to. Maybe there were only fourteen people in the world who had my job, maybe when we have fewer carriers, there will only be twelve.

But I will always be one of them.